AF614790

Management of Penile Cancer

Daniel J. Culkin
Editor

Management of Penile Cancer

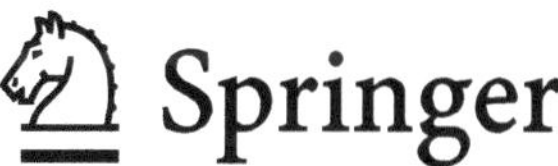

Editor
Daniel J. Culkin, MD, FACS
Department of Urology
University of Oklahoma Health Sciences Center
Oklahoma City, OK
USA

ISBN 978-1-4939-0460-0 ISBN 978-1-4939-0461-7 (eBook)
DOI 10.1007/978-1-4939-0461-7
Springer New York Heidelberg Dordrecht London

Library of Congress Control Number: 2014936598

Printed on acid-free paper

Springer is part of Springer Science+Business Media (www.springer.com)

Preface

Penile cancer presents many challenges to the clinician. In more advanced stages it requires resection that is devastating to the patient. It results in a loss of intimacy for the couple and deterioration of self-image. In the early stages resection can be minimized with excellent cosmetic results. Lymph node dissection is known to be therapeutic but is associated with significant morbidity, some of which is temporary and some of which is permanent. If the disease is identified early, the burden of the treatment is certainly less and the outcomes are much improved.

This highlights the importance of education of the public and the primary care physician. Self-examination and good hygiene will aid in early detection and prevention. Education of the primary care physician on the importance of a thorough genitourinary exam for all male patients will also contribute to the accomplishment of early detection. Infections with human papillomavirus are common in penile cancer as they are with cervical cancer which further supports the vaccination of both adolescent girls and boys. Unfortunately throughout the world, there are socioeconomic barriers that hinder the implementation of these strategies.

Standardization of practice as it relates to penile cancer is essential. Minimization of the adverse events in association with the interventions cannot be overemphasized. Narrowing the margin of resection for the primary cancer in appropriately selected patients and tailoring the lymph node dissection with the assistance of lymphoscintigraphy and dynamic sentinel lymph node biopsy can greatly reduce the burden of treatment. The utilization and referral of these patients to centers of excellence will greatly assist in these efforts as well. The multidisciplinary approach provides a thorough examination of all treatments available and most assuredly provides a more comprehensive discussion of available treatments and clinical trials. For that reason there are chapters dedicated to medical oncology as well as radiation oncology.

The purpose of this text is to provide a comprehensive information to direct evidence-based management of penile cancer not only for the urologic oncologist, the medical oncologist, and the radiation oncologist but also for the primary care physician. Hopefully it will be utilized by training programs for these disciplines as well.

A significant effort was made to include a large number of gross and microscopic pathology pictures to aid the primary care physician in the identification of early and premalignant lesions and also illustrations and photographs of innovative surgical approaches for the surgical oncologist.

Oklahoma City, OK, USA Daniel J. Culkin

Contents

Contributors

Özer Algan, MD Department of Radiation Oncology, Stephenson Cancer Center, University of Oklahoma Health Sciences Center, Oklahoma City, OK, USA

Gilda Alves, PhD Laboratório de Genética Aplicada, Serviço de Hematologia, Instituto Nacional de Câncer, Rio de Janeiro, Brazil

Nabil K. Bissada, MD Department of Urology, VA Medical Center, Oklahoma University, Oklahoma City, OK, USA

Olivier Bouchot, MD, PhD Department of Urologic Clinic, University Hospital, Nantes, France

Catherine M. Corbishley, BSc, MB ChB, FRCPath Department of Cellular Pathology, St George's Healthcare NHS Trust, London, UK

Juanita Crook, MD, FRCPC Department of Radiation Oncology, Cancer Center for the Southern Interior, British Columbia Cancer Agency, University of British Columbia, Kelowna, BC, Canada

Antonio L. Cubilla, MD Department of Pathology, Instituto de Patología e Investigación, Asunción, Paraguay

Daniel J. Culkin, MD, FACS Department of Urology, University of Oklahoma Health Sciences Center, Oklahoma City, OK, USA

Rosa S. Djajadiningrat, MD Department of Urology, Netherlands Cancer Institute, Amsterdam, The Netherlands

María José Fernández, PhD Laboratorio de Computación Científica y Aplicada, Facultad Politécnica, Universidad Nacional de Asunción, Ciudad Universitaria, San Lorenzo, Paraguay

Oliver W. Hakenberg, MD, PhD Department of Urology, University of Rostock, Rostock, Germany

Simon Horenblas, MD, PhD, FEBU Department of Urology, Netherlands Cancer Institute, Amsterdam, The Netherlands

Mohamed H. Kamel, MD, FACS, FRCS Department of Urology, University of Arkansas for Medical Sciences, Little Rock, AR, USA

Asheesh Kaul, MBBS, BSc, MRCS Department of Urology, St. George's Hospital, London, UK

Antonio Augusto Ornellas, MD, PhD Department of Urology, Instituto Nacional de Câncer, Rio de Janeiro, Brazil

Lance Pagliaro, MD Department of Genitourinary Medical Oncology, The University of Texas MD Anderson Cancer Center, Houston, TX, USA

Curtis Pettaway, MD Urology, Surgery Division, The University of Texas MD Anderson Cancer Center, Houston, TX, USA

Chris Protzel, MD Department of Urology, University of Rostock, Rostock, Germany

Jérôme Rigaud, MD, PhD Department of Urology Clinic, University Hospital, Nantes, France

Diego Fernando Sánchez, MD Department of Pathology, Facultad de Ciencias Médicas, Universidad Nacional de Asunción, Asunción, Paraguay

Aline Barros dos Santos Schwindt, MD, MSc Department of Pathology, Instituto Nacional de Câncer, Rio de Janeiro, Brazil

Joel Slaton, MD Department of Urology, University of Oklahoma Health Science Center, Oklahoma City, OK, USA

Massimiliano Spaliviero, MD Department of Urology, University of Oklahoma Health Sciences Center, Oklahoma City, OK, USA

Erik van Werkhoven, MSc Biometrics, Netherlands Cancer Institute, Amsterdam, The Netherlands

Nicholas A. Watkin, MA, MChir, BM, BCL, FRCS Department of Urology, St. Georges Hospital, London, UK

Chapter 1
Introduction to the Management of Penile Cancer

Daniel J. Culkin

The diagnosis and management of penile carcinoma presents many challenges. The purpose of this book is to centralize the most current information in an easily accessible source to reduce practice variability in the detection and management of penile cancer. The first part of the book deals with the epidemiology and natural history; the pathology of penile cancer detailing the clinical, morphologic, and outcome features of each tumor type that highlights the pathologic risk factors; the genetic pathologic mechanisms of penile cancer utilizing genetic and proteomic approaches that identify potential genetic and circulating tumor markers; and an overview of prognostic factors for penile cancer. Next, there is a critical review of current and newer imaging techniques for the detection, clinical staging, and surveillance of penile cancer with a critical assessment of their utility in each of these applications.

The next part of the book deals with the treatment of penile cancer with a critical analysis of the results constantly weighing the risks and benefits of these interventions. The diagnosis and management of premalignant penile lesions affords the greatest opportunity to reduce the incidence of penile cancer with excellent cosmetic results with the utilization of more current penile-sparing surgical techniques. These techniques have reduced the burden of older more aggressive extirpative approaches. The first two chapters of this part provide a description of these penile-sparing surgical techniques with a critical review of these results. The surgical treatment of locally advanced penile carcinoma with a personalized approach to the extent of the lymph node dissection is next followed by a critical analysis of the contemporary experience of Netherlands Cancer Institute.

Other interventions that are utilized in the treatment of penile cancer for primary, adjunctive, neo-adjunctive roles include radiotherapy and chemotherapy. The role

D.J. Culkin, MD, FACS
Department of Urology, University of Oklahoma Health Sciences Center, 920 Stanton L. Young Blvd., WP3150, Oklahoma City, OK 73104, USA
e-mail: daniel-culkin@ouhsc.edu

D.J. Culkin (ed.), *Management of Penile Cancer*,
DOI 10.1007/978-1-4939-0461-7_1, © Springer Science+Business Media New York 2014

of radiotherapy along with a discussion and description of techniques, appropriate patient selection, as well as a critical analysis of the results follows. Then an overview of the biologically active agents for penile cancer and their utilities are discussed with a critical analysis of the results.

Penile cancer in the Western world is rare with only a little over 1,500 new cases diagnosed in the USA in 2012. Data complied with such an experience abounds with treatment variability making any conclusion from retrospective analysis doubtful. Attempts at clinical trials have been futile within the USA for these reasons. Where prevalence is high, health systems may suffer from economic constraints and capabilities may not match the demands for prevention, education, and centralization and standardization of care for a malignancy that in some geographic locales represents 20 % of the male cancers.

In spite of these obstacles to progress in the treatment of penile cancer, much has been learned over the recent past. Penile cancer in the USA is declining although racial and economic variables identify issues. Even though a similar incidence is noted for African Americans and Whites, African Americans have more advanced stages of disease at diagnosis and SEER data reveals a lower percentage of lymph node dissections. The discussion of epidemiology by Spaliviero and Culkin provides an excellent review of current incidences and mortality of penile cancer as well as the geographic variability and racial and social variables.

Drs. Fernández, Sánchez, and Cubilla highlight the importance of the pathologist in this team approach for the detection and treatment of penile cancer. This information is directed to the clinical and academic pathologist. They highlight the important knowledge of penile anatomy, the macroscopic and microscopic features of the anatomical layers, and anatomical routes of cancer spread for appropriate pathologic staging. The accuracy of the *spread features* translates to a reliable identification of pathologic risk factors and assists in the prediction of lymph node metastasis and outcome. These include tumor site of origin, tumor growth pattern, histological grade, depth of invasion (in mm.), anatomical level of invasion, histological subtypes, irregular front invasion, vascular and perineural invasion, positive surgical margins, urethral invasion, and HPV presence. These features have identified three risk groups. Another strategy for the stratification of risk is that of the *prognosis index* which uses information from the anatomical level of invasion, tumor grade, and perineural invasion. Also Dr. Cubilla and coauthors address the topic of HPV infection and the utility of vaccination for prevention. The bimodal pathway for penile carcinogenesis (HPV related and non-HPV related) has directed the construction of a new classification for penile precancerous lesions (e.g., penile intraepithelial neoplasia or PeIN). These include differentiated (HPV negative) and undifferentiated (HPV positive). This is an excellent overview of the anatomical considerations, histological classification, pathologic factors and risk groups, and the role of HPV in penile cancer and PeIN.

Drs. Ornellas, Alves, and Schwindt provide an overview of the genetics and pathology of penile carcinoma. Both carcinogens and oncoviruses have been identified as etiologic factors for penile cancer. Although conventional cytogenetics has identified four karyotypes for penile cancer, the poor widespread use is related to the technical challenges due to low mitotic index, contamination of tissue cultures, and large areas of necrosis. The frequency of DNA aneuploidy, MYC numerical aberrations, and c-myc protein expression all correlate with clinical and pathologic features as well as HPV infection. Also MYC gains, tumor progression, and poor outcomes have been correlated as well. The gain or upregulation of the 5p15 region, which includes the hTERT gene which is the area that codes for the protein telomerase, may be responsible for stabilizing the telomeres of chromosomes. Regarding p53 function, tumor embolization and the expression of p53 were found to be independent predictors of metastases, and the expression of both PCNA and Ki-67 is a predictor of lymph node metastases. Telomerase activity and the expression of Bcl-2 and Bax have been identified in tissue adjacent to the tumor suggesting that there is an oncogenic influence of the tumor on adjacent tissues. Mutations of RAS and PIK3CA being mutually exclusive suggest that these pathways if deregulated may be sufficient for the development of and progression of penile cancer.

Dr. Slaton takes on the task of risk stratification and integration of prognostic markers into nomograms that have been built on clinical parameters to strengthen the prognostic capability and allow a more personalized approach to the penile cancer patient. The utility of combining all these prognostic variables to include genetic aberrations, circulating protein markers, and anatomical spread features and building new nomograms that are all inclusive can be a useful clinical protocol design and personalized medicine.

In the next chapter, Drs. Bouchot and Rigaud discuss and critically analyze the available data for imaging and clinical staging of penile carcinoma. The authors stress that history and a thorough physical exam will not be replaced by imaging. Regarding the primary tumor, the goal is to accurately assess the local extent of the tumor so as to guide the limits of resection. It is particularly important to identify infiltration of the tunica albuginea. Ultrasound and MRI in conjunction with a vasoactive intracavernosal injection are useful for the identification of corpora cavernosal invasion. Of note there is very little evidence to support the superiority of penile ultrasound over a thorough physical exam. Regarding MRI T1 and T2 tumors are hypointense and enhance with gadolinium. The authors stress the importance of the vasoactive penile injection. MRI indications are widening especially for the preselection of penile-sparing surgical candidates. Imaging for assessment of regional lymph nodes includes ultrasound, ultrasound-directed biopsy or fine needle aspiration cytology (FNAC) of inguinal lymph node, as well as a critical analysis of the dynamic sentinel lymph node biopsy in light of current data.

For the surgical treatise of the management of penile cancer, Drs. Kaul, Corbishley, and Watkin provide a thorough review of premalignant lesions that includes appropriate diagnosis and management. The appropriate diagnosis is essential for the selection of the best intervention. Then Drs. Bissada and Kamel review their experiences with penile-sparing surgery for penile cancer that includes appropriate patient selection and follow-up care. The surgical approaches include a laser ablation, Moh's micrographic surgery, circumcision, glansectomy, as well as partial penectomy. The contemporary experience of the Netherlands Cancer Institute with penile carcinoma is then provided by Drs. Djajadiningrat, van Werkhoven, and

Horenblas. Of note their results are not readily achievable at all centers as it relates to imaging such as the dynamic SLN biopsy and the tailored lymph node dissection. Drs. Pettaway and Pagliaro provide a critical analysis of the clinically node-negative patient as well as the patient with advanced inguinal metastases.

Another very useful modality for the treatment of penile cancer both as a primary treatment and as an adjuvant intervention is radiation. Drs. Algan and Crook provide a critical analysis of the different techniques, including brachytherapy as well as external beam radiation therapy, and provide guidance for appropriate patient selection, intervention, and follow-up.

The rarity of this malignancy has presented challenges to the medical oncologist as far as drug development. In spite of these challenges, biological activity of several agents has been identified. The role of chemotherapy as a primary and adjuvant treatment is reviewed by Drs. Protzel and Hakenberg.

Future Directions

The contributors to this volume provide the platform by which the management of penile cancer can now be standardized. The importance of establishing centers of excellence to achieve the best clinical results although intuitive may be impractical considering unique socioeconomic barriers that may occur regionally, nationally, and internationally.

Recognizing these barriers is the first step in developing the instruments for their destruction. Thinking in terms of incremental advances in knowledge in this advanced age of information access, genetic sequencing, and clinical research design may be shortsighted.

The goal for penile cancer should be its *prevention and/or the cure*. Because of the rarity within the USA, the approach requires patient-centric strategies. Cancer is a lethal attack on the public and it presents a life or death situation. The delivery of results that translate to meaningful impact on the disease burden is our responsibility. To this goal, incremental progress fails in some ways to accomplish this process. Competition for resources through traditional funding mechanisms in the USA will be futile for a malignancy that is rare in that country. Innovation and seeking alternative strategies are essential.

Strategies for *education, prevention, and early detection* will deliver the fastest and most impactful results from a public health vantage. The development of vaccines for the prevention of neoplastic transformation from HPV infections has had strong potential to reduce penile cancer and HPV-related condyloma. For instance, recent widespread use of HPV vaccines in girls has reduced HPV strains responsible for cervical cancer by 50 %.

The development of *regional centers of excellence* that can serve as referral centers and can provide a multidisciplinary management of penile cancer provides the opportunity to standardize interventions and improve outcomes. NIH-sponsored comprehensive cancer centers are such a model in the USA.

Basic science research is required to improve the understanding of *genetic, genomic, proteomic, and metabolomic alterations* that can identify targets to guide drug development and provide a *personalized medicine* approach for targeted therapeutics. Also, these discoveries may result in the identification of markers for detection or prognosis that can provide selection criteria for interventions and perhaps identify persons that are at risk for neoplastic transformation. Such approaches are already underway in penile cancer; clues provided by similar approaches that are being explored in HPV-related head and neck squamous cancers may assist in this process.

Regarding the development of personalized medicine, every surgical resection must include specimen acquisition and preparation to allow genetic sequencing proteomic and genomic discovery for this rare malignancy. Also, the development of international registries and universal information exchange will surely provide "leapfrogging" advances over incremental change.

International collaboration offers great promise to identify at-risk populations and provides samples that are robust enough to answer lifesaving questions. Utilization of preexisting networks such as the National Cancer Center Network and Medical Research Council for joint research can expedite this process.

Chapter 2
Epidemiology and Natural History

Massimiliano Spaliviero and Daniel J. Culkin

Abbreviations

AAPC	Average Annual Percentage Change
ASR	Age-Standardized Rate
CI	Confidence Interval
CIS	Carcinoma In Situ
HPV	Human Papilloma Virus
HR	Hazard Ratio
LS	Lichen Sclerosus
OR	Odds Ratio
PIN	Penile Intraepithelial Neoplasia
PUVA	Ultraviolet A Photochemotherapy
RR	Relative Risk
SCC	Squamous Cell Carcinoma
SEER	Surveillance Epidemiology, and End Results
SRR	Standardized Rate Ratio

M. Spaliviero, MD (✉) • D.J. Culkin, MD, FACS
Department of Urology, University of Oklahoma Health Sciences Center,
920 Stanton L. Young Blvd., WP3150, Oklahoma City, OK 73104, USA
e-mail: max.spaliviero@gmail.com; daniel-culkin@ouhsc.edu

D.J. Culkin (ed.), *Management of Penile Cancer*,
DOI 10.1007/978-1-4939-0461-7_2,

Epidemiology

Invasive penile cancers, which for the majority (approximately 95 %) are squamous cell carcinomas (SCC), originate from the squamous mucosal epithelium that covers the glans, the coronal sulcus, and the inner preputial surfaces [1]. The estimated global burden of new cases of penile cancer in 2008 was of about 22,000 cases. The proportion of cases attributable to human papillomavirus (HPV) infection was 50 % [2]. The highest incidence of penile SCC occurs in the sixth and seventh decade (mean *age* 60 years), although up to 25 % of patients may be younger than 50 years of age at diagnosis [3, 4]. The disease may also occur in younger men although it is rare before the age of 40 and exceedingly uncommon in adolescents and children [5]. Patient's age correlates with tumor subtype: basaloid and warty carcinomas are more common in patients of approximately 50 years of age, whereas verrucous and pseudohyperplastic carcinomas are mostly diagnosed in older patients (around 70 years) [6].

Penile cancer is uncommon in Western countries such as the United States, Canada, and European countries where it accounts for 0.4–0.6 % of all malignancies. As shown in Table 2.1, the age-standardized rate (ASR) of penile cancer, which is approximately zero among Israeli Jews [7], varies between *geographical regions* of low incidence (ASR $\leq$1 per 100,000 men) and regions of high incidence (ASR $\geq$2 per 100,000 men), such as tropical and subtropical regions of Brazil (ASR = 2.3–3.7), Thailand (ASR = 2.2), and African countries, such as Uganda (ASR = 2.8), where penile cancer is the most commonly diagnosed cancer in men (10–20 % of all tumors) [8]. Different racial and ethnic groups with their different socioeconomic statuses, religions, sexual practices, and other habits, including smoking and poor genital hygiene, might influence the exposure to risk factors and ultimately result in different incidence of penile cancer in the various areas of the world [9, 10]. The geographical region (endemic versus nonendemic) of origin also appears to influence the distribution patterns of penile precancerous lesions: differentiated penile intraepithelial neoplasia (PIN) in the squamous epithelium adjacent to invasive tumors was found to be significantly ($p < 0.00001$) more prevalent (65.0 % versus 19.8 %, respectively) in high-incidence regions; isolated lesions showing warty and/or basaloid features were predominant (35.0 % versus 80.2 %, respectively) in low-incidence regions [11]. The geographical area and the ethnic/racial group of origin as well as the socioeconomic status and the religious beliefs are associated with tumor stage, metastatic rate, and cancer-specific mortality rates [12].

Hernandez and colleagues assessed *incidence and mortality* in 4,967 American men diagnosed with histologically confirmed invasive penile SCC between 1998 and 2003 using population-based data from the National Cancer Institute's Surveillance, Epidemiology and End Results (SEER) program, the Centers for Disease Control and Prevention's National Program for Cancer Registries, and the National Center for Health Statistics [9]. Overall, median age at presentation was 68 years old. A steady increase of the average, age-adjusted annual incidence of penile SCC, from 13.8 % in patients younger than 50 years to 26.4 % in patients 70–79 years

Table 2.1 Lowest and highest age-standardized incidence rates of penile cancer in geographical areas of the world

Region	Number of cases	Age-standardized incidence (per 100,000)
Africa		
Algeria, Setif	0	–
Tunisia, Centre, Sousse	0	–
Zimbabwe, Harare: African	19	0.9
Uganda, Kyadondo County	25	*2.8*
America, Central and South		
Chile, Valdivia	6	*0.7*
France, La Martinique	9	*0.7*
Brazil, Brasilia	80	*3.7*
America, North		
Canada, Northwest Territories	0	–
USA, California, Los Angeles County: Filipino	0	–
USA, California, Los Angeles County: Japanese	0	–
USA, California, Los Angeles County: Korean	0	–
Canada, Prince Edward Island	1	*0.2*
USA, California, Greater San Francisco Bay Area: Chinese	3	*0.2*
USA, Ohio: Black	8	*0.2*
USA, New Mexico: non-Hispanic White	10	*0.2*
USA, New Mexico: American Indian	7	*1.8*
Asia		
Israel	19	*0.1*
Thailand, Songkhla	58	*2.2*
Europe		
Italy, Brescia Province	4	*0.2*
Spain, Murcia	57	*1.4*
Oceania		
USA: Hawaii: Chinese	0	–
USA: Hawaii: Hawaiian	0	–
USA: Hawaii: Japanese	3	*0.2*
Australia, Northern Territory	4	*1.1*

Adapted from Curado et al. [8]

old, was observed during the study period. Despite an overall incidence of less than 1 % (ASR = 0.81), Hispanic ethnicity and residence in Southern regions and in areas of the United States with low socioeconomic status correlated with considerable disparities in invasive penile cancer incidence. In fact, excess incidence of invasive penile cancer was 72 % higher in Hispanics compared with non-Hispanics, comparable between White and Black men, and approximately twofold lower in Asians/Pacific Islanders. Lower rates of circumcised Mexican Americans compared to non-Hispanic Whites were considered as one of the reasons for excess risk of penile SCC among Hispanics. Risk factors for excess mortality included residence in the Southern and in regions of the United States with low socioeconomic status in addition to the Black race. Of note, certain histologic and anatomic site differences related to race and ethnicity were observed.

Using the SEER database, Rippentrop and coworkers analyzed the associations between different demographic variables and the prevalence, presentation, and survival of patients with penile SCC in the US population [13]. No difference in the incidence of penile cancer in the African-American and White men was noted. However, time to death in patients with regional disease and relative risk (RR) of death from penile cancer in the African-American and White population was significantly different despite similar overall cancer prevalence in the two groups. In the authors' opinion, the presence of an underlying pathologic difference between the two racial categories or the impact of lower socioeconomic factors and decreased access to health care contributed to a delay in diagnosis that resulted in higher disease stages at presentation in African-Americans. The overall worse prognosis for African-Americans compared with Whites appeared to be related to (a) more aggressive disease, (b) more advanced disease due to decreased access to health care or a delay in seeking medical attention, and (c) less frequently performed or reported lymphadenectomy in the Black population.

The improvement in hygienic standards and socioeconomic status in recent years has possibly led to some decline in incidence in many countries including the United States [10, 14–18], where approximately 1,570 new cases of penile cancers were diagnosed and 310 cancer-related deaths were projected, respectively, in 2012 [19]. Other studies have shown a stable incidence of invasive penile cancer [20]. Although Pukkala and Weiderpass did not find an impact of social class variation on the incidence of penile cancer in Finland [21], Colon-Lopez et al. showed that socioeconomic factors continue to hold an impact on incidence and mortality in developing countries [22]. Analyzing the Puerto Rico Cancer Registry and the US SEER database, Puerto Rican men were found to have an approximately threefold higher incidence of penile cancer as compared to non-Hispanic White Americans (standardized rate ratio [SRR]: 3.33; 95 % confidence interval [CI]: 2.80, 3.95) and non-Hispanic Black Americans (SRR: 3.04; 95 % CI: 2.21, 4.36). The incidence of penile cancer in Puerto Rican men was also more than two times higher than that US Hispanic men (SRR: 2.59; 95 % CI: 1.99, 3.43). In a similar fashion, the cancer-specific mortality in Puerto Rican men was higher than in all other ethnic/racial groups included in the study. Furthermore, Puerto Rican men in the lowest socioeconomic position index had 70 % higher incidence of penile cancer as compared with those PR men in the highest socioeconomic position index (SRR: 1.70; 95 % CI: 0.97, 2.87). However, only the low educational component of the socioeconomic position was significantly ($p < 0.05$) associated with higher penile cancer incidence (SRR: 2.18; 95 % CI: 1.42, 3.29).

Although most of the reported studies found a declining incidence of penile cancer in recent years, a few studies reported an increasing incidence of carcinoma in situ (CIS), high-grade PIN, and penile cancer [20, 23]. In the Netherlands, the overall age-standardized incidence of penile SCC increased from 1.4 to 1.5 per 100,000 person-years with an average annual percentage change (AAPC) of 1.3 % (95 % CI: 0.1 %, 2.6 %). This appeared to be the result of earlier diagnosis and therefore increased incidence rate of penile CIS from 0.1 to 0.3 with an AAPC of 4.5 % (95 % CI: 2.0 %, 6.9 %) [20]. In Denmark, the overall age-standardized incidence rate of penile cancer increased from 1.0 to 1.3 per 100,000 men-years in 1978–1979 to 2006–2008, representing an AAPC of 0.8 % (95 % CI: 0.17 %, 0.37 %). In the same study, the incidence of PIN increased significantly in 1998–1999 to 2006–2008 with an AAPC of 7.1 % (95 % CI: 3.3 %, 11.1 %) [23]. In the authors' opinion, the high prevalence of HPV and the low circumcision rates in Denmark partly explained the results of their study.

Number of sexual partners, marital status, and cohabitation seem to correlate with the risk of developing penile cancer. Rippentrop et al. showed that married patients sought care earlier than unmarried patients, thus presenting with disease at a lower stage (CIS or localized disease) and having a significantly stage-by-stage longer time to cancer death. Married patients were also more likely to pursue more aggressive treatment of their condition. On multivariated analysis, however, no difference in prevalence or RR of death was noted in married or unmarried individuals [13]. Ulff-Moller et al. examined the incidence trends of invasive penile SCC and the impact of marital and cohabitation status on the risk of developing the disease [24]. A total of 1,292 cases of invasive penile SCC in Denmark during 65.6 million person-years between 1978 and 2010 were studied. The average incidence rate (1.05 cases per 100,000 person-years) and the world age-standardized incidence rate (p-trend = 0.41) remained stable during the studied period. The risk of developing invasive penile SCC in single-living and unmarried Danish men increased with the number of prior cohabitations. Unmarried (hazard ratio [HR] 1.37; 95 % CI: 1.13, 1.66), divorced (HR 1.49; 95 % CI: 1.24, 1.79), or widowed (HR 1.36; 95 % CI: 1.13, 1.63) patients were at increased risk of invasive penile SCC when compared to married men. Single-living men were at increased risk of invasive penile SCC compared to men in opposite-sex cohabitation (HR 1.43; 95 % CI: 1.26, 1.62). Risk increased with increasing numbers of prior opposite-sex (p-trend = 0.02) and same-sex (p-trend < 0.001) cohabitations. Greater exposure to HPV secondary to less stable sexual relations might explain the findings in the study subgroups.

Etiology

The etiology of penile cancer is *multifactorial* [12, 25, 26]. In a review of scientific publications on penile cancers between 1996 and 2000, phimosis (inability to fully retract the foreskin), chronic inflammatory conditions (i.e., balanoposthitis, lichen sclerosus et atrophicus), and treatment with psoralen and ultraviolet A photochemotherapy (PUVA) were identified as strong risk factors associated with an odds ratio (OR) greater than 10 [25]. Other risk factors, such as poor hygiene, history of smoking, multiple sexual partners, and history of genital warts, have been identified.

Phimosis is present in up to one half of patients with penile cancer. Although preventive circumcision has been suggested in patients with phimosis living in areas with high incidence of penile cancer [27], adult circumcision failed to show a protective effect since men never circumcised or circumcised after the neonatal period had, respectively, a 3.2 and 3.0 times higher risk compared to men circumcised as neonates [26]. In a population-based case–control study conducted in western Washington State between 1979 and 1998, men not circumcised during childhood resulted at increased risk of invasive (OR = 2.3; 95 % CI: 1.3, 4.1) but not in situ (OR = 1.1; 95 % CI: 0.6, 1.8) penile cancer [28]. Approximately 35 % of men with penile cancer who had not been circumcised in childhood and 7.6 % of controls reported a history of phimosis (OR = 7.4; 95 % CI: 3.7, 15.0). Phimosis was found to be strongly associated with development of invasive penile cancer (OR = 11.4; 95 % CI: 5.0, 25.9) in men not circumcised in childhood. The risk of invasive penile cancer in men with no phimosis and not having been circumcised in childhood was not elevated (OR = 0.5; 95 % CI: 0.1, 2.5). On the contrary, neonatal circumcision is associated with a threefold decreased risk of invasive penile cancer since it protects against *phimosis*, poor penile hygiene, and retention of desquamated epidermal cells and urinary products resulting in *chronic inflammation* of the glans and prepuce. Nonetheless, 20 % of penile cancer patients had been circumcised neonatally [25, 28]. Interestingly, Schoen and colleagues determined that the level of protective effect of neonatal circumcision for CIS is not as high as that for invasive penile cancer [29]. Of 89 men with invasive penile cancer whose circumcision status was known, 2 (2.3 %) had been circumcised as newborns and 87 (97.7 %) were not circumcised. Of 118 men with CIS whose circumcision status was known, 16 (15.7 %) had been circumcised as newborns.

Lichen sclerosus (LS), an unusual chronic mucocutaneous condition of the penis preferentially involving the foreskin but also the glans, coronal sulcus, and urethra, was found to cause phimosis and to be associated with the usual, verrucous, papillary, and pseudohyperplastic subtypes of invasive penile carcinoma in 30–50 % of patients [12, 30]. In a retrospective study from Italy, Nasca and colleagues reported penile invasive SCC or premalignant lesions in 9 of 86 men (9.3 %) with a history of penile LS after a mean lag time of 18 (range, 10–34) years. The transition from LS to frank neoplastic foci was histologically evident in all cases of SCC [31]. Powell and coworkers retrospectively found histological or clinical evidence of LS in 11 of 20 patients with SCC of the penis [32]. SCC was well differentiated in seven of the eight cases with histologic evidence of LS in the excision specimen. Only 3 SCCs were well differentiated among the 12 cases with no evidence of LS, although a history of LS sometimes preceding the SCC by 10 years was identified in the records of 7 of these 12 patients. Of the ten deceased patients in this study, seven died from metastatic disease. The authors concluded that the association between SCC of the penis and LS was present even in the patients in whom the clinical presentation of LS or the need for circumcision preceded the SCC by many years. A large retrospective study from Paraguay assessed the anatomic distribution and prevalence of LS in patients with SCC of the penis [30]. The penectomy and circumcision specimens from 207 patients with carcinoma and giant condylomas were examined, and 68 (33 %) patients were found with evidence of LS; however, the true association was felt to be likely underestimated. The preferential anatomic site of LS was the foreskin, although involvement was noted at the level of the glans and coronal sulcus, including the urethra. The gross and microscopic findings suggested that LS may represent preneoplastic condition for at least some types of penile cancers, in particular those not related to HPV. Evidence of LS was found in 28 % of 155 patients with penile carcinoma studied prospectively by Pietrzak and colleagues [33]. Prowse et al. investigated the role of HPV infection and expression of the tumor suppressor protein $p16^{INK4A}$ in the pathogenesis of penile cancer [34]. In 26 penile SCCs and 20 independent penile LS, HPV DNA was found in 54 % of penile SCCs and 33 % of penile LS patients. Strong immunostaining for $p16^{INK4A}$ correlated with HPV 16/18 infection in both penile LS and penile SCC. Penile SCC margins were also associated with penile LS in 13 of 26 lesions. HPV was detected in 7 of the 13 SCC cases associated with LS and in 6 of the 11 SCC lesions not involving LS. Barbagli and coworkers evaluated the presence of premalignant or malignant lesions in 130 patients with LS involving the male genitalia. Eleven (8.4 %) men with genital LS showed premalignant or malignant histopathological features including 7 (64 %) with SCC. Based on all these studies, it has been estimated that the risk of malignant transformation of penile LS is similar to vulval lichen sclerosus (4–8 %) [35].

Stern reported on the risk of genital tumors in 892 patient with psoriasis treated with oral methoxsalen (8-methoxypsoralen) and *PUVA* [36]. In his 12.3-year prospective study, 30 genital neoplasms in 14 (1.6 %) patients were identified between 1976 and 1989. Compared to expected morbidity (based on population incidence data), patients treated with PUVA had a standard morbidity ratio of 95.7 (95 % CI: 43.8, 181.8) for invasive SCC of the penis and scrotum and 58.8 (95 % CI: 26.9, 111.7) for invasive and in situ penile tumors. When compared to the general population or patients exposed to low levels of PUVA, the incidence of invasive SCC in patients exposed to high levels of PUVA was 286 times and 16.3 times higher, respectively ($p<0.001$ for both comparisons). After controlling for the level of exposure to PUVA, patients exposed to high levels of ultraviolet B radiation were found to have a risk of genital tumors 4.6 times higher than that in other patients (95 % CI: 1.4, 15.1). Considering the strong dose-dependent increase in the risk of genital tumors associated with exposure to PUVA and ultraviolet B radiation, the author recommended the use of genital protection (e.g., shielding) in men exposed to PUVA or other forms of ultraviolet radiation. In a subsequent update of this experience nearly 10 years later, the development of genital cancer in ten new cohort patients confirmed the persistence of the risk associated with PUVA exposure despite the increased use of genital protection and the decreased use or the discontinuation of PUVA. Men previously unaffected by such tumors developed cancer in the decade starting nearly 15 years after initial exposure to PUVA, with an overall risk of invasive scrotal and penile SCC since enrollment 81.7 times (95 % CI: 52.1, 122.6) higher than that expected in the general population. Multivariate analyses revealed the highest genital tumor risk among men with high-dose exposure to both PUVA and topical tar/ultraviolet B, with an incidence rate ratio of 4.5 (95 % CI: 1.3, 16.1) compared with the low-dose exposure group. Another study by Perkins et al. showed a greater than 300-fold increase in genital tumors in 130 patients with psoriasis treated with PUVA [37].

The attributable fraction of penile cancers related to *human papillomavirus* is estimated to be 47 % (95 % CI: 44.4, 49.6) [38]. HPV DNA, especially high-risk genotype HPV-16, was identified in 70 and 100 % of PIN lesions and 40–50 % of cases invasive penile cancers [12, 25, 39]. Other HPV genotypes, such as −18, −31, and −33, are associated with both CIS and invasive penile cancer [40]. A systematic review of the major studies reporting on the HPV prevalence among the different histological types of penile cancer in 1,466 patients between 1986 and 2008 showed a global HPV prevalence of 47 % [38]. The two most frequent HPV genotypes were −16 (60 %) and −18 (13 %) and associated with the basaloid and warty SCC most frequently, although the prevalence of the keratinizing and nonkeratinizing subtypes was also of approximately 50 %. A history of multiple sexual partners and a self-reported history of condyloma were associated with a three to fivefold increased penile cancer risk; however, cervical cancer was not consistently associated with cancer of the penis in the male partner [25, 26].

Hellberg and colleagues identified *tobacco smoking* as one of the risk factors significantly associated with penile cancer [41]. Light smokers had a relative risk of 0.98 (95 % CI: 0.68, 1.42), whereas the relative risk in smokers of more than ten cigarettes a day was 1.53 (95 % CI: 1.00, 2.35). Harish and Ravi studied the role of tobacco in the form of cigarettes, chewing tobacco, and snuff in SCC of the penis in a total of 503 patients and age-matched controls [42]. Compared with controls, cigarette smoking ($p=0.002$), tobacco chewing ($p<0.001$), and the use of snuff ($p=0.004$) associated with penile carcinoma. A relationship between dose and response was observed for both cigarette smoking and tobacco chewing. Active smokers have a consistent, dose-dependent, 2.8 times higher risk of penile cancer than men who never smoked [25, 26]. In another study, cigarette smoking was associated with a 4.5-fold higher risk (95 % CI: 2.0, 10.1) of invasive penile cancer [28]. The exact role of smoking in the development of the disease is unknown; however, the increased risk is probably related to the presence of systemic carcinogenic metabolites [12].

Penile trauma, tears, and rashes have been reported as additional risk factors for the development of penile cancer [26]. Bissada et al. reported the development of penile SCC in circumcision scars on the penile shaft of 15 patients after mutilating circumcision [43].

Natural History

Carcinoma of the penis usually develops in a stepwise fashion over a period of years with a series of events extending from a preneoplastic lesion to SCC that can be found on the glans (48–60 %%), the inner foreskin (21 %), the glans and inner foreskin (9 %), the coronal sulcus (6 %), or the shaft (<2 %) [3, 44]. Diagnosis, histologic characteristics, role in the pathogenesis of penile cancer, and management of premalignant lesions will be discussed in other chapters of this book. The exact site of origin of penile cancer may be difficult to identify when the tumor is locally advanced and affects multiple compartments at presentation [1]. The glans is more likely to be involved by high-grade tumor variants, e.g., basaloid, sarcomatoid, and adenosquamous, whereas unusual tumors arising in the foreskin or coronal sulcus (verrucous or papillary type) are usually of lower grade [3]. Other primary malignant epithelial, soft tissue, or lymphoid tumors are exceedingly rare; however, the penis can also be the site for metastatic tumors.

Penile cancer presents clinically with a penile lesion, which may consist in an area of induration, a papule, a papillary and exophytic mass, or a flat and ulcerating lesion. PIN usually presents as a flat to slightly raised, pearly whitish to reddish area with irregular borders. In some cases, pigmented papules, erythematous plaques, or ulceration might be seen [45]. Usual SCC has a superficial spreading pattern and extends horizontally through the glans, the coronal sulcus, or foreskin. Extensive ulceration is a common finding in basaloid and sarcomatoid carcinoma tumors that also have a vertical growth pattern frequently invading into deep penile erectile tissues. Verruciform tumors are predominantly exophytic papillomatous low-grade tumors, although they may invade into the corpus spongiosum and the corpora cavernosa. Mixed patterns of growth can be observed, typically in the mixed or hybrid verrucous and the warty-basaloid carcinomas [3, 46, 47].

The most common symptoms are related to the primary lesion and include pruritus and burning sensation under the foreskin, discharge, history of injury, bleeding, pain, voiding symptoms, and lymph node enlargement [44]. Multiple patient factors, including underestimation of the significance of the lesion, embarrassment, guilt, fear, personal neglect, and ignorance, may result in more than 1 year delay in diagnosis in 15–20 % of patients [48]. Also, the presence of phimosis may prevent the early identification of a lesion silently growing and progressing on the glans until erosion through the prepuce, and symptoms, such as foul odor, discharge, and possibly bleeding, occur prompting sought of medical attention.

Growth of the lesion progresses gradually to involve the glans, the shaft, and the corpora. The growth rates of papillary/exophytic and flat/ulcerative lesion are similar, although earlier nodal involvement and related lower 5-year survival rates have been reported for flat, ulcerative lesions [49]. Also, increased incidence of metastasis and poorer survival rates have been reported for large (>5 cm) lesions and extensive (>75 %) involvement of the penile shaft [50, 51]. Until penetration of Buck's fascia occurs, the corporal bodies are protected from tumoral invasion. However, once the natural barrier represented by Buck's fascia is broken and the tunica albuginea has been involved as well, invasion of the vascular corpora and potential vascular dissemination of disease occurs. The involvement of bladder and urethra is rare [52].

Regional femoral and iliac nodes are the earliest sites of metastatic dissemination from penile cancer [53]. The lymphatics from the prepuce join with those from the skin of the shaft and drain in the superficial inguinal nodes. The lymphatics of the glans join those from the corporal bodies and drain in the superficial inguinal nodes as well. The superficial inguinal nodes (external to the fascia lata) drain to the deep inguinal nodes, which are deep to the fascia lata. The rates of inguinal lymph node metastasis vary according to the cancer subtype, from 50 to 75 % for sarcomatoid, basaloid, and adenosquamous carcinomas to infrequent for mixed, warty, and papillary carcinomas to absent in verrucous carcinoma [3]. Next, the drainage is to the pelvic nodes (external and internal iliacs and obturator) [54]. Penile lymphatic drainage is bilateral to both inguinal areas due to multiple cross-connections present at all levels of drainage. No evidence of skip drainage was observed in penile lymphangiographic studies by Cabanas and coworkers [55]. Metastases in the regional lymph nodes result in node enlargement with cutaneous and vascular involvement leading to skin ulceration with infection and necrosis and vascular erosion causing life-threatening sepsis and hemorrhage from the femoral vessels [53, 56].

Once metastatic disease involves the pelvic lymph nodes, further spread, which occurs late in the course of the diseases in 1–10 % of cases [50–52, 57], involves distant sites, including para-aortic lymph nodes, lungs, liver, bone, and brain. Distant metastases are uncommon in the absence of regional node metastases [53]. In a study on 333 penile SCC, Guimaraes et al. reported a recurrence rate of 22 % [3]. Usual, mixed, papillary, and warty carcinomas recurred locoregionally, whereas the more likely to recur sarcomatoid, basaloid, and adenosquamous types relapsed systemically. Patients with verrucous carcinoma did not recur. In their cohort, the 10-year survival of patients with verrucous, adenosquamous, mixed, papillary, and warty carcinoma was higher (90–100 %) than that (78 %) of patients with SCC and basaloid carcinoma. Leijte and coworkers conducted a study on 700 penile cancer patients managed from 1956 to 2007 [57]. Of the 205 (29 %) patients that relapsed, 74.1 % recurred within 2 years and 92 % recurred within 5 years of diagnosis. In this cohort, local recurrence occurred in 18.6 %, regional recurrence in 9.3 %, and metastatic recurrence in 1.4 % of patients, respectively.

Despite systemic chemotherapy, once disseminated disease occurs, survival is usually measured in months [58]. The prognosis of patients with untreated penile cancer, for whom autoamputation usually occurs, is even worse, with the majority of patients dying of disease within 2 years of the diagnosis. Although no cases of spontaneous remission have been reported, sporadically patients with advanced local disease and regional lymph node metastases reached long-term survival [50].

The natural history model for penile cancer routes of spread (local intrapeneal, regional and systemic nodes, regional skin, liver, lungs, heart, and other multiple sites) was confirmed by the autopsy findings of Chaux and colleagues in 14 patients with penile SCC [59]. Local/regional recurrence was found in 5 of the 9 patients who died from disseminated disease. Local recurrence sites were the corpus cavernosum, Buck's fascia and urethra, regional skin, and prostate. Metastatic sites were lymph nodes (64 %), liver (50 %), lungs (43 %), heart (36 %), adrenals, bone and skin (3 cases each), thyroid and brain (2 cases each), and pancreas, spleen, and pleura (1 case each). The different tumor profiles, such as low-grade superficial tumors with usual and warty subtypes versus high-grade deeply invasive basaloid or hybrid verrucous/sarcomatoid carcinomas, correlated with cancer-specific survival.

References

1. Velazquez E, Chaux A, Cubilla A. Histologic classification of penile intraepithelial neoplasia. Semin Diagn Pathol. 2012;29:96.
2. Forman D, de Martel C, Lacey CJ, et al. Global burden of human papillomavirus and related diseases. Vaccine. 2012;30 Suppl 5:F12.

3. Guimarães G, Cunha I, Soares F, et al. Penile squamous cell carcinoma clinicopathological features, nodal metastasis and outcome in 333 cases. J Urol. 2009;182:528.
4. Hegarty P, Kayes O, Freeman A, et al. A prospective study of 100 cases of penile cancer managed according to European Association of Urology guidelines. BJU Int. 2006;98:526.
5. Narasimharao K, Chatterjee H, Veliath A. Penile carcinoma in the first decade of life. Br J Urol. 1985;57:358.
6. Chaux A, Cubilla A, editors. Diagnosis, epidemiology, and pathology of penile cancer. Baltimore: Lippincot Williams & Wilkins; 2011. p. 803–10.
7. Arya M, Kalsi J, Kelly J, et al. Malignant and premalignant lesions of the penis. BMJ. 2013(346).
8. Curado MP, Edwards B, Shin HR, Storm H, Ferlay J, Heanue M, Boyle P, et al., editors. Cancer incidence in five continents, IARC scientific publication no. 160, vol. IX. Lyon: IARC; 2007.
9. Hernandez B, Barnholtz-Sloan J, German R, et al. Burden of invasive squamous cell carcinoma of the penis in the United States, 1998–2003. Cancer. 2008;113:2883.
10. Barnholtz-Sloan J, Maldonado J, Pow-sang J, et al. Incidence trends in primary malignant penile cancer. Urol Oncol. 2007;25:361.
11. Soskin A, Vieillefond A, Carlotti A, et al. Warty/basaloid penile intraepithelial neoplasia is more prevalent than differentiated penile intraepithelial neoplasia in nonendemic regions for penile cancer when compared with endemic areas: a comparative study between pathologic series from Paris and Paraguay. Hum Pathol. 2012;43:190.
12. Bleeker M, Heideman D, Snijders P, et al. Penile cancer: epidemiology, pathogenesis and prevention. World J Urol. 2009;27:141.
13. Rippentrop JM, Joslyn SA, Konety BR. Squamous cell carcinoma of the penis: evaluation of data from the surveillance, epidemiology, and end results program. Cancer. 2004;101:1357.
14. Vatanasapt V, Martin N, Sriplung H, et al. Cancer incidence in Thailand, 1988–1991. Cancer Epidemiol Biomarkers Prev. 1995;4:475.
15. Maiche A. Epidemiological aspects of cancer of the penis in Finland. Eur J Cancer Prev. 1992;1:153.
16. Frisch M, Friis S, Kjaer S, et al. Falling incidence of penis cancer in an uncircumcised population (Denmark 1943–90). BMJ. 1995;311:1471.
17. Parkin D, Nambooze S, Wabwire-Mangen F, et al. Changing cancer incidence in Kampala, Uganda, 1991–2006. Int J Cancer. 2010;126:1187.
18. Parkin D, Whelan S, Ferlay J, et al., editors. Cancer incidence in five continents, vol. VIII. Lyon: IARC Scientific Publications; 2002.
19. Siegel R, Naishadham D, Jemal A. Cancer statistics, 2012. CA Cancer J Clin. 2012;62:10.
20. Graafland N, Verhoeven R, Coebergh J, et al. Incidence trends and survival of penile squamous cell carcinoma in the Netherlands. Int J Cancer. 2011;128:426.
21. Pukkala E, Weiderpass E. Socio-economic differences in incidence rates of cancers of the male genital organs in Finland, 1971–95. Int J Cancer. 2002;102:643.
22. Colón-López V, Ortiz A, Soto-Salgado M, et al. Penile cancer disparities in Puerto Rican men as compared to the United States population. Int Braz J Urol. 2012;38:728.
23. Baldur-Felskov B, Hannibal CG, Munk C, et al. Increased incidence of penile cancer and high-grade penile intraepithelial neoplasia in Denmark 1978–2008: a nationwide population-based study. Cancer Causes Control. 2012;23:273.
24. Ulff-Moller CJ, Simonsen J, Frisch M. Marriage, cohabitation and incidence trends of invasive penile squamous cell carcinoma in Denmark 1978–2010. Int J Cancer. 2013;133:1173.
25. Dillner J, von Krogh G, Horenblas S, et al. Etiology of squamous cell carcinoma of the penis. Scand J Urol Nephrol Suppl. 2000;205:189.
26. Maden C, Sherman K, Beckmann A, et al. History of circumcision, medical conditions, and sexual activity and risk of penile cancer. J Natl Cancer Inst. 1993;85:19.
27. Velazquez E, Bock A, Soskin A, et al. Preputial variability and preferential association of long phimotic foreskins with penile cancer: an anatomic comparative study of types of foreskin in a general population and cancer patients. Am J Surg Pathol. 2003;27:994.

28. Daling J, Madeleine M, Johnson L, et al. Penile cancer: importance of circumcision, human papillomavirus and smoking in in situ and invasive disease. Int J Cancer. 2005;116:606.
29. Schoen E, Oehrli M, Colby C, et al. The highly protective effect of newborn circumcision against invasive penile cancer. Pediatrics. 2000;105:E36.
30. Velazquez E, Cubilla A. Lichen sclerosus in 68 patients with squamous cell carcinoma of the penis: frequent atypias and correlation with special carcinoma variants suggests a precancerous role. Am J Surg Pathol. 2003;27:1448.
31. Micali G, Nasca M, Innocenzi D. Penile cancer among patients with genital lichen sclerosus. Sex Transm Infect. 2001;77:226.
32. Powell J, Robson A, Cranston D, et al. High incidence of lichen sclerosus in patients with squamous cell carcinoma of penis. Br J Dermatol. 2001;145:85.
33. Pietrzak P, Hadway P, Corbishley C, et al. Is the association between balanitis xerotica obliterans and penile carcinoma underestimated? BJU Int. 2006;98:74.
34. Prowse D, Ktori E, Chandrasekaran D, et al. Human papillomavirus-associated increase in p16INK4A expression in penile lichen sclerosus and squamous cell carcinoma. Br J Dermatol. 2008;158:261.
35. Clouston D, Hall A, Lawrentschuk N. Penile lichen sclerosus (balanitis xerotica obliterans). BJU Int. 2011;108(Suppl):14.
36. Stern R. Genital tumors among men with psoriasis exposed to psoralens and ultraviolet A radiation (PUVA) and ultraviolet B radiation. The Photochemotherapy Follow-up Study. N Engl J Med. 1990;322:1093.
37. Perkins W, Lamont D, MacKie R. Cutaneous malignancy in males treated with photochemotherapy. Lancet. 1990;336:1248.
38. Miralles-Guri C, Bruni L, Cubilla A, et al. Human papillomavirus prevalence and type distribution in penile carcinoma. J Clin Pathol. 2009;62:870.
39. Grulich A, Jin F, Conway E, et al. Cancers attributable to human papillomavirus infection. Sex Health. 2010;7:244.
40. Wiener J, Walther P. The association of oncogenic human papillomaviruses with urologic malignancy. The controversies and clinical implications. Surg Oncol Clin N Am. 1995;4:257.
41. Hellberg D, Valentin J, Eklund T, et al. Penile cancer: is there an epidemiological role for smoking and sexual behaviour? Br Med J (Clin Res Ed). 1987;295:1306.
42. Harish K, Ravi R. The role of tobacco in penile carcinoma. Br J Urol. 1995;75:375.
43. Bissada N, Morcos R, el-Senoussi M. Post-circumcision carcinoma of the penis. I. Clinical aspects. J Urol. 1986;135:283.
44. Pow-Sang M, Ferreira U, Pow-Sang J, et al. Epidemiology and natural history of penile cancer. Urology. 2010;76(2 Suppl 1):S2.
45. Chaux A, Pfannl R, Lloveras B, et al. Distinctive association of p16INK4a overexpression with penile intraepithelial neoplasia depicting warty and/or basaloid features: a study of 141 cases evaluating a new nomenclature. Am J Surg Pathol. 2010;34:385.
46. Cubilla A, Reuter V, Velazquez E, et al. Histologic classification of penile carcinoma and its relation to outcome in 61 patients with primary resection. Int J Surg Pathol. 2001;9:111.
47. Cubilla A, Lloveras B, Alejo M, et al. The basaloid cell is the best tissue marker for human papillomavirus in invasive penile squamous cell carcinoma: a study of 202 cases from Paraguay. Am J Surg Pathol. 2010;34:104.
48. Narayana A, Olney L, Loening S, et al. Carcinoma of the penis: analysis of 219 cases. Cancer. 1982;49:2185.
49. Ornellas A, Seixas A, Marota A, et al. Surgical treatment of invasive squamous cell carcinoma of the penis: retrospective analysis of 350 cases. J Urol. 1994;151:1244.
50. Beggs J, Spratt JJ. Epidermoid carcinoma of the penis. J Urol. 1964;91:166.
51. Staubitz W, Lent M, Oberkircher O. Carcinoma of the penis. Cancer. 1955;8:371.
52. Riveros M, Gorostiaga R. Cancer of the penis. Arch Surg. 1962;85:377.
53. Pettaway C, Lynch DJ, Davis J. Tumors of the penis. In: Wein A, editor. Campbell-Walsh urology, vol. 1. Philadelphia: Saunders Elsevier; 2007. p. 959–92.

54. Dewire D, Lepor H. Anatomic considerations of the penis and its lymphatic drainage. Urol Clin North Am. 1992;19:211.
55. Cabanas R. Anatomy and biopsy of sentinel lymph nodes. Urol Clin North Am. 1992;19:267.
56. Burgers J, Badalament R, Drago J. Penile cancer. Clinical presentation, diagnosis, and staging. Urol Clin North Am. 1992;19:247.
57. Leijte J, Kirrander P, Antonini N, et al. Recurrence patterns of squamous cell carcinoma of the penis: recommendations for follow-up based on a two-centre analysis of 700 patients. Eur Urol. 2008;54:161.
58. Syed S, Eng T, Thomas C, et al. Current issues in the management of advanced squamous cell carcinoma of the penis. Urol Oncol. 2003;21:431.
59. Chaux A, Reuter V, Lezcano C, et al. Autopsy findings in 14 patients with penile squamous cell carcinoma. Int J Surg Pathol. 2011;19:164.

Chapter 3
Pathology, Risk Factors, and HPV in Penile Squamous Cell Carcinoma

María José Fernández, Diego Fernando Sánchez, and Antonio L. Cubilla

Anatomy for Pathological Staging

The structural complexity of penile anatomy requires a basic knowledge for appropriate handling of specimens for pathological staging. Tumors may originate in any of the three penile anatomical compartments which are the glans, coronal sulcus, and foreskin (Fig. 3.1a). The majority originates in the glans, some in the foreskin inner mucosa, and rare tumors are exclusive of the coronal sulcus. Large tumors involve more than one site or all sites, and it is not possible to identify their site of origin. The determination of tumor site is important because glans and foreskin harbor different anatomical layers resulting in specific pathological staging methods for each site [1]. Another reason is that there may be variable biological factors influencing pathogenesis of glans and foreskin tumors. Like in sites with transitional epithelia, such as the cervix and anal canal, poorly differentiated HPV-related carcinomas are more likely to develop around the glans, where urethral-meatal mucosae merge (central tumors), whereas lower-grade keratinizing carcinomas are more prevalent in the foreskin (peripheral tumors). Foreskin tumors are mostly HPV unrelated and usually associated with lichen sclerosus [2].

There is a correlation of tumor depth or thickness and prognosis [3]. The TNM staging system is based on the extent of tumor invasion into anatomical levels [1]. It is important for the pathologist to be familiar with penile anatomical levels. They are

M.J. Fernández, PhD
Laboratorio de Computación Científica y Aplicada, Facultad Politécnica, Universidad Nacional de Asunción, Ciudad Universitaria, San Lorenzo, Paraguay

D.F. Sánchez, MD
Department of Pathology, Facultad de Ciencias Médicas, Universidad Nacional de Asunción, Asunción, Paraguay

A.L. Cubilla, MD (✉)
Department of Pathology, Instituto de Patología e Investigación, Martín Brizuela 325, Asunción, Paraguay
e-mail: antoniocubillaramos@gmail.com

D.J. Culkin (ed.), *Management of Penile Cancer*,
DOI 10.1007/978-1-4939-0461-7_3, © Springer Science+Business Media New York 2014

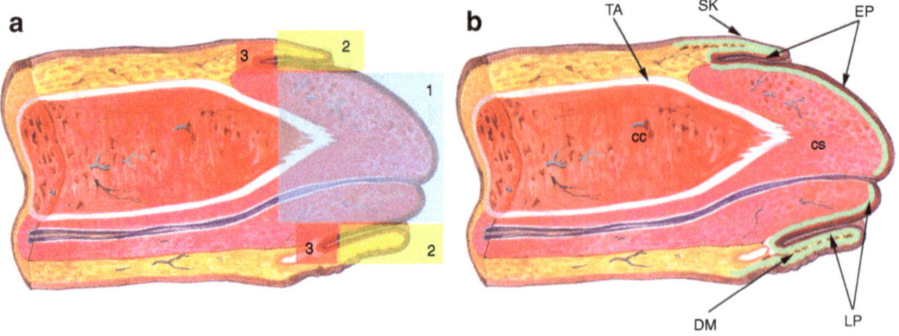

Fig. 3.1 Penile anatomy. (**a**) Anatomical compartments: *1* is glans, *2* is foreskin, and *3* represents coronal sulcus. (**b**) Anatomical levels in the glans are *EP* (epithelium), *LP* (lamina propria), *CS* (corpus spongiosum), *CC* (corpus cavernosum), and *TA* (tunica albuginea). Foreskin levels are EP, LP, *DM* (dartos muscle), and *SK* (skin)

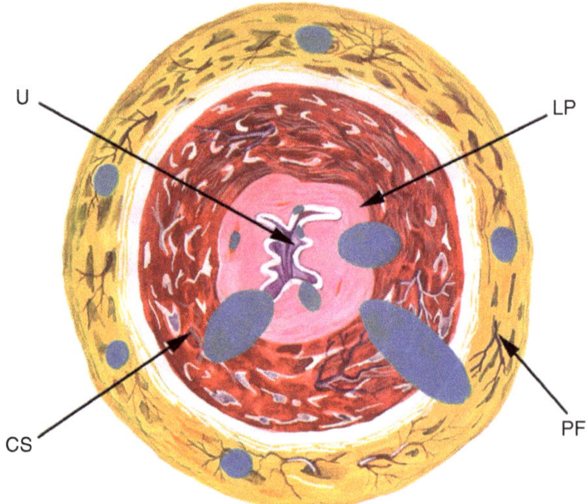

Fig. 3.2 Positive surgical margins. Frequent sites of tumor involvement in urethral and periurethral tissues. Each *blue dot* represents the affected site in a different patient. Urethral epithelium and penile fascia are the most commonly involved anatomical sites in the urethra. *U* urethra, *LP* lamina propria, *CS* corpus spongiosum, *PF* penile fascia

in the glans, squamous epithelium, lamina propria (LP), corpus spongiosum (CS), and corpora cavernosa (CC). The latter are subdivided by the tunica albuginea, which is considered part of the corpus cavernosum. In the foreskin, the levels are squamous epithelium, lamina propria, dartos muscle, and outer skin (Fig. 3.1b) [4, 5]. Anatomical levels for coronal sulcus tumors are not well established, considering the rarity of tumors originating at this site [5]. For the evaluation of resection margins, anatomical sites commonly involved by carcinoma should be identified. In one study, the most common site was demonstrated to be the penile urethral margin with its underlying lamina propria and surrounding corpus spongiosum, penile

Table 3.1 Pathological classification of invasive SCCs

Frequent subtypes	Rare subtypes
Usual SCC	Carcinoma cuniculatum
Verrucous carcinoma	Papillary-basaloid carcinoma
Basaloid carcinoma	Sarcomatoid carcinoma
Warty (condylomatous) carcinoma	Pseudohyperplastic carcinoma
Papillary carcinoma	Pseudoglandular carcinoma
Warty-basaloid carcinoma	Adenosquamous carcinoma
Mixed squamous cell carcinomas	Mucoepidermoid carcinoma

(Buck) fascia, and skin of shaft (Fig. 3.2) [6]. There is some criticism of the current pathological TNM staging system. Currently, a T2 is given to tumors invading either corpus spongiosum or corpus cavernosum. We and others think that tumor invasion of each anatomical level, CS and CC, should be given a different T, considering the variable prognosis of tumors in each invasion category [7–9].

Subtypes of Invasive Squamous Cell Carcinomas

About half of penile neoplasms are conventional squamous cell carcinomas (Usual SCCs). There are, however, various subtypes with distinct clinical, morphological, and outcome features (Table 3.1) [2, 10]. Well known is the *verrucous carcinoma* (Fig. 3.3a), recognized in the oral mucosa by Dr. Lauren Ackerman [11]. They are exophytic verruciform tumors which on cut surface show a white tumor with a distinct broad base separating it from the stroma [12]. Microscopically, they are papillomatous, acanthotic, keratinizing, and extremely differentiated neoplasms. There are three pathological variants, the classical or pure, by definition noninvasive; the microinvasive (in lamina propria), both without metastatic potential; and the mixed or hybrid, with metastatic potential in up to 20–25 % of the cases [2].

Carcinoma cuniculatum is a variant of verrucous carcinoma characterized by a distinctive labyrinthine growth pattern simulating rabbits' burrows (Fig. 3.3b). Similar tumors have been originally described in the plantar region of the foot [13]. Tumor tracts and sinuses are present, often with foreskin fistula formation. No nodal metastases have been reported [14].

Basaloid carcinomas are distinctive and aggressive penile tumors. The gross appearance of the cut surface is characteristic: a solid, tan, firm moderately to deeply invasive neoplasm with yellow foci of necrosis. Microscopically there is a nesting pattern, often confluent, each nest with a solid or necrotic (comedonecrosis) center (Fig. 3.3c). Keratinization, when present, is abrupt and non-gradual. Cells are small or intermediate, basophilic, spindle, or pleomorphic, with many apoptotic and mitotic figures. Vascular and perineural invasion are frequent. Metastasis is present in more than 50 % of the cases [15].

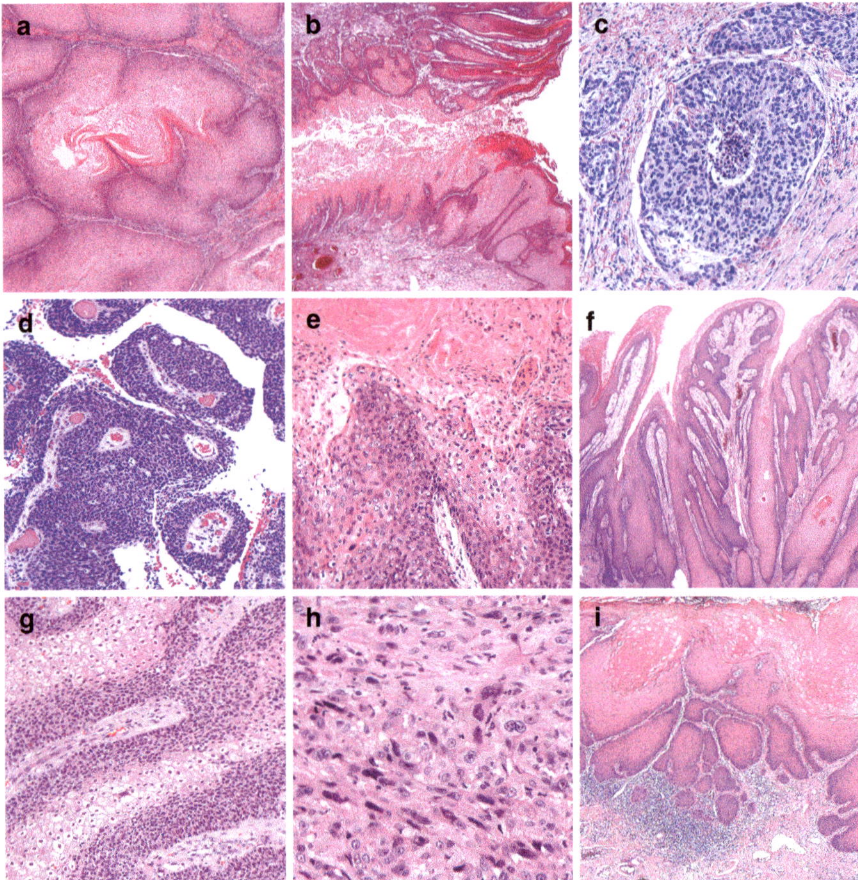

Fig. 3.3 Subtypes of invasive squamous cell carcinomas. (**a**) *Verrucous carcinoma*: extremely differentiated, acanthotic, keratinizing carcinoma. There is a sharp delineation between tumor and underlying stroma. (**b**) *Cuniculatum*: deeply penetrating low-grade hyperkeratotic tumor. Tumor "burrows" into underlying tissues. Note the verrucous features of the tumor. (**c**) *Basaloid*: there is a nesting pattern of growth. Each nest is composed of basophilic small neoplastic cells. There is central necrosis (comedonecrosis). (**d**) *Papillary-basaloid*: note the condylomatous papillae with a central fibrovascular core. Cells are basophilic and uniformly small. (**e**) *Warty (condylomatous)*: there is hyperkeratosis and papillomatosis. The papillae are typically condylomatous with a central fibrovascular core and pleomorphic koilocytosis. (**f**) *Papillary, NOS*: hyperkeratosis and papillomatosis. Papillae are irregular and composed of well-differentiated squamous cells. No koilocytosis is present. (**g**) *Warty-basaloid*: tumor invasive nest with both koilocytic (clear) and basaloid (*blue*) cells. (**h**) *Sarcomatoid*: there are spindle and giant cell features simulating a sarcoma. (**i**) *Pseudohyperplastic*: extremely well-differentiated SCC with infiltration of preputial lamina propria. The lesion simulates pseudoepitheliomatous squamous hyperplasia

The *papillary-basaloid carcinoma*, a variant of basaloid carcinomas which may simulate urothelial tumors, has been recently reported. The surface is exophytic and villous. Microscopically the papillae resemble condylomatous papillae, but unlike warty carcinomas composed of keratinized pleomorphic koilocytosis, the cells are uniformly small and basaloid (Fig. 3.3d). Urothelial immunohistochemical markers are negative. Patients with purely exophytic and minimally invasive tumors do well, but if deeply invasive, they carry a potential for nodal metastasis [16].

Warty (condylomatous) carcinomas are verruciform neoplasms with a characteristic cobblestone appearance. The cut surface shows an exoendophytic tumor. Histologically, the tumor at low power resembles condylomas. At high power cells are malignant. The papilla is arborescent with a central fibrovascular core. The cells are keratinized, pleomorphic, and with koilocytosis (Fig. 3.3e). The interface between tumor and stroma is jagged. The differential diagnosis with giant condylomas (Buschke-Lowenstein tumor) may be problematic especially in those atypical. Low-risk HPV by polymerase chain reaction (PCR) or a negative $p16^{INK4a}$ immunohistochemical stain would favor a giant condyloma. Prognosis in warty carcinomas is in general good, but occasional nodal metastasis may occur, mainly in deeply invasive carcinomas [17].

Papillary carcinoma, a verruciform tumor, is diagnosed after the exclusion of verrucous and warty carcinomas. Grossly they are exophytic and large. The cut surface shows a jagged interface between tumor and stroma. Microscopically, there is papillomatosis and low-grade histology (Fig. 3.3f). Unlike verrucous carcinomas, acanthosis is not prominent, and the interface of the tumor and stroma is jagged. Unlike warty carcinoma, no koilocytosis is observed. Prognosis is excellent, with infrequent metastases, providing corpora cavernosa is not invaded [18].

Warty-basaloid carcinomas (Fig. 3.3g) are heterogeneous exoendophytic neoplasms. Histologically, mixed features of warty and basaloid carcinomas are noted. Frequently, condylomatous features are present at the surface, and basaloid carcinoma features in the deeper invasive component. In fewer cases, there is a mixture of warty and basaloid features in the invasive tumor (Fig. 3.3g) without papillomatous surface. Metastatic rates are higher than in warty carcinoma but lower than in basaloid carcinoma [19].

Sarcomatoid carcinomas are biphasic epithelial spindle cell neoplasms. Macroscopically, they may be polypoid or hemorrhagic and necrotic. Histologically, they are sarcomatoid spindle and giant cell tumors (Fig. 3.3h) and may simulate malignant fibrous histiocytoma, leiomyosarcoma, rhabdomyosarcoma, fibrosarcoma, or osteosarcoma. Diagnostic clues are tumor location in glans and not in corpora cavernosa (where most sarcomas occur) [2], presence of areas of invasive carcinoma, or foci of penile intraepithelial neoplasia (PeIN). Immunohistochemical stains with high-molecular-weight cytokeratins and p63 are useful for diagnosis. Nodal metastasis and tumor-related death are common [20]. It is the penile carcinoma with the worst prognosis.

Pseudohyperplastic carcinomas are unusual and affect mainly the foreskin of older individuals with long-standing lichen sclerosus. They are extremely differentiated tumors simulating pseudoepitheliomatous hyperplasia (Fig. 3.3i), often multicentric or spread superficially. Secondary tumors may harbor verrucous or papillary features making diagnosis of tumor type difficult. Pseudohyperplastic carcinomas rarely invade beyond lamina propria. In relation with their low grade and superficiality, the prognosis is excellent [21].

Pseudoglandular carcinomas resemble adenocarcinomas. There are acantholytic or adenoid features secondary to central necrosis of tumor nests. There may be a honeycomb polycystic appearance. These tumors are usually of high grade with a high metastatic rate [22].

Mixed squamous cell carcinomas are heterogeneous neoplasms in which more than 2 of the previously described features are present. Common mixtures are verrucous SCC, warty-basaloid, and others.

Surface adenosquamous carcinoma is a rare tumor composed of squamous cell and adenocarcinoma. Glandular differentiation is usually focal and the squamous component predominates. About a dozen cases have been reported [10, 23–25]. The tumor originates in the glans central/perimeatal region and has a tendency for deep infiltration. Most tumors are high grade, with frequent vascular and perineural invasion. The glandular component is positive for mucin stains and CEA.

Mucoepidermoid carcinoma of the penis is an exceedingly rare tumor histologically similar to its cervical counterpart. The neoplasia is composed of cells with squamous and mucinous differentiation and, unlike adenosquamous carcinomas, without well-defined glandular or ductal structures. CEA and mucin stains are positive [26, 27].

Pathological Prognostic Factors: Risk Groups

Pathological Prognostic Factors

Routes of cancer spread: There is a predictable pattern of local, regional, and systemic spread in penile carcinomas. Early invasion is in lamina propria. It follows infiltration of preputial dartos and/or corpus spongiosum. Later and more significant invasion is in skin of the foreskin or corpora cavernosa. Urethral invasion occurs in either early or advanced stages and should not be an indicator of late stage. Intrapenile satellitosis (i.e., nodules of carcinoma separated from the main tumor mass) is a late phenomenon indicative of aggressive behavior [6, 28]. Regional invasion also follows a pattern starting with the sentinel lymph node, usually in the upper inner inguinal quadrant [29], although some tumors metastasize directly to deep inguinal nodes. Skip metastasis to pelvic nodes is most unusual [30]. Penile carcinoma is considered a locoregional disease, but widespread dissemination occurs in 20–40 % of patients. Death from cancer usually occurs within 2–3 years of initial diagnosis [10]. Metastatic sites at autopsy are the lymph nodes (pelvic, retroperitoneal, and mediastinal), liver, lungs, bone, and myocardium [31].

A small biopsy is usually not sufficient for a proper evaluation of all pathological prognostic factors. Histological subtype and tumor grade can be assessed in 70 % of the cases, but tumor depth and vascular invasion are correctly determined in only

9 and 11 % of the cases (as compared with the resected specimen) [32]. Resection specimens such as circumcisions, glansectomies, or penectomies are recommended for the identification of pathologic prognostic factors. The number of tissue sections determines the accuracy of pathologic evaluation and the proper identification of prognostic factors. A detailed protocol for handling circumcisions and penectomies and a check list for prognostic factors are in the manual of the College of American Pathologists [1].

Inguinal nodal metastasis is the single most important adverse prognostic factor. Reported pathological factors related to prognosis are tumor site of origin, tumor growth pattern, histological grade, depth of invasion or thickness in mm, anatomical levels of invasion, histological subtypes, irregular front of invasion, vascular and perineural invasion, positive surgical margins and urethral invasion, HPV, and other molecular factors [3].

Anatomical location: Sites of the primary tumor may have prognostic significance. Tumors exclusive of the foreskin are associated with better prognosis than those exclusive of glans. Tumors in the foreskin tend to be superficial, highly keratinized, associated with lichen sclerosus, and of lower grade, whereas those of the glans tend to be deeper, of higher grade, and associated with HPV. Carcinomas of the foreskin show a lower frequency of regional metastasis [33].

Patterns of growth (Fig. 3.4): Tumors with a *superficial spreading* growth pattern show a lower incidence of groin metastasis. Tumor recurrence in glans may occur in circumcised patients with superficially spreading tumors due to subclinical microscopic tumors left at the time of original surgery. *Verruciform* tumors have excellent prognosis despite their occasional large size and deep invasion mainly due to their low-grade histology. Tumors with *vertical growth* pattern have the worst prognosis with a high metastatic rate. *Multicentric* tumors are defined as independent noncontinuous foci of carcinoma affecting one or more than one anatomical compartments; they are usually superficial and of low-grade histology [34, 35].

Histological grade: Histologic grade predicts metastasis in penile cancer, but reproducibility of grading systems may be problematic. For this reason it is advisable to select an adequate grading method. Tumor heterogeneity (more than a grade present in the same tumor) should be considered. We use a simple 3-tier system that emphasizes grading both extremes of the differentiation spectrum, well differentiated (grade 1) and poorly differentiated (grade 3) (Fig. 3.5). In the grade two category are the remaining tumors [36, 37].

Depth of invasion: Depth of invasion and tumor thickness are significant pathological prognostic factors related to patients' outcome. Tumors invading less than 5 mm are at low risk for metastasis. Tumors invading more than 10 mm show a high incidence of nodal metastasis (about 80 %). Tumors invading 5–10 mm are problematic to predict. In these instances, perineural invasion (PNI) and histologic grade are helpful features to take into account [37].

Anatomical levels of invasion: The TNM staging system is based on the progressive tumor invasion of anatomical levels [38]. Tumor involvement of anatomical levels correlates with inguinal metastasis. Stage pTis is carcinoma in situ, and pTa

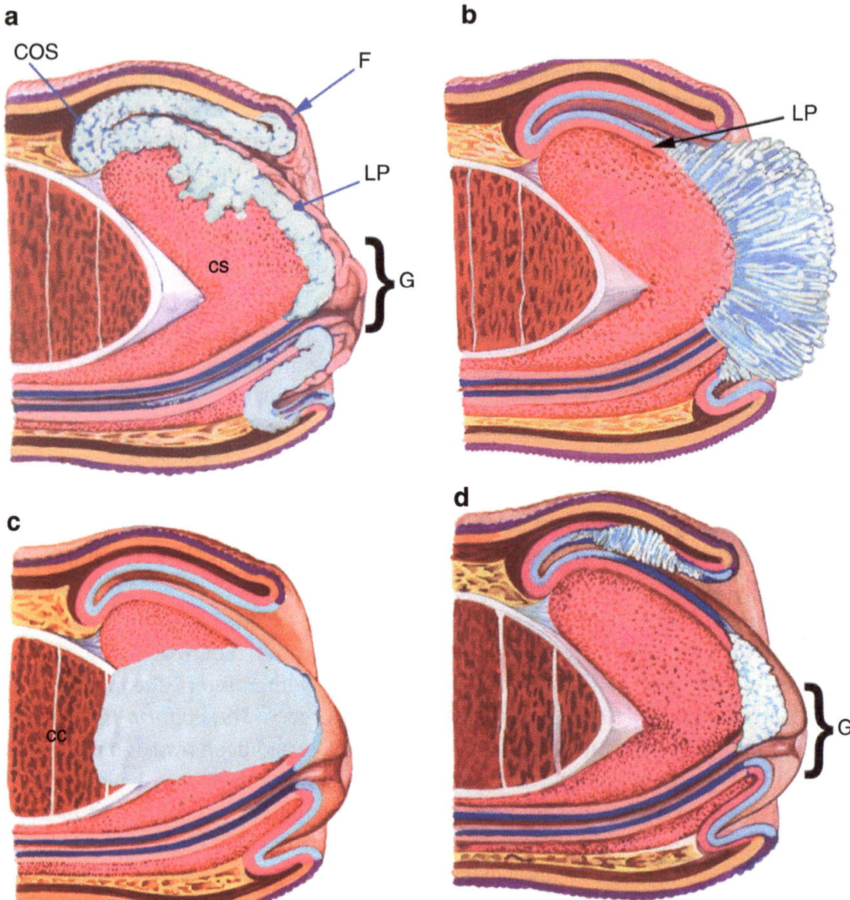

Fig. 3.4 Growth pattern (tumors depicted in *light blue*). (**a**) In *superficially spreading* carcinoma tumor grows horizontally involving lamina propria (*LP*) and superficial corpus spongiosum (*CS*) of multiple contiguous anatomical sites. *G* glans, *COS* coronal sulcus, *F* foreskin. (**b**) In *verruciform* tumors there is an exophytic and papillomatous growth. Invasion is superficial into lamina propria (*LP*). (**c**) *Vertical growth*: tumor deeply infiltrates into corpus cavernosum (*CC*). (**d**) In *multicentric* tumors, neoplastic growth affects discontinuously more than one anatomical compartment

corresponds to noninvasive verrucous carcinoma. pT1 invades lamina propria, and pT2 indicates invasion of corpus spongiosum or corpus cavernosum. Tumors invading penile urethra are staged as pT3, and tumors extending to adjacent organs are staged as pT4. Lumping the erectile tissues (corpus spongiosum and corpus cavernosum) into a single pT stage may not be appropriate because of the wide space separating LP from corpus cavernosum (about 10–13 mm) [4]. Tumors superficially invading the corpus spongiosum show a lower metastatic rate, whereas tumors invading deep corpus spongiosum show a higher metastatic rate, similar to those invading corpus cavernosum [7].

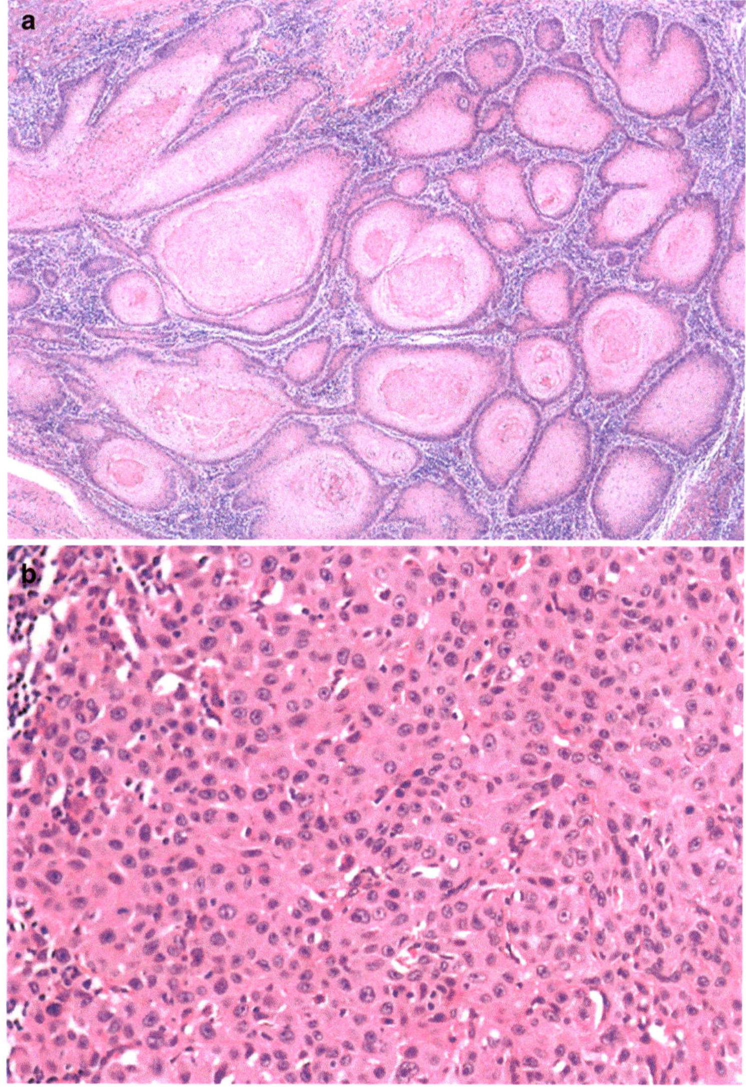

Fig. 3.5 Histological grade. (**a**) Extremely well-differentiated (*grade I*) keratinizing infiltrating SCC. Atypias are minimal. (**b**) Poorly differentiated (*grade III*) nonkeratinizing SCC growing in solid sheets

Histological subtypes: There is a broad correlation of histologic subtypes of SCC and rates of regional or systemic dissemination in univariate analysis. This is less significant on multivariate analysis [10]. Tumors associated with excellent prognosis are verrucous, papillary, warty, pseudohyperplastic, and cuniculatum carcinomas [2]. The high-risk group for metastasis comprises basaloid, sarcomatoid, adenosquamous, pseudoglandular, and poorly differentiated SCCs [39]. The intermediate category of metastatic risk includes the usual SCC, some mixed neoplasms, and pleomorphic variants of warty carcinomas [10]. In a study of 72 patients, histopathology classification was a significant predictor of lymph node metastasis [40].

Front of tumor invasion: The irregular invasion of small strands of cells was designated as the infiltrative front as opposed to the pushing front (large cell blocks with well-defined tumor borders). Patients with infiltrative tumor front demonstrated in one study to do worse than those with the pushing front [41].

Vascular invasion: Vascular invasion, lymphatic or venous, adversely affects prognosis of penile cancer. In an outcome study of 375 surgical resections, *lymphatic invasion* was an independent predictor of nodal metastasis [3]. Common sites of lymphatic invasion include the lamina propria underneath the squamous or urethral epithelium and the penile fascia [6]. *Venous invasion* is less frequent and appears in more advanced cases, mainly related to invasion of corpora spongiosa and cavernosa. Both lymphatic and vascular embolizations were found to be significant predictors of metastasis [42]. The pathological distinction of lymphatic and venular structures may be problematic and immunostains may be useful.

Perineural invasion (PNI) was the most significant single predictor of mortality in a study of 375 resected specimens [10]. In another evaluation of 134 patients with tumors invading from 5 to 10 mm, PNI and histologic grade were the most significant independent predictors of nodal metastasis [37]. For this reason PNI is part of our Prognostic Index (see below).

Resection margins and urethral involvement: Positive resection margins adversely affect prognosis in patients with penile SCCs [6]. Urethral involvement by cancer has been reported as an adverse prognostic factor [38, 43]. Invasion of the anterior urethra occurs in 25 % of cases, and it is not necessarily associated with a poor outcome as a pT3 classification would suggest [44]. Urethral invasion as an adverse prognostic factor should be reevaluated.

Presence of HPV: HPV status has proven to be a significant prognostic factor for survival and therapeutic response in certain head and neck SCCs [45], and a similar trend can reasonably be expected in penile carcinomas. Although HPV has been associated with high-grade tumors [46], the impact on outcomes is unclear. Some reports have not shown any survival difference, but others have reported HPV to be significantly associated with a favorable prognosis [47, 48]. A recent evaluation disclosed a better disease-specific 5-year survival in high-risk HPV-positive comparing with HPV-negative tumors (93 vs. 78 %). In multivariate analysis, the HPV status was identified as an independent predictor for disease-specific mortality [49]. In addition, a study indicated the presence of $p16^{INK4a}$, a tumor suppressor associated with the presence of high-risk HPV, in penile carcinomas as a survival advantage [50]. Therefore, it has been suggested that high-risk HPV penile tumors comprise a distinct clinical and molecular entity and that survival of patients with HPV-positive carcinomas may be related to a lower degree of gross genetic alterations.

Other molecular prognostic factors: A number of immunohistochemical markers of interest in the potential prediction of biologic behavior have been investigated in penile cancer, including the cell cycle-associated proteins Ki-67, p53, and $p16^{INK4a}$ [51, 52]. Ki-67 is a marker of cell proliferation that has been used to predict malignant behavior. p53 is a tumor suppressor protein that is often mutated in cancers, leading to its accumulation in malignant cells. However, the HPV E6 protein inactivates p53; therefore, its expression in HPV-related tumors is thought to be downregulated, at least in squamous cell carcinomas of the gynecologic tract [52]. However, overexpression of p53 on immunohistochemistry has been found in both HPV-positive and HPV-negative patients [50, 52, 53]. This supports the notion that these pathways of carcinogenesis are not mutually exclusive. Finally, p16^{INK4a} is a tumor suppressor protein known to accumulate in HPV-related tumors in response to Rb inactivation by the viral E7 protein [54]. Overexpression of p16^{INK4a} can be used as a reliable marker for the presence of high-risk HPV DNA and as a tool in the differential diagnostic of penile subtypes. p16^{INK4a}-positive tumors more likely exhibit a basaloid and/or warty morphology, whereas the negative cases tend to correspond to well-differentiated, keratinizing, low-grade variants of penile SCC [55]. Other suggested markers are E-cadherin, MMP-9 (matrix metalloproteinase-9), annexins I and IV, and decreased KAI1/CD82, a metastasis suppressor gene [56–60]. A focus of current research is to identify additional prognostic biomarkers in penile cancer.

Pathological Risk Groups for Prediction of Inguinal Metastasis and Outcome

The dynamic sentinel node biopsy is considered the best clinical instrument for detection of early nodal metastasis [61]. Before a wider dissemination of this method, not available in underdeveloped countries where penile cancer abounds, other methods more dependent of pathological findings were devised. A combination of prognostic significant factors forms the stratification risk groups. The better-known systems by Solsona et al. [62] and Hungerhuber et al. [63] are based on the combination of histologic grade and depth of invasion. A third system, which we use in our clinical practice for all invasive penile cancers, combines anatomical level of invasion, tumor grade, and perineural invasion [7]. There are three risk categories in all systems: low, intermediate, and high.

Solsona et al. [62] series comprises 33 patients with penile cancer. Patients with pT1 stage and grade 1 tumors are in the low-risk category. The high-risk category is for patients with stages pT2/pT3 and grades 2 or 3 tumors, whereas the intermediate group encompassed the remaining patients. Inguinal metastases appeared in 0, 33, and 83 % of the low-, intermediate-, and high-risk categories. Surveillance is proposed for the low -risk and lymphadenectomy for the high-risk group. They recognized the difficulty for an optimal approach for patients in the intermediate group.

Hungerhuber et al. [63] series was of 56 patients with inguinal lymphadenectomy. Patients with grades 1 or 2 and stage pT1 tumors were in the low-risk category. Patients with grade 3 tumors were in the high-risk group and the remaining in the intermediate category. Inguinal metastases were found in 8, 29, and 75 % of the patients in the low-, intermediate-, and high-risk groups. They recommended prophylactic lymphadenectomy for patients in the high-risk group and surveillance for those in the low-risk category. For the problematic intermediate group, authors suggested the dynamic sentinel lymph node biopsy [30].

The third system, named "*Prognostic Index*," was validated in a series of 193 patients with penile cancer [7]. Risk groups were based on scores obtained by the addition of numerical values given to histologic grade, deepest anatomical level involved by cancer, and presence of PNI. For histologic grades, the numerical values were 1, 2, and 3 points for well-, moderately, and poorly differentiated carcinomas. Values for anatomical levels were 1 point for lamina propria, 2 points for corpus spongiosum or dartos, and 3 points for corpus cavernosum or preputial skin. PNI was evaluated as follows: absence of PNI, 0 points, and presence of PNI, 1 point. Scores ranged from 2 to 7 points. Using this system, the inguinal metastatic rate was 0 % for the low-risk group (scores 2 and 3), 20 % for the intermediate-risk group (score 4), and 64 % for the high-risk group (scores 5–7). In addition, scores obtained with this system were also useful to predict survival. Patients with scores 2–4 had a 5-year survival rate of 95 %. The survival rate of patients with scores 5 and 6 was 65 %, whereas the score 7 was associated with a survival rate of 45 %. This method requires a resected specimen and a thorough pathological evaluation. It needs to be tested in patients with nonpalpable inguinal lymph nodes.

Nomograms to predict patient outcome have been recently designed. The first includes eight clinical and pathologic variables [64] selected from a multivariate analysis performed on 175 patients from 11 institutions. The following data were used: clinical stage of lymph nodes, microscopic growth pattern, histologic grade, vascular invasion, and invasion of corpus spongiosum, corpus cavernosum, and urethra. The model showed good prognostic accuracy and calibration. The probability of nodal metastasis, as predicted by the nomogram, was close to the actual incidence of metastasis observed at follow-up. A second nomogram was devised using the same clinical and pathologic factors with similar outcomes [65]. The third nomogram was based on a multivariate and regression analysis of pathologic data from 134 uniformly surgically treated patients with penile cancer most of them in the intermediate-risk category. PNI and histological grade were the strongest predictors of mortality in tumors measuring 5–10 mm in thickness. A nomogram was accordingly constructed using PNI and histological grade [37]. The probability of metastasis in grade 1 tumors without PNI was near zero; in tumors with grade 1 and PNI, the probability was 18 %. Grade 2 tumors without PNI had a probability of metastasis of about 40 %, but when PNI was present, it rose to 70 %. For grade 3 tumors without PNI, the probability of metastasis was 55 %; with PNI, the probability of metastasis was 80 %.

HPV in Penile Carcinomas

General Features

Penile cancers are likely to be initiated by interference with the cellular p14ARF/MDM2/p53 and/or p16^{INK4a}/cyclin D/Rb pathways, either by viral or nonviral mechanisms. This may lead to uncontrolled cell division and reduced apoptosis and may trigger a state of chromosomal instability that further drives the carcinogenic process. More common molecular events in late-stage penile carcinogenesis include altered expression of genes involved in disease progression, invasion, angiogenesis, and metastasis. HPV was found to be an important factor in penile cancer pathogenesis [46]. Epidemiological research has classified 15 genotypes of HPV as high risk, based on their association with cervical cancer, HPV-16, HPV-18, HPV-31, HPV-33, HPV-35, HPV-39, HPV-45, HPV-51, HPV-52, HPV-56, HPV-58, HPV-59, HPV-68, HPV-73, and HPV-82, and three types as probably high risk, HPV-26, HPV-53, and HPV-66 [66].

Kurman seminal study established the association of HPV with morphology indicating the correlation of the virus with histological subtypes of vulvar squamous cell carcinomas [67]. Gregoire also found, using cases from New York and Paraguay, a preferential detection of HPV in penile carcinomas of basaloid and mixtures of warty and basaloid morphology. Other tumors, such as verrucous, papillary NOS, and usual squamous cell carcinomas, are less frequently associated with the virus [46]. Despite the geographical coexistence of high incidence rates of cervical and penile cancer, it was noted that penile tumors pathologically resemble vulvar rather than cervical carcinomas. Penile HPV-positive carcinomas are, however, identical to cervical cancers. Near 100 % of cervical SCCs are HPV related [68], whereas it is found in about one third to one half of penile and vulvar cancers [69, 70]. For these reasons, a dual pathogenesis has been postulated for these tumors [46, 71]. Prevalence rates vary widely in the literature from 20 to 80 % with an average detection rate of 48 % [72, 73]. Variations in HPV detection rate may be related to (1) geographical prevalence differences of environmental factors (sexual habits, socioeconomic status, and/or cultural practices), (2) technical problems resulting in failures in the detection of HPV DNA by using inappropriate methods or testing the sample only once, (3) poor DNA preservation or degradation of tissue samples (DNA detection using PCR is highly sensitive, and tissue fixation for more than 24 h and the use of non-buffered formalin reduce the chances of detection), and (4) lack of experience or use of variable morphologic criteria for tumor classification resulting in low concordance rates when comparing series. Patients with HPV-positive tumors are about 10 years younger than those with HPV-negative tumors.

HPV Genotypes in Invasive Penile Carcinomas

HPV was detected in 64 (32 %) of 202 invasive penile SCCs in our recent study. Cases were classified according to the method published in 2011 by the Armed Forces Institute of Pathology Atlas of Tumor Pathology [2]. A single genotype was identified in most cases (48 cases; 75 %) [74]. High-risk genotypes were prevalent and specifically HPV-16 was the most common genotype (72 %) followed by HPV-18 (6 %). HPV-16 was frequent in basaloid and warty-basaloid carcinomas, although a greater variety of single genotypes (16, 6, 45, 11, and 18) were detected in usual SCCs (Table 3.2). Surprisingly, low-risk genotypes were also found in association with invasive carcinomas. Histological types associated with low-risk genotypes were 2 usual SCCs (HPV-6 and HPV-11) and 2 warty-basaloid carcinomas (HPV-6). Warty-basaloid carcinomas were more likely to be associated with multiple

Table 3.2 HPV-type prevalence distribution in penile carcinomas

Genotype	Frequency (%)
HPV-16	18.3
HPV-18	6.3
HPV-6/11	3.8
HPV-31	0.5
HPV-45	0.5
HPV-33	0.4
HPV-52	0.3
Other types[a]	1.2
Any type	47.0

Adapted by permission from BMJ Publishing Group Limited, Miralles-Guri et al. [73], copyright 2009

[a]Includes HPV-68 (0.2 %); HPV-34 (0.14 %); HPV-35 (0.14 %); HPV-53 (0.14 %); HPV-54 (0.14 %); HPV-74 (0.14 %); HPV-22 (0.07 %); HPV-39 (0.07 %); HPV-51 (0.07 %); and HPV-70 (0.07 %)

Table 3.3 HPV-related invasive squamous cell carcinomas

Subtypes	% HPV+
Papillary-basaloid	90
Warty-basaloid	82
Basaloid	76
Warty	39

infections (33 %) than warty (29 %), basaloid (16 %), or usual (11 %) carcinomas. In 6 of 13 tumors with multiple viral infections, the presence of both low- and high-risk HPVs was detected [74].

In a systematic literature review based on 31 studies including 1,466 penile carcinomas cases, the contribution of the HPV genotypes varied as follows: HPV-16 (60.23 %), HPV-18 (13.35 %), HPV-6/HPV-11 (8.13 %), HPV-31 (1.16 %), HPV-45 (1.16 %), HPV-33 (0.97 %), HPV-52 (0.58 %), and other types (2.47 %) [73]. An overall pooled estimate showed that HPV prevalence was found within a range from 24.5 % in verrucous SCC to 76 % in basaloid SCC, with an overall average percentage of 47 %. A recent study documented the very unusual association of low-risk HPV genotypes with various carcinomas from the anogenital region including the penis [75].

HPV and Histologic Subtypes of SCC

Higher HPV detection is observed in warty-basaloid (82 %), basaloid (76 %), and warty carcinomas (39 %) [74]. Among the HPV-positive basaloid carcinomas, there is a papillary variant resembling urothelial carcinomas [16] (Table 3.3). It was puzzling that despite classical morphological features [17], some warty carcinomas were negative for HPV. HPV is detected less frequently in usual (24 %), sarcomatoid (17 %), mixed (19 %), and papillary (15 %) carcinomas.

Table 3.4 High-risk HPV infection and p16^{INK4a} positivity in subtypes of invasive SCC

Subtype	No. cases	HPV+ (%)	p16^{INK4a}+ (%)	Concordance index (95 % CI)
Basaloid	40	29 (72.5)	34 (85)	78 (62–89)
Warty	28	10 (36)	8 (29)	86 (67–96)
Usual	95	16 (17)	10 (11)	83 (74–90)
Papillary	13	2 (15)	0 (0)	85 (55–98)
Sarcomatoid	6	1 (17)	0 (0)	83 (36–100)
Verrucous	8	0 (0)	0 (0)	100 (63–100)
Others[a]	7	0 (0)	0 (0)	100 (59–100)
Total	197	58 (29)	52 (26)	84 (78–89)

Modified from Cubilla et al. [55]

[a]Includes cuniculatum (2 cases), pseudoglandular (2 cases), and pseudohyperplastic (3 cases). CI indicates confidence intervals. Low-risk HPV-positive tumors excluded (5 cases)

HPV is not or rarely present in verrucous, pseudohyperplastic, pseudoglandular, and cuniculatum carcinomas. In the mixed category, the highest HPV positivity is present in squamous, warty, and/or basaloid carcinomas, whereas those tumors without W/B features, typically hybrid verrucous carcinomas, do not show evidence of HPV infection. Table 3.4 summarizes in detail the prevalence of HPV infection according to SCC subtypes [74].

Cell Types and HPV

Attention has been paid to the relation of tumor architecture and presence of HPV, but there are a limited number of studies evaluating cell types [69, 74]. We devised a classification of tumors in three cell types, small nonkeratinized basaloid (blue cell), koilocytic (clear cell), and larger eosinophilic, keratinized (pink cells). HPV was found in association of 72 % of tumors with predominant basaloid cells, 47 % of predominantly koilocytic cells, and only 19 % of tumors composed mostly of pink cells. The association of HPV in basaloid cells was significant in univariate and multivariate analyses. The association of HPV and koilocytes, diagnostic tissue hallmark of warty carcinomas, was marginally significant on univariate and not significant on multivariate analyses. The increasing low frequency or negativity of HPV was also associated with an increase in the proportion of maturing, keratinizing, differentiated squamous cells. Cell type appears to be more important than histological tumor configuration to predict presence of HPV [74].

The Value of p16^{INK4a} in the Classification of Subtypes of SCCs

The immunostain p16^{INK4a} may be used as a surrogate for HPV detection [55] (Fig. 3.6). Comparing virus detection by PCR and p16^{INK4a}, there is an overall concordance of 84 %. In a recent study, p16^{INK4a} positive tumors were present in 53

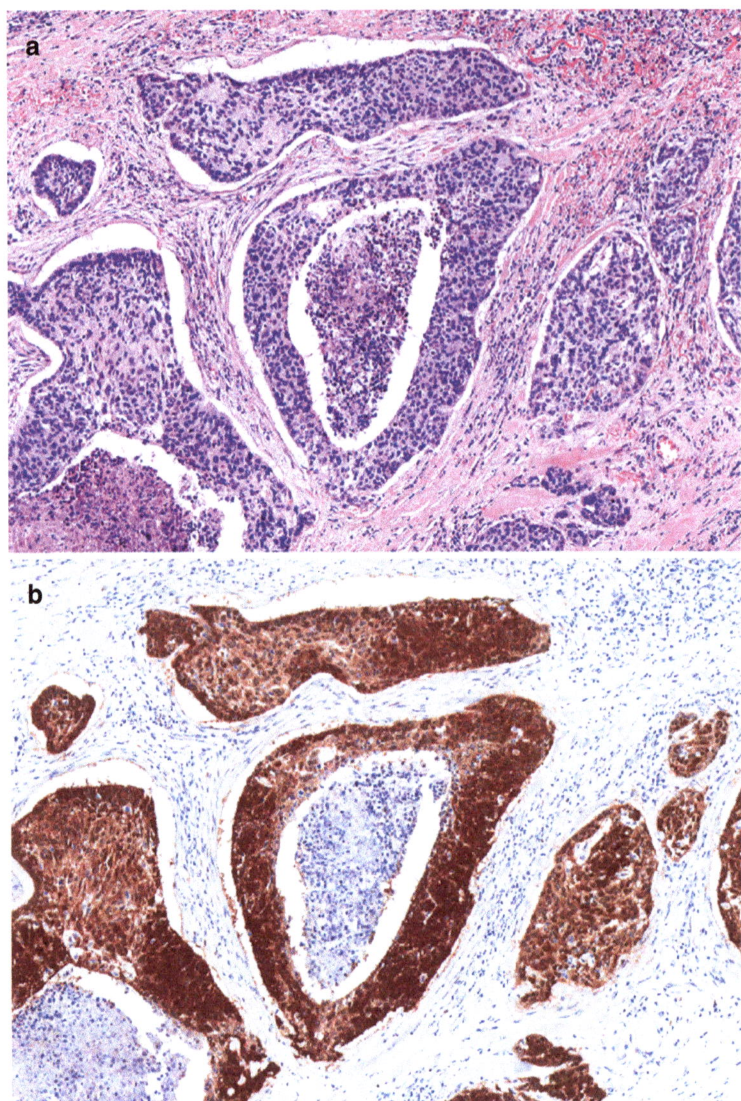

Fig. 3.6 p16^{INK4a} positivity. p16^{INK4a}-positive carcinoma: (**a**) infiltrating basaloid carcinoma with (**b**) strong positivity for p16^{INK4a}

(26 %) of 202 penile SCCs. Highest positivity was in basaloid or mixed basaloid carcinomas. Intermediate ratios were present in warty and usual carcinomas. Papillary, sarcomatoid, verrucous, cuniculatum, and pseudohyperplastic carcinomas were p16^{INK4a} negative (Table 3.4). Overexpression of p16^{INK4a} on immunohistochemistry can also be used as a prognostic marker and as a tool in the differential diagnostic of penile cancer [49, 50].

Table 3.5 Penile intraepithelial neoplasia (PeIN)

Differentiated	Undifferentiated
Classical	Basaloid
Hyperplasia-like	Warty
Pleomorphic	Warty-basaloid

Penile Intraepithelial Neoplasia (PeIN)

General Features

Penile precancerous lesions are among the oldest of such lesions to be historically recognized. To our knowledge first were Paget [76] and Tarnowsky [77]. In 1893, Fournier and Darier described the lesions in detail with the designation of "epithe-liome papillaire." Thomson's "psoriasis praeputialis" referred to epithelial changes found adjacent to ten invasive SCCs of the penis in 1897. Even now, psoriasis is a lesion which can be confused with differentiated PeIN. Better known are the terms erythroplasia of Queyrat (1911), who characterized the mucosal lesions [78, 79] and, Bowen disease, the later after the description of 2 cases of cutaneous carcinomas that were morphologically similar to those described by Queyrat, but localized in the extragenital skin. By extension, premalignant lesions of the skin of the penile shaft were also named as Bowen disease. Other terminologies for penile precancerous lesions were low- and high-grade squamous intraepithelial lesions; mild, moderate, and severe dysplasia; PIN I-II-III; or, like in WHO system, PIN III [80, 81].

Histologic Classification

As it was shown above, there is a consistent association of tumor morphology and presence of HPV in invasive penile carcinomas. Tumors composed of basaloid ("blue") cells are often HPV positive, whereas HPV is rare in tumors with eosinophilic ("pink") cells. A new nomenclature of penile precancerous lesions was proposed based on these observations. Precursor lesions can be also categorized as HPV related and HPV unrelated. The classification consists of two categories, differentiated and undifferentiated PeIN. The latter is subdivided in warty, basaloid, and warty-basaloid subtypes [2, 82, 83] (Table 3.5). Differentiated PeIN is commonly associated with usual SCC and their low-grade keratinizing variants, whereas warty or basaloid PeINs are seen adjacent to invasive warty or basaloid carcinomas. In our experience in our geographical region with a higher frequency of penile cancer (2–4 × 100,000 habitants), differentiated PeIN is a frequent precursor lesion of penile carcinomas. It is important to emphasize the difficulty of the diagnosis in some cases of differentiated PeIN, due to its minimal atypias. Sometimes immunohistochemical markers may be necessary. The second type of PeIN (the undifferentiated,

HPV-related type) shows distinctive morphologic changes and it is easier to categorize; then, it is most commonly diagnosed by pathologists. It corresponds to older terminology of Queyrat's erythroplasia and Bowen disease, terms we consider obsolete.

Clinical and Demographic Features

Patients with PeIN are usually 10 years younger than those with invasive carcinomas. They may present with a solitary or multifocal PeIN, or lesions may be found in association with invasive carcinomas. The noninvasive presentation is typical in countries with low incidence of penile cancer and diagnosis at earlier stages, whereas the presentation with invasive cancers is common in countries with high incidence of penile cancer. Differentiated PeIN is more prevalent in countries with high incidence of penile cancer, and undifferentiated PeIN is frequent in regions with low incidence of penile cancer [84]. In our experience, about two thirds of penile precursor lesions corresponded to differentiated PeIN [84]. In a survey of precancerous lesion from high-risk patients (phimotic) living in a geographical region with high risk for penile cancer, differentiated PeIN was found in 20 % of 116 consecutive circumcision specimens. Most differentiated PeINs were associated with lichen sclerosus [85].

Morphologic Features

Lesions are grossly white, pink to dark brown, or black-pigmented maculae or plaques. Surface is flat or, rarely, villous. Contours vary from sharply delineated to irregular. At cut surface, a linear white thickening of penile mucosa can be observed. Differentiated and undifferentiated PeIN cannot be clearly distinguished from one another based on macroscopic examination alone, but white leukoplakia-like lesions tend to be differentiated, and reddish or dark pigmentation is more typical of undifferentiated HPV-related lesions. Microscopically, *differentiated PeIN* (Fig. 3.7a) shows acanthosis, hyperkeratosis/orthokeratosis, and parakeratosis. Rete ridges may be flat or more typically elongated. Abnormal maturation is seen, characterized by enlarged keratinocytes with abundant eosinophilic cytoplasm, vesicular nuclei, and occasional prominent nucleoli mainly at the base but often present up to two upper thirds of epithelia. Intraepithelial keratin pearl formation, prominent intercellular bridges (spongiosis and, sometimes, acantholysis), and atypical basal cells with hyperchromatic nuclei are also noted. The surface of differentiated PeIN is usually flat, rarely papillary, and it is commonly adjacent to invasive SCCs. In a study, more than half of the cases of differentiated PeIN were associated with lichen sclerosus. In another study, lichen planus was associated with differentiated PeIN [86]. In *basaloid PeIN* (Fig. 3.7c), the cells are small to intermediate in size, round to ovoid basophilic nuclei, and immature with high nuclear/cytoplasmic ratio. Parakeratosis is frequent. Koilocytes within the parakeratotic surface can be noted, but they are not prominent. Apoptosis and mitosis are prominent. *Warty PeIN* (Fig. 3.7e) is characterized by acanthosis with a typical papillary or spiky surface and atypical parakeratosis. Cellular pleomorphism and pleomorphic koilocytosis are common. *Warty-basaloid PeIN* (Fig. 3.7g) shows mixed features of warty and basaloid types. They tend to have a spiking surface with koilocytes on the upper part of the epithelium, whereas the lower half of the epithelium is composed predominantly of small basaloid cells. Rarely, a warty or basaloid PeIN can be found in the same specimen associated with differentiated PeIN. There are cases in which the lesion is difficult to classify under the proposed system and we designated them as unclassified PeIN.

Immunohistochemical Features

p16^{INK4a} is usually positive in undifferentiated PeIN and negative in differentiated PeIN (Fig. 3.7b, d, f, h). In a study, the sensitivity of p16^{INK4a} for discriminating subtypes of PeIN was 82 %, with a specificity of 100 % and accuracy of 95 % [86]. p16^{INK4a} overexpression seems to be useful for discriminating differentiated, warty, basaloid, and warty-basaloid PeIN. An immunohistochemical triple panel of p16^{INK4a} /p53/Ki-67 determines the profile of penile precancerous lesions, including that of squamous hyperplasia, sometimes problematic to be distinguished from differentiated PeIN. Differentiated PeIN is usually p16^{INK4a} negative and Ki-67 positive,

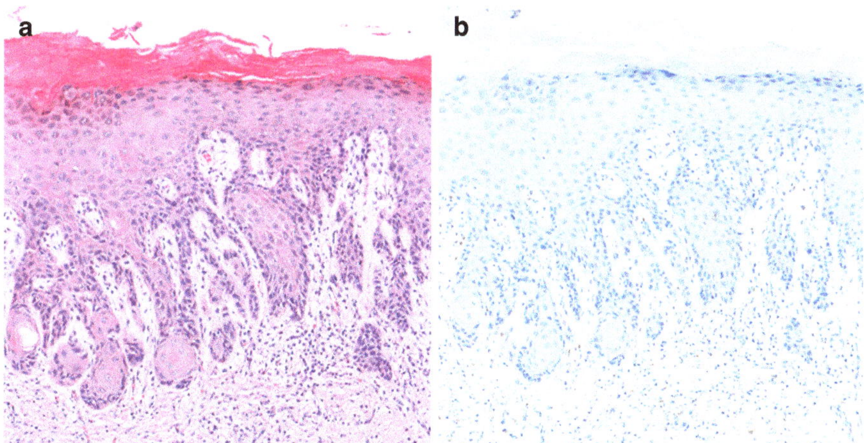

Fig. 3.7 PeIN subtypes. (**a**) Differentiated PeIN with a p16^{INK4a}-negative pattern (**b**). (**c**) Basaloid PeIN with a full-thickness p16^{INK4a}-positive pattern (**d**). (**e**) Warty PeIN with a spotty (negative) p16^{INK4a} pattern (**f**). (**g**) Warty-basaloid PeIN, note the strong positive p16^{INK4a} pattern in the blue basaloid cells (**h**)

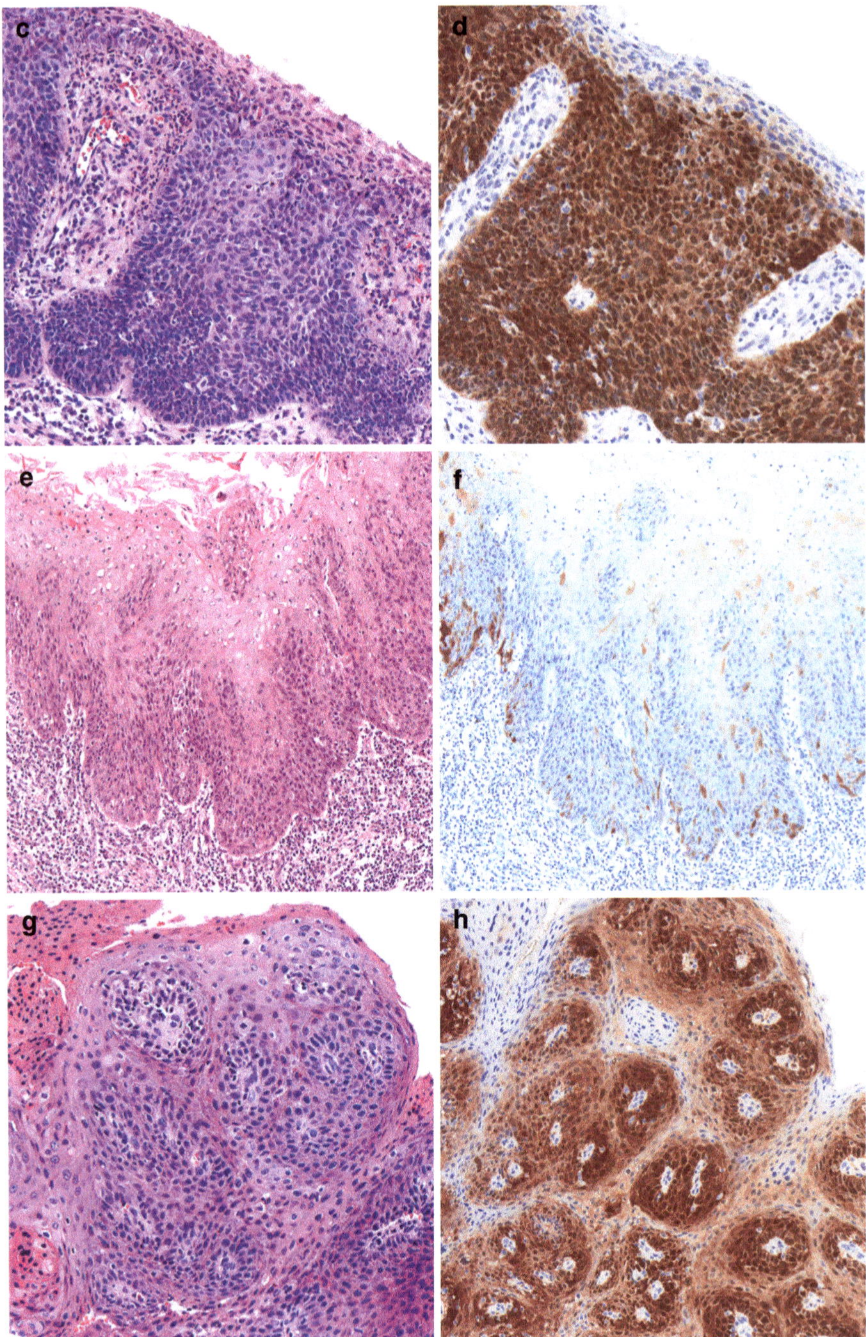

Fig. 3.7 (continued)

with variable p53 positivity. Basaloid and warty PeINs are consistently $p16^{INK4a}$ and Ki-67 positive, with variable p53 positivity. Positive Ki-67 and $p16^{INK4a}$ positivity practically exclude the diagnosis of squamous hyperplasia. $P16^{INK4a}$ positive exclude the diagnosis of differentiated PeIN.

Summary

The knowledge of penile anatomy is important because the identification of pathological risk factors and tumor staging depends of tumor sites (glans vs foreskin) as well as the invasion of specific anatomical levels. It is known that patients with tumors exclusively affecting the foreskin carry a better prognosis than those with primary neoplasm in the glans. There is a gradual increase in tumor regional metastasis and patient specific death according to invasion of penile anatomical levels (in the glans the lamina propria, corpus spongiosum, and corpus cavernosum and in the foreskin lamina propria, dartos, and dermis).

The majority of penile neoplasms are usual SCCs, but there is a broad spectrum of different subtypes with distinct pathological and outcome features. From the point of view of prognosis, subtypes of penile SCC can be grouped in those of low risk of metastasis and mortality (verrucous, pseudohyperplastic, papillary, and cuniculatum), intermediate risk (usual, warty, mixed), and high risk (basaloid, warty-basaloid, and sarcomatoid).

In addition to histological subtypes, there are other pathological factors that should be taken into account for tumor staging and prognosis: anatomical location, pattern of growth, histological grade, depth of invasion, anatomical level of invasion, front of tumor invasion, vascular and/or perineural invasion, resection margin, and urethral involvement. Prognostic risk group construction is based on the significance of the combination of some of these factors.

There is an association between tumor morphology and HPV status. A preferential detection of HPV is found in penile carcinomas of basaloid and mixtures of warty and basaloid morphology. Other tumors, such as verrucous, papillary NOS, and usual squamous cell carcinomas, are less frequently associated with the virus. Despite the consistent association of HPV with high-grade tumors, the impact of HPV infection on outcomes remains unclear. There are other molecular markers that have been used to classify and predict malignant behavior, including p16INK4, Ki-67, and p53. Overexpression of p16INK4 is associated with high-risk HPV.

Precursor lesions have been categorized as HPV related and HPV unrelated. There are two categories of penile intraepithelial neoplasia (PeIN): differentiated (HPV negative) and undifferentiated (HPV positive). The latter is subdivided in basaloid, warty, and warty-basaloid subtypes, each with distinctive morphology and HPV genotypes.

References

1. Velazquez EF, Amin MB, Epstein JI, Grignon DJ, Humphrey PA, Pettaway CA, Members of the Cancer Committee, College of American Pathologists, et al. Protocol for the examination of specimens from patients with carcinoma of the penis. Arch Pathol Lab Med. 2010; 134(6):923–9.
2. Epstein JH, Cubilla AL, Humphrey PA. Tumors of the prostate gland, seminal vesicles, penis, and scrotum, Atlas of tumor pathology. Washington, D.C: Armed Forces Institute of Pathology; 2011. p. 405–612.
3. Cubilla AL. The role of pathologic prognostic factors in squamous cell carcinoma of the penis. World J Urol. 2009;27:169–77.
4. Cubilla AL, Piris A, Pfannl R, Rodriguez I, Aguero F, Young RH. Anatomic levels: important landmarks in penectomy specimens: a detailed anatomic and histologic study based on examination of 44 cases. Am J Surg Pathol. 2001;25:1091–4.
5. Velazquez EF, Barreto JE, Cubilla AL. Chapter 38. Penis and distal urethra. In: Mills SE, editor. Histology for pathologists. 4th ed. Philadelphia: Lippincott Williams & Wilkins; 2012. p. 1027–42.
6. Velazquez EF, Soskin A, Bock A, Codas R, Barreto JE, Cubilla AL. Positive resection margins in partial penectomies: sites of involvement and proposal of local routes of spread of penile squamous cell carcinoma. Am J Surg Pathol. 2004;28:384–9.
7. Chaux A, Caballero C, Soares F, Guimarães GC, Cunha IW, Reuter V, et al. The prognostic index: a useful pathologic guide for prediction of nodal metastases and survival in penile squamous cell carcinoma. Am J Surg Pathol. 2009;33:1049–57.
8. Graafland NM, Lam W, Leijte JA, Yap T, Gallee MP, Corbishley C, et al. Prognostic factors for occult inguinal lymph node involvement in penile carcinoma and assessment of the high-risk EAU subgroup: a two-institution analysis of 342 clinically node-negative patients. Eur Urol. 2010;58:742–7.
9. Longpre MJ, Lange PH, Kwon JS, Black PC. Penile carcinoma: lessons learned from vulvar carcinoma. J Urol. 2013;189:17–24.
10. Guimaraes GC, Cunha IW, Soares FA, et al. Penile squamous cell carcinoma clinicopathological features, nodal metastasis and outcome in 333 cases. J Urol. 2009;182:528–34.
11. Ackerman LV. Verrucous carcinoma of the oral cavity. Surgery. 1948;23:670–8.
12. Johnson DE, Lo RK, Srigley J, Ayala AG. Verrucous carcinoma of the penis. J Urol. 1985;133:216–8.
13. Kathuria S, Rieker J, Jablokow VR, Van den Broek H. Plantar verrucous carcinoma (epithelioma cuniculatum): case report with review of the literature. J Surg Oncol. 1986;31:71–5.
14. Barreto JE, Velazquez EF, Ayala E, Torres J, Cubilla AL. Carcinoma cuniculatum: a distinctive variant of penile squamous cell carcinoma: report of 7 cases. Am J Surg Pathol. 2007; 31:71–5.
15. Cubilla AL, Reuter VE, Gregoire L, Ayala G, Ocampos S, Lancaster WD, et al. Basaloid squamous cell carcinoma: a distinctive human papilloma virus-related penile neoplasm: a report of 20 cases. Am J Surg Pathol. 1998;22:755–61.
16. Cubilla AL, Lloveras B, Alemany L, Alejo M, Vidal A, Kasamatsu E, et al. Basaloid squamous cell carcinoma of the penis with papillary features: a clinicopathologic study of 12 cases. Am J Surg Pathol. 2012;36:869–75.
17. Cubilla AL, Velazquez EF, Reuter VE, Oliva E, Mihm Jr MC, Young RH. Warty (condylomatous) squamous cell carcinoma of the penis: a report of 11 cases and proposed classification of 'verruciform' penile tumors. Am J Surg Pathol. 2000;24:505–12.
18. Chaux A, Soares F, Rodríguez I, Barreto J, Lezcano C, Torres J, et al. Papillary squamous cell carcinoma, not otherwise specified (NOS) of the penis: clinicopathologic features, differential diagnosis, and outcome of 35 cases. Am J Surg Pathol. 2010;34:223–30.
19. Chaux A, Tamboli P, Ayala A, Soares F, Rodríguez I, Barreto J, et al. Warty-basaloid carcinoma: clinicopathological features of a distinctive penile neoplasm. Report of 45 cases. Mod Pathol. 2010;23:896–904.

20. Velazquez EF, Melamed J, Barreto JE, Aguero F, Cubilla AL. Sarcomatoid carcinoma of the penis: a clinicopathologic study of 15 cases. Am J Surg Pathol. 2005;29:1152–8.
21. Cubilla AL, Velazquez EF, Young RH. Pseudohyperplastic squamous cell carcinoma of the penis associated with lichen sclerosus. An extremely well-differentiated, nonverruciform neoplasm that preferentially affects the foreskin and is frequently misdiagnosed: a report of 10 cases of a distinctive clinicopathologic entity. Am J Surg Pathol. 2004;28:895–900.
22. Cunha IW, Guimaraes GC, Soares F, Velazquez E, Torres JJ, Chaux A, et al. Pseudoglandular (adenoid, acantholytic) penile squamous cell carcinoma: a clinicopathologic and outcome study of 7 patients. Am J Surg Pathol. 2009;33:551–5.
23. Cubilla AL, Ayala MT, Barreto JE, Bellasai JG, Noel JC. Surface adenosquamous carcinoma of the penis. A report of three cases. Am J Surg Pathol. 1996;20:156–60.
24. Jamieson NV, Bullock KN, Barker TH. Adenosquamous carcinoma of the penis associated with balanitis xerotica obliterans. Br J Urol. 1986;58:730–1.
25. Masera A, Ovcak Z, Volavsek M, Bracko M. Adenosquamous carcinoma of the penis. J Urol. 1997;157:2261.
26. Froehner M, Schöbl R, Wirth MP. Mucoepidermoid penile carcinoma: clinical, histologic, and immunohistochemical characterization of an uncommon neoplasm. Urology. 2000;56:154.
27. Layfield LJ, Liu K. Mucoepidermoid carcinoma arising in the glans penis. Arch Pathol Lab Med. 2000;124:148–51.
28. Chaux A, Reuter V, Lezcano C, Velazquez EF, Torres J, Cubilla AL. Comparison of morphologic features and outcome of resected recurrent and nonrecurrent squamous cell carcinoma of the penis: a study of 81 cases. Am J Surg Pathol. 2009;33:1299–306.
29. Cabanas RM. The concept of the sentinel lymph node. Recent Results Cancer Res. 2000;157:109–20.
30. Leijte JA, Kroon BK, Valdés Olmos RA, Nieweg OE, Horenblas S. Reliability and safety of current dynamic sentinel node biopsy for penile carcinoma. Eur Urol. 2007;52:170–7.
31. Chaux A, Reuter V, Lezcano C, Velazquez E, Codas R, Cubilla AL. Autopsy findings in 14 patients with penile squamous cell carcinoma. Int J Surg Pathol. 2011;19:164–9.
32. Velazquez EF, Barreto JE, Rodriguez I, Piris A, Cubilla AL. Limitations in the interpretation of biopsies in patients with penile squamous cell carcinoma. Int J Surg Pathol. 2004; 12:139–46.
33. Oertell J, Duarte S, Ayala J, Chaux A, Velazquez EF, Cubilla AL. Squamous cell carcinoma (SCC) exclusive of the foreskin: distinctive association with low grade variants, multicentricity and lichen sclerosus [abstract]. Mod Pathol. 2002;15:175A.
34. Cubilla AL, Barreto J, Caballero C, Ayala G, Riveros M. Pathologic features of epidermoid carcinoma of the penis. A prospective study of 66 cases. Am J Surg Pathol. 1993; 17:753–63.
35. Villavicencio H, Rubio-Briones J, Regalado R, Chéchile G, Algaba F, Palou J. Grade, local stage and growth pattern as prognostic factors in carcinoma of the penis. Eur Urol. 1997;32:442–7.
36. Chaux A, Torres J, Pfannl R, Barreto J, Rodriguez I, Velazquez EF, et al. Histologic grade in penile squamous cell carcinoma: visual estimation versus digital measurement of proportions of grades, adverse prognosis with any proportion of grade 3 and correlation of a Gleason-like system with nodal metastasis. Am J Surg Pathol. 2009;33:1042–8.
37. Velazquez EF, Ayala G, Liu H, Chaux A, Zanotti M, Torres J, et al. Histologic grade and perineural invasion are more important than tumor thickness as predictor of nodal metastasis in penile squamous cell carcinoma invading 5 to 10 mm. Am J Surg Pathol. 2008;32:974–9.
38. Edge SB, Byrd DR, Compton C, Fritz AG, Greene FL, Trotti A. AJCC cancer staging manual. New York: Springer; 2009.
39. Cubilla AL, Reuter V, Velazquez E, Piris A, Saito S, Young RH. Histologic classification of penile carcinoma and its relation to outcome in 61 patients with primary resection. Int J Surg Pathol. 2001;9:111–20.
40. Dai B, Ye DW, Kong YY, Yao XD, Zhang HL, Shen YJ. Predicting regional lymph node metastasis in Chinese patients with penile squamous cell carcinoma: the role of histopathological classification, tumor stage and depth of invasion. J Urol. 2006;176:1431–5.

41. Guimarães GC, Lopes A, Campos RS, Zequi Sde C, Leal ML, Carvalho AL, et al. Front pattern of invasion in squamous cell carcinoma of the penis: new prognostic factor for predicting risk of lymph node metastases. Urology. 2006;68:148–53.
42. Ficarra V, Zattoni F, Cunico SC, Galetti TP, Luciani L, Fandella A, Gruppo Uro-Oncologico del Nord Est (Northeast Uro-Oncological Group) Penile Cancer Project, et al. Lymphatic and vascular embolizations are independent predictive variables of inguinal lymph node involvement in patients with squamous cell carcinoma of the penis: Gruppo Uro-Oncologico del Nord Est (Northeast Uro-Oncological Group) Penile Cancer data base data. Cancer. 2005;103:2507–16.
43. Novara G, Galfano A, De Marco V, Artibani W, Ficarra V. Prognostic factors in squamous cell carcinoma of the penis. Nat Clin Pract Urol. 2007;4:140–6.
44. Velazquez EF, Soskin A, Bock A, Codas R, Cai G, Barreto JE, et al. Epithelial abnormalities and precancerous lesions of anterior urethra in patients with penile carcinoma: a report of 89 cases. Mod Pathol. 2005;18:917–23.
45. Westra WH. The morphologic profile of HPV-related head and neck squamous carcinoma: implications for diagnosis, prognosis, and clinical management. Head Neck Pathol. 2012;6 Suppl 1:S48–54.
46. Gregoire L, Cubilla AL, Reuter VE, Haas GP, Lancaster WD. Preferential association of human papillomavirus with high-grade histologic variants of penile-invasive squamous cell carcinoma. J Natl Cancer Inst. 1995;87:1705–9.
47. Bezerra AL, Lopes A, Santiago GH, Ribeiro KC, Latorre MR, Villa LL. Human papillomavirus as a prognostic factor in carcinoma of the penis: analysis of 82 patients treated with amputation and bilateral lymphadenectomy. Cancer. 2001;91:2315–21.
48. Lont AP, Kroon BK, Horenblas S, Gallee MP, Berkhof J, Meijer CJ, et al. Presence of high-risk human papillomavirus DNA in penile carcinoma predicts favorable outcome in survival. Int J Cancer. 2006;119:1078.
49. Gunia S, Erbersdobler A, Hakenberg OW, Koch S, May M. p16(INK4a) is a marker of good prognosis for primary invasive penile squamous cell carcinoma: a multi-institutional study. J Urol. 2012;187:899–907.
50. Bethune G, Campbell J, Rocker A, Bell D, Rendon R, Merrimen J. Clinical and pathologic factors of prognostic significance in penile squamous cell carcinoma in a North American population. Urology. 2012;79:1092–7.
51. Guimarães GC, Leal ML, Campos RS, de ZequiS C, da Fonseca FP, da Cunha IW, et al. Do proliferating cell nuclear antigen and MIB-1/Ki-67 have prognostic value in penile squamous cell carcinoma? Urology. 2007;70:137–42.
52. Stankiewicz E, Kudahetti SC, Prowse DM, Ktori E, Cuzick J, Ambroisine L, et al. HPV infection and immunochemical detection of cell-cycle markers in verrucous carcinoma of the penis. Mod Pathol. 2009;22:1160–8.
53. Lam KY, Chan KW. Molecular pathology and clinicopathologic features of penile tumors: with special reference to analyses of p21 and p53 expression and unusual histologic features. Arch Pathol Lab Med. 1999;123:895–904.
54. Smeets SJ, Hesselink AT, Speel EJ, Haesevoets A, Snijders PJ, Pawlita M, et al. A novel algorithm for reliable detection of human papillomavirus in paraffin embedded head and neck cancer specimen. Int J Cancer. 2007;121:2465–72.
55. Cubilla AL, Lloveras B, Alejo M, Clavero O, Chaux A, Kasamatsu E, et al. Value of p16(INK)^{4}(a) in the pathology of invasive penile squamous cell carcinomas: a report of 202 cases. Am J Surg Pathol. 2011;35:253–61.
56. Zhu Y, Zhou XY, Yao XD, Dai B, Ye DW. The prognostic significance of p53, Ki-67, epithelial cadherin and matrix metalloproteinase-9 in penile squamous cell carcinoma treated with surgery. BJU Int. 2007;100:204–8.
57. Campos RS, Lopes A, Guimarães GC, Carvalho AL, Soares FA. E-cadherin, MMP-2, and MMP-9 as prognostic markers in penile cancer: analysis of 125 patients. Urology. 2006; 67:797–802.

58. Protzel C, Kakies C, Kleist B, Poetsch M, Giebel J. Down-regulation of the metastasis suppressor protein KAI1/CD82 correlates with occurrence of metastasis, prognosis and presence of HPV DNA in human penile squamous cell carcinoma. Virchows Arch. 2008;452:369–75.
59. Protzel C, Knoedel J, Zimmermann U, Woenckhaus C, Poetsch M, Giebel J. Expression of proliferation marker Ki67 correlates to occurrence of metastasis and prognosis, histological subtypes and HPV DNA detection in penile carcinomas. Histol Histopathol. 2007;22:1197–204.
60. Protzel C, Richter M, Poetsch M, Kakies C, Zimmermann U, Woenckhaus C, et al. The role of annexins I, II and IV in tumor development, progression and metastasis of human penile squamous cell carcinomas. World J Urol. 2011;29:393–8.
61. Horenblas S. Sentinel lymph node biopsy in penile carcinoma. Semin Diagn Pathol. 2012;29:90–5.
62. Solsona E, Iborra I, Rubio J, Casanova JL, Ricos JV, Calabuig C. Prospective validation of the association of local tumor stage and grade as a predictive factor for occult lymph node micrometastasis in patients with penile carcinoma and clinically negative inguinal lymph nodes. J Urol. 2001;165:1506–9.
63. Hungerhuber E, Schlenker B, Karl A, Frimberger D, Rothenberger KH, Stief CG, et al. Risk stratification in penile carcinoma: 25-year experience with surgical inguinal lymph node staging. Urology. 2006;68:621–5.
64. Ficarra V, Zattoni F, Artibani W, Fandella A, Martignoni G, Novara G, et al. Nomogram predictive of pathological inguinal lymph node involvement in patients with squamous cell carcinoma of the penis. J Urol. 2006;175:1700–4.
65. Kattan MW, Ficarra V, Artibani W, Cunico SC, Fandella A, Martignoni G, et al. Nomogram predictive of cancer specific survival in patients undergoing partial or total amputation for squamous cell carcinoma of the penis. J Urol. 2006;175:2103–8.
66. Muñoz N, Bosch FX, de Sanjosé S, Herrero R, Castellsagué X, Shah KV, International Agency for Research on Cancer Multicenter Cervical Cancer Study Group, et al. Epidemiologic classification of human papillomavirus types associated with cervical cancer. N Engl J Med. 2003;348:518–27.
67. Kurman RJ, Toki T, Schiffman MH. Basaloid and warty carcinomas of the vulva. Distinctive types of squamous cell carcinoma frequently associated with human papillomaviruses. Am J Surg Pathol. 1993;17:133–45.
68. Boyle P, Levin B, editors. Cervical cancer. World cancer report 2008. Lyon: International Agency for Research on Cancer; 2008. p. 418–23.
69. Krustrup D, Jensen HL, van den Brule AJ, Frisch M. Histological characteristics of human papilloma-virus–positive and –negative invasive and in situ squamous cell tumours of the penis. Int J Exp Pathol. 2009;90:182–9.
70. Toki T, Kurman RJ, Park JS, Kessis T, Daniel RW, Shah KV. Probable nonpapillomavirus etiology of squamous cell carcinoma of the vulva in older women: a clinicopathologic study using in situ hybridization and polymerase chain reaction. Int J Gynecol Pathol. 1991; 10:107–25.
71. Rubin MA, Kleter B, Zhou M, Ayala G, Cubilla AL, Quint WG, et al. Detection and typing of human papillomavirus DNA in penile carcinoma: evidence for multiple independent pathways of penile carcinogenesis. Am J Pathol. 2001;159:1211–8.
72. Backes DM, Kurman RJ, Pimenta JM, Smith JS. Systematic review of human papillomavirus prevalence in invasive penile cancer. Cancer Causes Control. 2009;20:449–57.
73. Miralles-Guri C, Bruni L, Cubilla AL, Castellsague X, Bosch FX, de Sanjose S. Human papillomavirus prevalence and type distribution in penile carcinoma. J Clin Pathol. 2009; 62:870–8.
74. Cubilla AL, Lloveras B, Alejo M, Clavero O, Chaux A, Kasamatsu E, et al. The basaloid cell is the best tissue marker for human papillomavirus in invasive penile squamous cell carcinoma: a study of 202 cases from Paraguay. Am J Surg Pathol. 2010;34:104–14.

75. Guimerà N, Lloveras B, Lindeman J, Alemany L, van de Sandt MM, Alejo M, et al. The occasional role of low risk human papillomaviruses 6, 11, 42, 44 and 70 in anogenital carcinoma defined by laser capture microdissection/PCR methodology. Results from a global study. Am J Surg Pathol. 2013;37:1299–310.
76. Paget J. On disease of the mammary areola preceding cancer of mammary gland. St Bartholomews Hosp Rep. 1874;10:87–9.
77. Tarnowsky VM. Congres des Medecins Busses. Moscow, January 19, 1891. Ann Dermatol Syphiligr. 1891;2:410.
78. Fournier A, Darier J. Epitheliome bénin syphiloïde de la verge (epithélioma papillaire). Bull Soc Fr Dermatol Syphiligr. 1893;4:324–8.
79. Queyrat A. Érythroplasie du gland. Bull Soc Fr Dermatol Syphiligr. 1911;22:378–82.
80. Cubilla AL, Meijer CJ, Young RH. Morphological features of epithelial abnormalities and precancerous lesions of the penis. Scand J Urol Nephrol Suppl. 2000;205:215–9.
81. Cubilla AL, Velazquez EF, Young RH. Epithelial lesions associated with invasive penile squamous cell carcinoma: a pathologic study of 288 cases. Int J Surg Pathol. 2004;12:351–64.
82. Chaux A, Velazquez EF, Amin A, Soskin A, Pfannl R, Rodríguez IM, et al. Distribution and characterization of subtypes of penile intraepithelial neoplasia and their association with invasive carcinomas: a pathological study of 139 lesions in 121 patients. Hum Pathol. 2012;43:1020–7.
83. Chaux A, Pfannl R, Rodríguez IM, Barreto JE, Velazquez EF, Lezcano C, et al. Distinctive immunohistochemical profile of penile intraepithelial lesions: a study of 74 cases. Am J Surg Pathol. 2011;35:553–62.
84. Soskin A, Vieillefond A, Carlotti A, Plantier F, Chaux A, Ayala G, et al. Warty/basaloid penile intraepithelial neoplasia is more prevalent than differentiated penile intraepithelial neoplasia in nonendemic regions for penile cancer when compared with endemic areas: a comparative study between pathologic series from Paris and Paraguay. Hum Pathol. 2012;43:190–6.
85. Oertell J, Caballero C, Iglesias M, Chaux A, Amat L, Ayala E, et al. Differentiated precursor lesions and low-grade variants of squamous cell carcinomas are frequent findings in foreskins of patients from a region of high penile cancer incidence. Histopathology. 2011;58:925–33.
86. Chaux A, Pfannl R, Lloveras B, Alejo M, Clavero O, Lezcano C, et al. Distinctive association of p16INK4a overexpression with penile intraepithelial neoplasia depicting warty and/or basaloid features: a study of 141 cases evaluating a new nomenclature. Am J Surg Pathol. 2010;34:385–92.

Chapter 4
Pathology and Genetics

Antonio Augusto Ornellas, Gilda Alves, and Aline Barros dos Santos Schwindt

Pathology

Squamous cell carcinoma of the penis (SCCP) has behaved similarly to squamous cell carcinoma in other parts of the skin. This tumor represents the most common malignant neoplasm that can be developed anywhere on the penis, affecting shaft and distal segment as glans, coronal sulcus, and foreskin. That distal sites shelter SCCP most frequently (Fig. 4.1).

Stage is important in the treatment of primary lesion. In a study with 196 patients, a local extension of the primary tumor into corpora cavernosa was found in 44.9 % of patients. The corpus spongiosum and urethra were involved in 21.4 and 35.2 % of cases, respectively [1].

Pathological factors with a known prognostic value, other than lymph node metastasis, are tumor thickness, grade, histological type, lymphovascular embolization, and stage [2, 3].

The rate of depth invasion is significantly high when the thickness is more than 5 mm. The histological grade of penile carcinoma, including SCCP usual type, should attend the protocol based on the American Joint Committee on Cancer, TNM, 7th edition [4]:

A.A. Ornellas, MD, PhD (✉)
Department of Urology, Instituto Nacional de Câncer,
Praça da Cruz Vermelha 23, Rio de Janeiro 20230-130, Brazil
e-mail: ornellasa@hotmail.com, asuint@gmail.com

G. Alves, PhD
Laboratório de Genética Aplicada, Serviço de Hematologia,
Instituto Nacional de Câncer, Rio de Janeiro, Brazil

A.B.dos S. Schwindt, MD, MSc
Department of Pathology, Instituto Nacional de Câncer, Rio de Janeiro, Brazil

D.J. Culkin (ed.), *Management of Penile Cancer*,
DOI 10.1007/978-1-4939-0461-7_4, © Springer Science+Business Media New York 2014

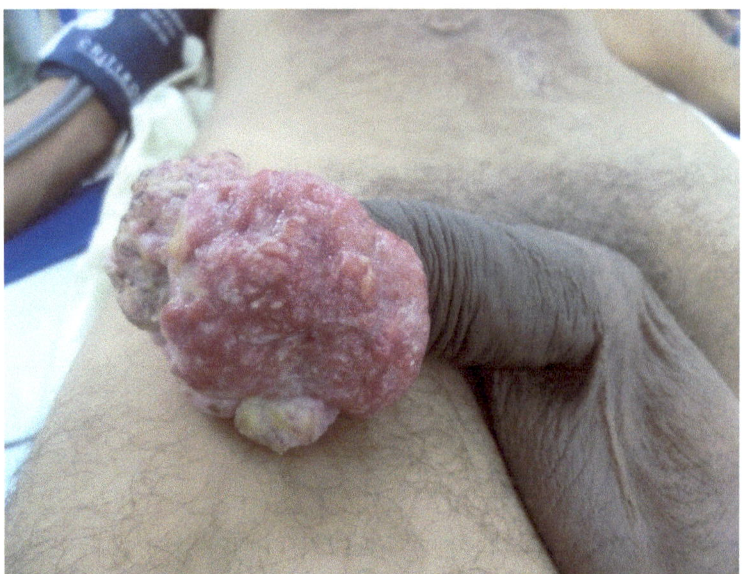

Fig. 4.1 Penile cancer. Exophytic lesion

(G1) Well-differentiated carcinoma, tumors with a minimal deviation from the morphology of normal/hyperplastic squamous epithelium (Fig. 4.2)

(G2) Moderately differentiated carcinoma constitutes the great part of the cases; tumors show a more disorganized growth as compared to grade 1 lesions, increased nucleus-cytoplasm ratio, evident mitoses, and, although present, less prominent keratinization (Fig. 4.3)

(G3) Poorly differentiated carcinomas are tumors showing any proportion of anaplastic cells, identified as solid sheets or irregular small aggregates, cords, or nests of cells with little or no keratinization, high nucleus-cytoplasm ratio, thick nuclear membranes, nuclear pleomorphism, clumped chromatin, prominent nucleoli, and numerous mitoses (Fig. 4.4)

A tumor should be graded according to the least differentiated component. Any proportion of grade 3 should be distinguished in the description. Patients with well-differentiated carcinoma have a higher 10-year survival rate than those with moderately and poorly differentiated carcinoma ($P<0.0001$ and $P=0.006$) [5].

Lymphovascular embolization and absent koilocytosis have proved to be independent prognostic factors for the risk of lymphatic metastasis. Patients with koilocytosis and without lymphovascular embolization had better 5-year survival [1].

SCCP can be seen as usual SCCP type or constituting the variant forms or subtypes sometimes associated with HPV. Basically the grossly usual SCCP shows itself either as a flat, an endophytic, or as an exophytic tumor (cauliflower

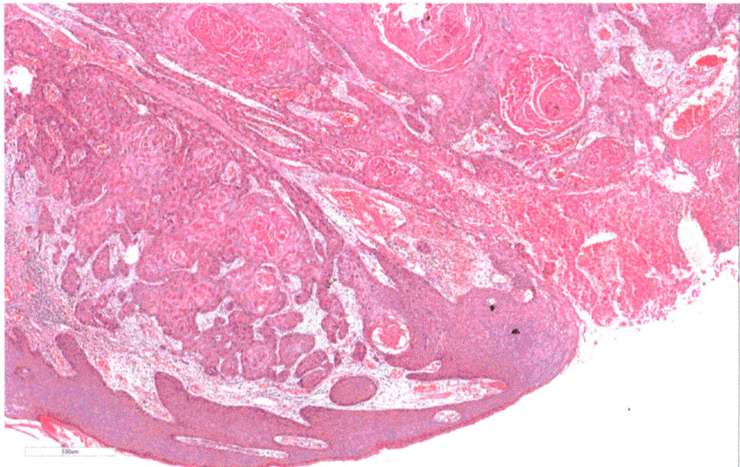

Fig. 4.2 Usual grade 1, well-differentiated SCC. Proliferation of mature epithelial cells with basal atypia forming nets. Abundant centralized keratin pearl

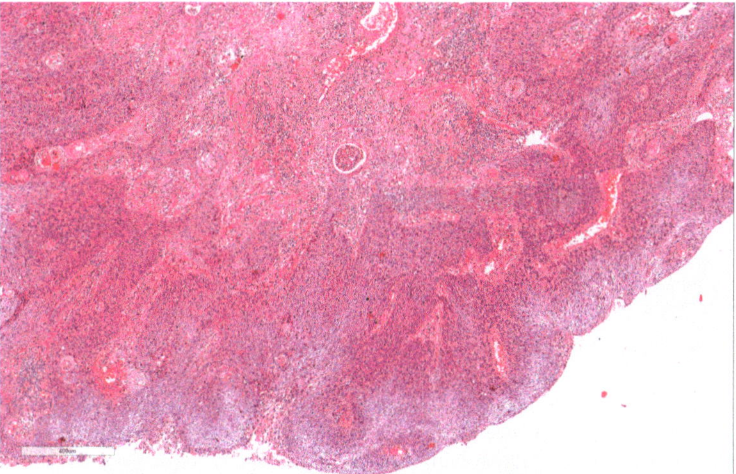

Fig. 4.3 Usual grade 2, moderately differentiated SCC. Less keratin and cell differentiation than grade 1. Irregular infiltrative borders, nuclear atypia, evident mitosis

appearance), white-gray and firm tumor with necrosis foci. Microscopically it consists of squamous cell proliferation that may infiltrate superficially or profoundly penile tissues and/or projecting outside itself with variable degrees of cytological atypia, mitotic figures, and keratin that can be seen as mild or prominent keratinized cell [6, 7].

Variations of squamous cell carcinoma or subtypes can be seen forming two groups: high-grade and low-grade groups. The high-grade tumors (basaloid and

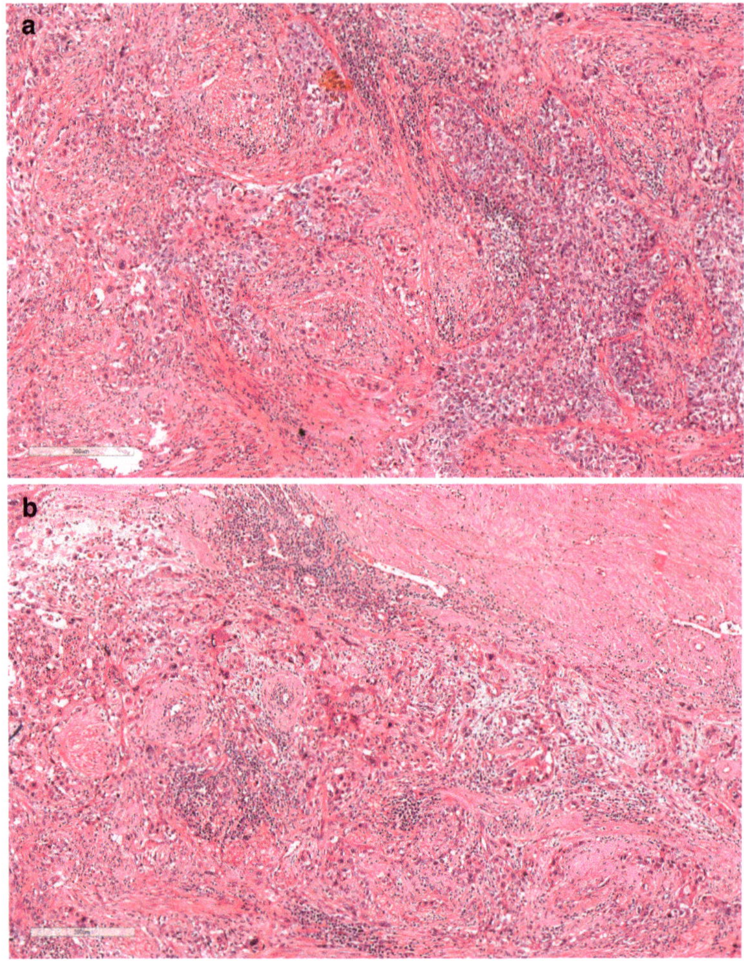

Fig. 4.4 (**a**) Usual grade 3, poorly differentiated SCC. Prominent stromal desmoplastic tissue involved solids nets and irregular small aggregates of anaplastic cells. Individual keratinized cells are present. (**b**) Usual grade 3, poorly differentiated SCC. Sheets, cords, and small aggregates of anaplastic squamous cells, isolated keratinized cells, nuclear pleomorphism, hyperchromatin, prominent nucleoli, and numerous mitoses

sarcomatoid) frequently are associated with deeper invasion, recurrence of tumors, lymph node metastasis, and significant mortality rate [8]. Low-grade variants (papillary, warty, and verrucous) have mild to moderate morbidity features and better survive rate [9]. The following are a short description of them:

Basaloid carcinoma (BC) is a high-grade subtype associated to HPV and can be seen as flat, endophytic, or papillar [10]. Macroscopic features are ulcerated lesion, flat or slightly elevated, and firm. Microscopy is infiltrated tumor made of cell nests with few cytoplasm and basophilic nuclei, centered by comedonecrosis. Nucleus is

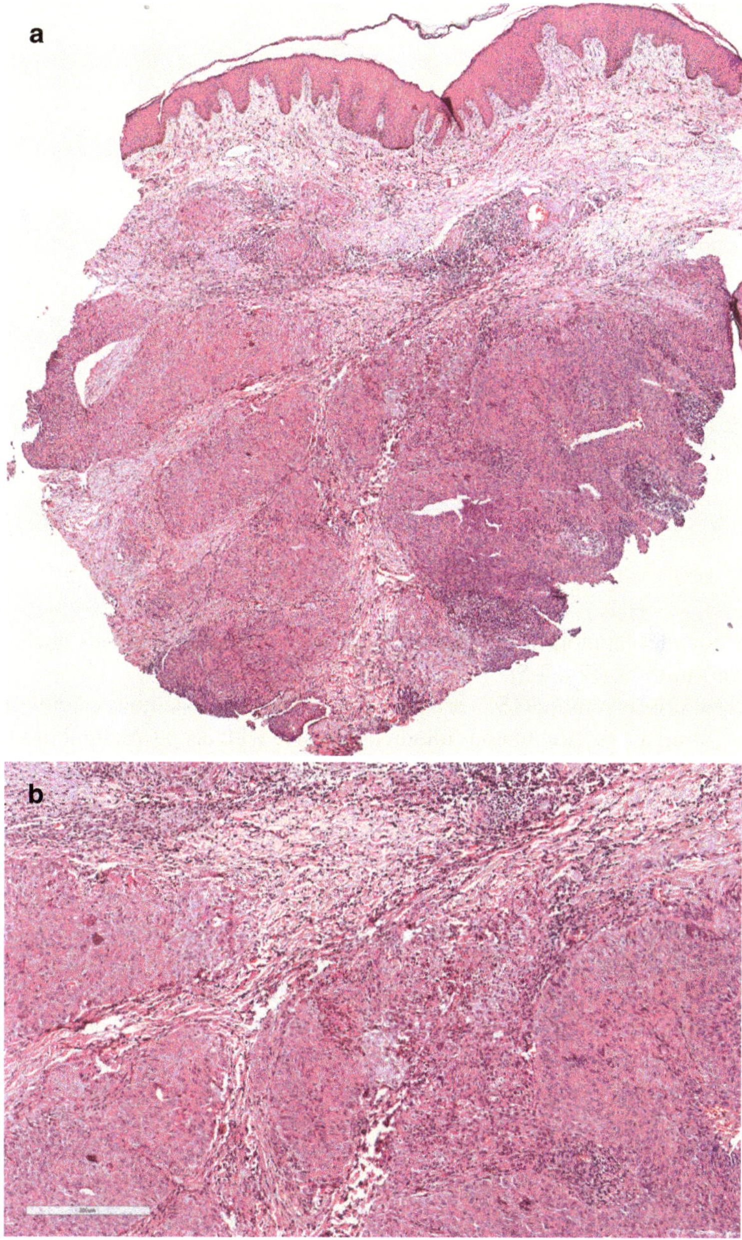

Fig. 4.5 (**a**) High-grade SCC, basaloid subtype (panoramic vision). Endophytic infiltrative tumor of basaloid cells. (**b**) High-grade SCC, basaloid variant group. Note irregularity of the tumor nets with ragged basal membrane showing its aggressiveness. Cells present poor cytoplasm, great oval or round basophilic nuclei with prominent nucleolus, and atypical mitoses. (**c**) Basaloid SCC subtype. Tumor shows papillary appearance. Comedonecrosis involved by basaloid cells

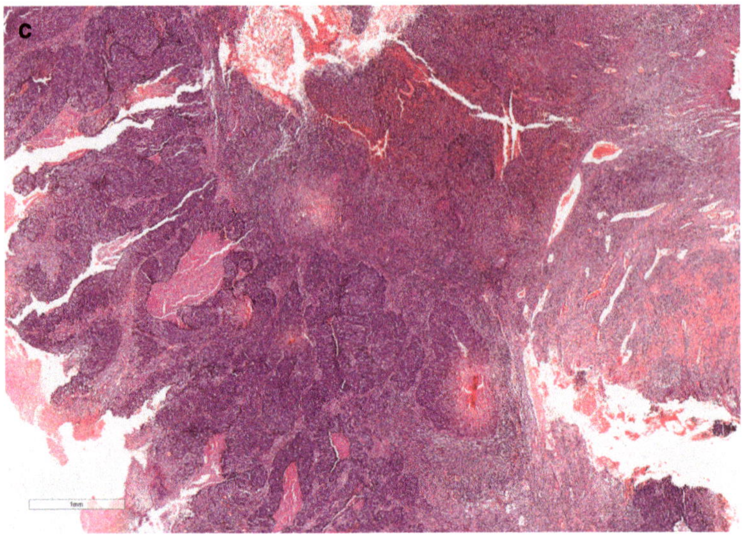

Fig. 4.5 (continued)

oval or round, pleomorphic and hyperchromatic, with inconspicuous nucleoli and numerous mitoses (Fig. 4.5).

Sarcomatoid carcinoma (SC) is a primary spindle-cell squamous carcinoma, rare in penis, similar to a sarcomatous tumor, aggressive with deep structural infiltration, poor prognosis, associated with lymphatic, and hematogenous spread (Fig. 4.6). Metastatic disease develops in a high percentage of cases. Distant tumor metastases occur mainly in lung, skin, bone, and pericardium and pleura [11, 12].

Warty carcinoma (WC) is a morphologically distinct verruciformis tumor with features of HPV-related lesions [13]. HPV attacks the squamous epithelium and produces nuclear atypia, binucleation, and koilocytosis (identified by a large halo around cellular nuclei) (Fig. 4.7).

Papillary carcinoma (PC) is a papillary well-differentiated carcinoma which can invade stromal tissue until deep structures but with rare lymph node involvement. The prognosis is good and tumor is associated with lichen sclerosus [9]. Grossly it is an exophytic white-gray and firm tumor. Microscopy is complex and simple papillae with fibrovascular core and hyperkeratosis.

Verrucous carcinoma (VC) is generally a large lesion (average 4 cm) with exophytic papillary growth, frequently softy, ulcerated sometimes purulent, and foul smelling tumor. Tumor can be seen anywhere on the penis, frequently on the glans and foreskin. A specific etiologic factor is not described. Microscopically, the presence of well-differentiated characteristics frequently makes hard differential diagnostics, mainly with condyloma accuminatum and well-differentiated SCC. Superficially, hyperkeratosis, acanthosis, and papillomatosis are seen, and it excavates through the normal tissue and slowly invades continuous structures (Fig. 4.8). Regional lymph node metastases are rare and distant metastases have not been reported [14].

Genetics

Introduction

Cancer is a disease caused by our own genes' deregulation. Cancer cells divide indefinitely as a consequence of a deep genetic expression turning. This occurs step by step or mutation by mutation until the cell reaches the point of no return, ignoring the cell cycle checkpoints. Environmental risk factors causing mutagenesis and the failure of the mechanisms of genome repair combine to promote mutations in the key genes that control the cell cycle progress.

The key genes in the carcinogenesis process are the proto-oncogenes and the tumor suppressor genes. In normal cells, proto-oncogenes are responsible for promoting the cell growth. When altered or mutated, they become oncogenes and then can contribute to indefinitely cell division. The tumor suppressor genes that are normally present in our cells can lose their capacity of controlling the processes of cell growth and cell death (called apoptosis) when they are mutated or deleted.

Damage in the key genes that control the cell cycle is caused by many factors. Carcinogens are a class of substances that are directly responsible for promoting cancer. Tobacco, asbestos, arsenic, radiation such as gamma and x-rays, the sun

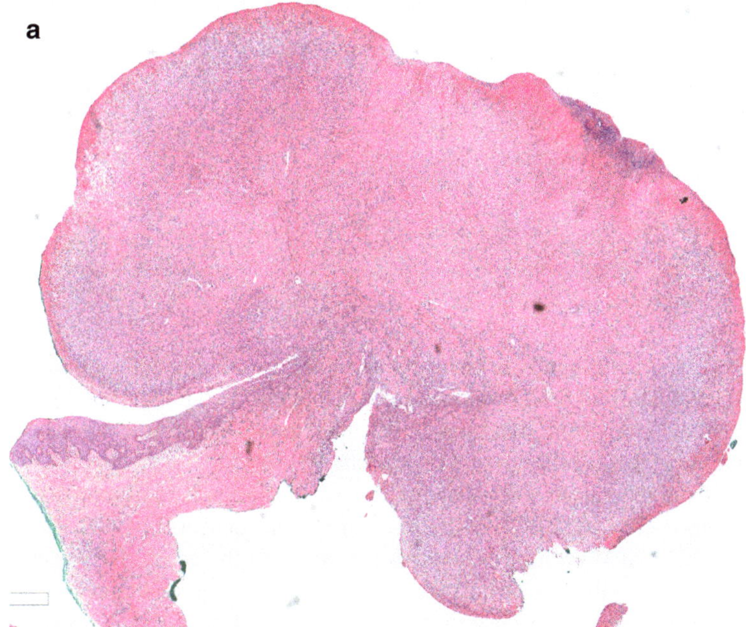

Fig. 4.6 (**a**) Spindle-cell carcinoma, high-grade group. Ulcerated tumor presents fusiform cells similar to those present in other sarcomatous tumors. (**b** and **c**) Sarcomatoid SCC. Groups of squamous and isolated brown cells were stained by 34BE12 keratin

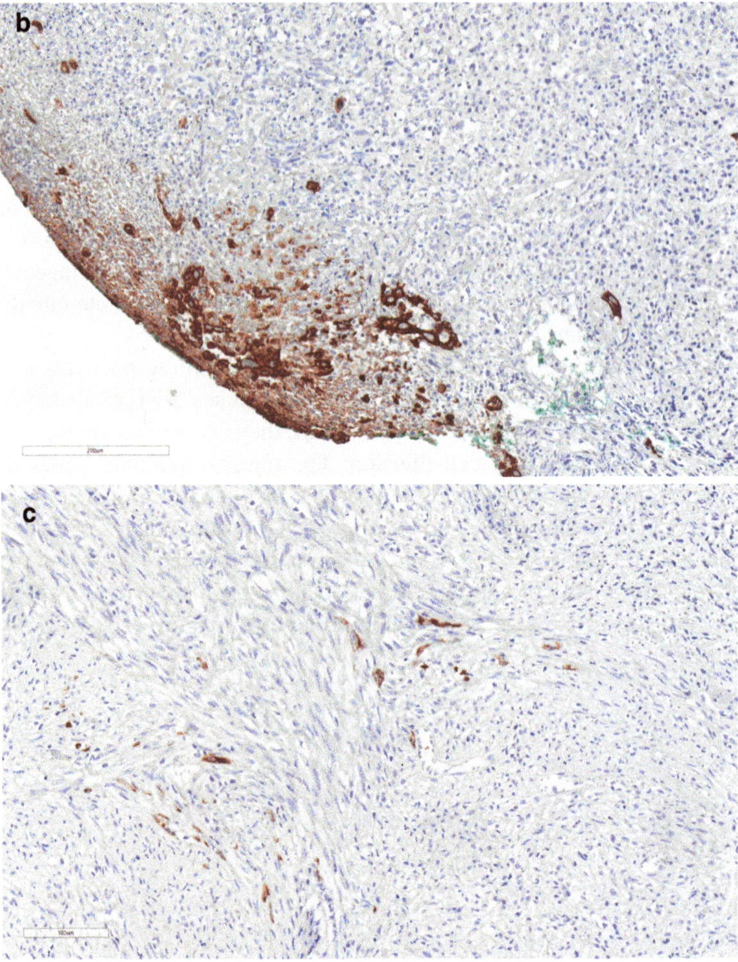

Fig. 4.6 (continued)

(UV rays), and compounds in car exhaust fumes are all examples of carcinogens [15–18]. When our bodies are exposed to carcinogens, free radicals are formed that try to steal electrons from other molecules in the body. These free radicals damage cells and affect their ability to function normally.

Apart from the carcinogens, oncoviruses such as human papillomavirus (HPV) and Epstein-Barr virus (EBV) can help to cause penile cancers [19, 20]. The mechanism by which HPV promotes cancer is not affecting the genes. HPV encodes for E6 and E7 proteins that are able to bind to two important tumor suppressor proteins, p53 and pRB, respectively, inactivating them [21]. EBV is widely distributed in human population; however, the exact role of EBV in the development of penile cancer is not understood. A possible cooperation between EBV and HPV in the process of penile carcinogenesis should be considered [20].

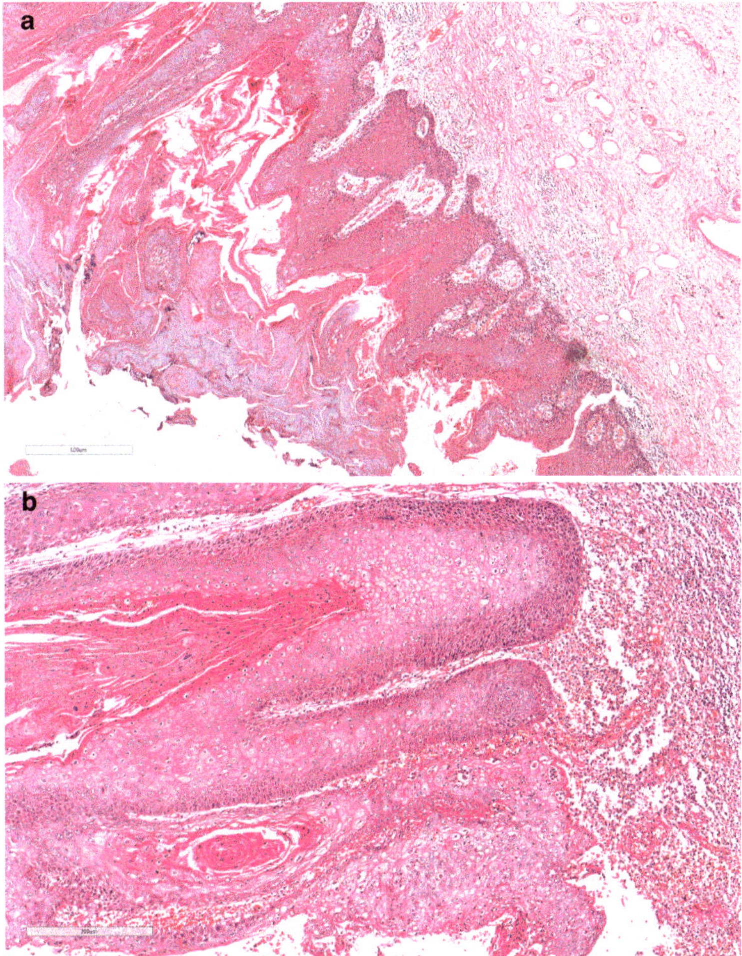

Fig. 4.7 (**a**) Warty carcinoma, low-grade variant. The keratin fills up the space between acanthotics cells columns with long and large papillae. (**b**) HPV-related warty carcinoma exhibiting darker band of basaloid tumor cells deep in the tumor and present area with clear cells and koilocytosis

Cytogenetics and Flow Cytometry Findings

Genes made of DNA are organized in a complex nuclear structure called chromosomes. A normal human cell contains 46 chromosomes. In cancer cells, chromosome rearrangements and the alteration of chromosome number can be detected with the application of cytogenetic techniques. Chromosomes in metaphase can be fixed on slides and can be observed under a microscope. The karyotype is the picture of the chromosomes from one metaphase that is arranged according to the standard classification.

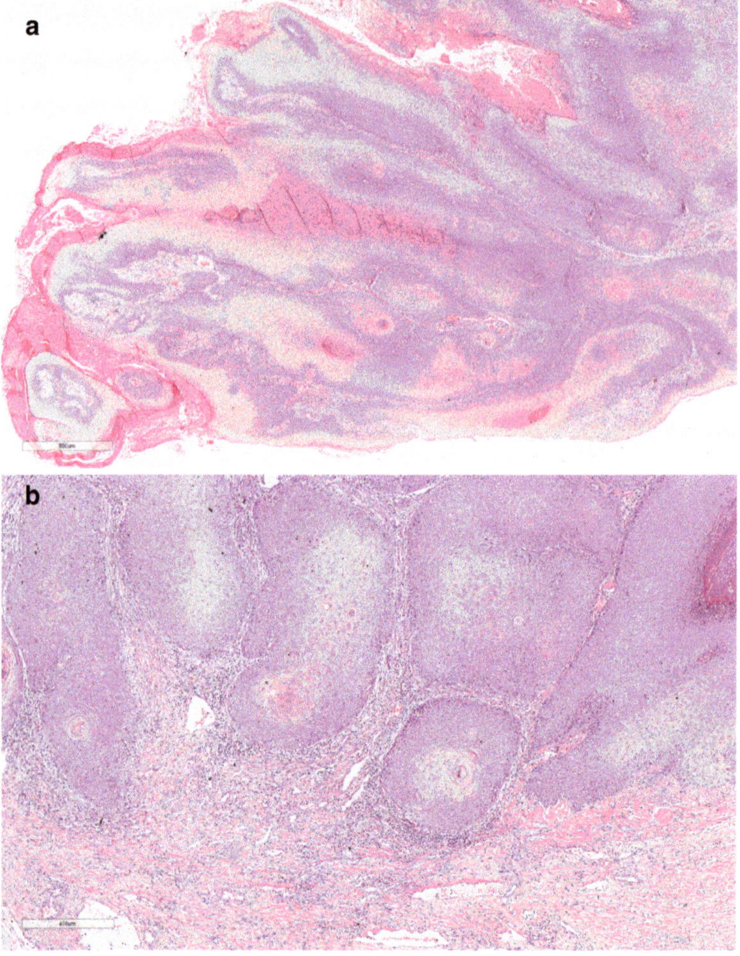

Fig. 4.8 (**a**) Verrucous carcinoma, low-grade variant. Tumor not associated with HPV represented by well-differentiated squamous cells with thin and long papillae containing fibrovascular cores and hyperkeratosis. (**b**) Verrucous carcinoma, low-grade variant. The round tumor board of squamous cell is present in stromal tissue configuring nest with single basal cells involved by inflammatory infiltrated. Inside keratinized material

In contrast to most tumors, publications about karyotype alterations in squamous cell carcinoma of the penis (SSCP) are uncommon. By conventional cytogenetics only four karyotypes were described for penile carcinoma. The rarity of karyotype description is due to technical difficulties related to the low mitotic index, contamination of primary cultures, and the occurrence of large areas of necrosis in the tumor.

The first SSCP karyotype description [22] was from a Chinese patient showing moderately differentiated SSCP (stage II). Several inguinal lymph nodes were palpable. Thirty metaphases showed the stemline karyotype 46,XY,del(2)(q33q36),der(4)

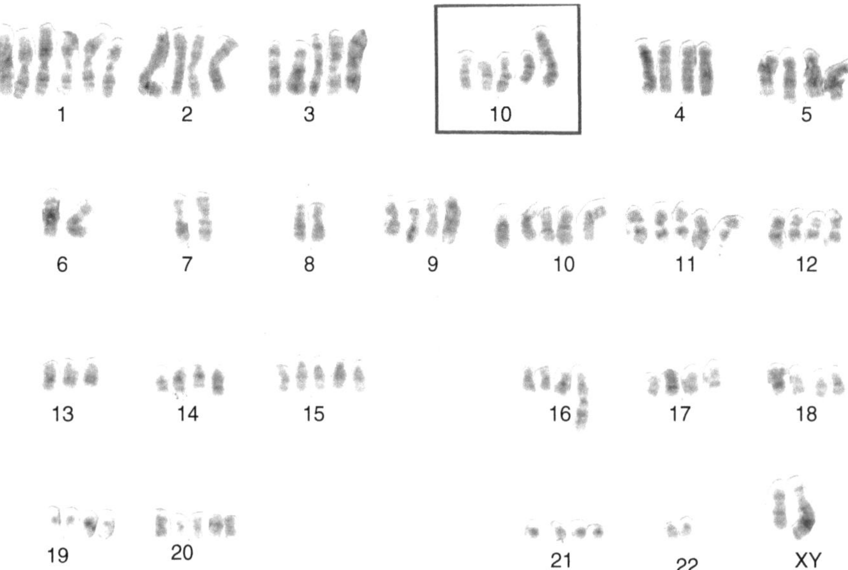

Fig. 4.9 Complete karyotype from the tumoral cells of a patient with poorly differentiated penile carcinoma, including a partial karyotype showing an isochromosome i (10) (q10) (From Ornellas et al. [23])

t(4;?)(p16;?),der(5;15)(q10;q10),der(8)t(8;?13)(q21;?),-13,- 13,-15,+3mar. Twelve cells had the stemline pattern with additional chromosome aberrations. Chromosomes 17, 22, and Y were usually lost, whereas chromosome 14 was frequently trisomic. Five to eight markers were observed in each cell of this population. Eight polyploid cells with poor chromosome spreading were also observed. The other three described karyotypes were from Brazilian cases. The next and second karyotype description [23] was obtained from an SSCP patient who presents an advanced poorly differentiated invasive carcinoma. Cytogenetic analysis of 11 cells obtained from fresh biopsy revealed a complex karyotype nearly tetraploid: 88, XY, + der. X, t (X; ?), (q28; ?), + del. (1), (p36), + 1, + 1, + 1, + 2, + 2, + 3, + 3, + 4, + 5, + 5, + 5, + 9, + 9, + 10, + 10, + 11, + 11, + 12, + 12, + 13, + 14, + 14, + 15, + 15, + 15, + der. 16, t (1; 16), (q24; p12), + 16, + 17, + 17, + 17, + 18, + 18, + 19, + 19, + 20, + 20, + 21, + 21, + mar 2, + mar 2 (Fig. 4.9). Polyploidy was confirmed by flow cytometry (Fig. 4.10). Besides the polyploidy, translocation involving chromosomes 1 and 16 and the appearance of additional genetic material on the X chromosome and isochromosome of the short arm of chromosome 10 were remarkable.

In contrast, the karyotypes of two early-stage SSCP patients showed no polyploidy [24]. One patient, with clinical stage T2N2MX, presented a moderately differentiated carcinoma of the penis, with a DNA pattern diploid. Cytogenetic analysis of 43 cells showed no cytogenetic alteration. The other patient, with clinical stage T3N1MX, presented also a moderately differentiated penile carcinoma. Cytogenetic

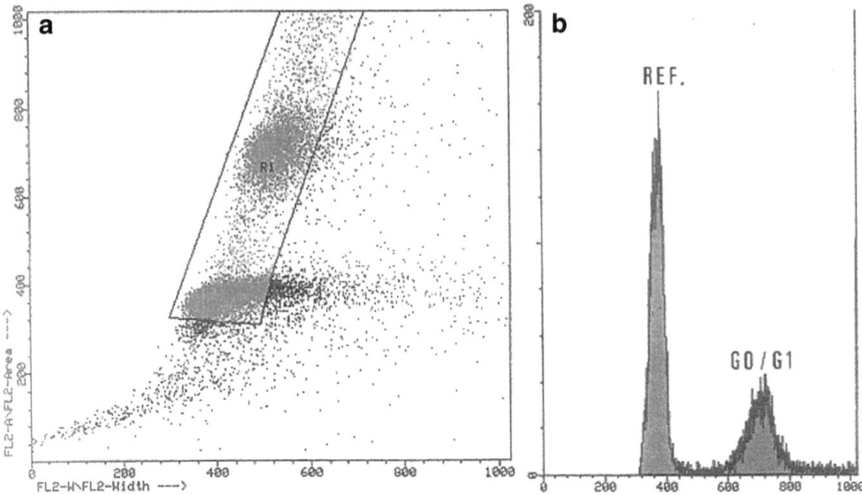

Fig. 4.10 Distribution pattern of the nuclear DNA content (near-tetraploid tumor). (**a**) Gated events displayed in identified singlet nucleus populations. (**b**) Singlet nucleus fluorescence intensity showing a near-tetraploid population and the diploid reference cells (From Ornellas et al. [23])

analysis of 11 cells showed an altered karyotype (49,XY, dup(1)(q21q32), i(1)(q10), -3, add(11)(q23), del (12)(p12),+i(18)(q10), +3 mar) with a DNA pattern hyperdiploid (Figs. 4.11 and 4.12). Although few, these karyotype descriptions suggest the possibility of the patients' present different tumors with different behaviors and that polyploidy could be a characteristic of advanced SSCP. Patient with normal karyotype had probably submicroscopic changes responsible for tumor development. In the future, a combination of cytogenetic, molecular, and histopathological stage and grade analyses will contribute to decisions on the classification of a particular solid tumor, leading to better predictive and prognostic information.

Flow cytometry is a technique for counting and examining microscopic particles, such as cells and chromosomes, by suspending them in a stream of fluid and passing them by an electronic detection apparatus. A chromosome counting performed by flow cytometry [25] from 90 SSCP patients showed that ploidy in these tumors is proportional to the degree of cellular differentiation. The frequency of DNA aneuploidy showed correlation with histological type of invasive squamous cell carcinoma of the penis. Preliminary analysis of these cases suggested that patients with high DNA index may be at increased risk of metastatic involvement and highlights that aneuploidy seems to be a risk factor for metastatic dissemination [25].

An original molecular cytogenetics study of penile carcinoma [26] was performed by comparative genomic hybridization (CGH). The CGH technique has a great advantage over conventional cytogenetics since it is not necessary to make the primary culture of tumor cells for obtaining slides with chromosome preparations. Only DNA extraction from the tissues is necessary. This technique generates a genomic map that leads to the discovery of chromosomal regions greatly amplified in tumors as well as regions in which there were large deletions. The procedure

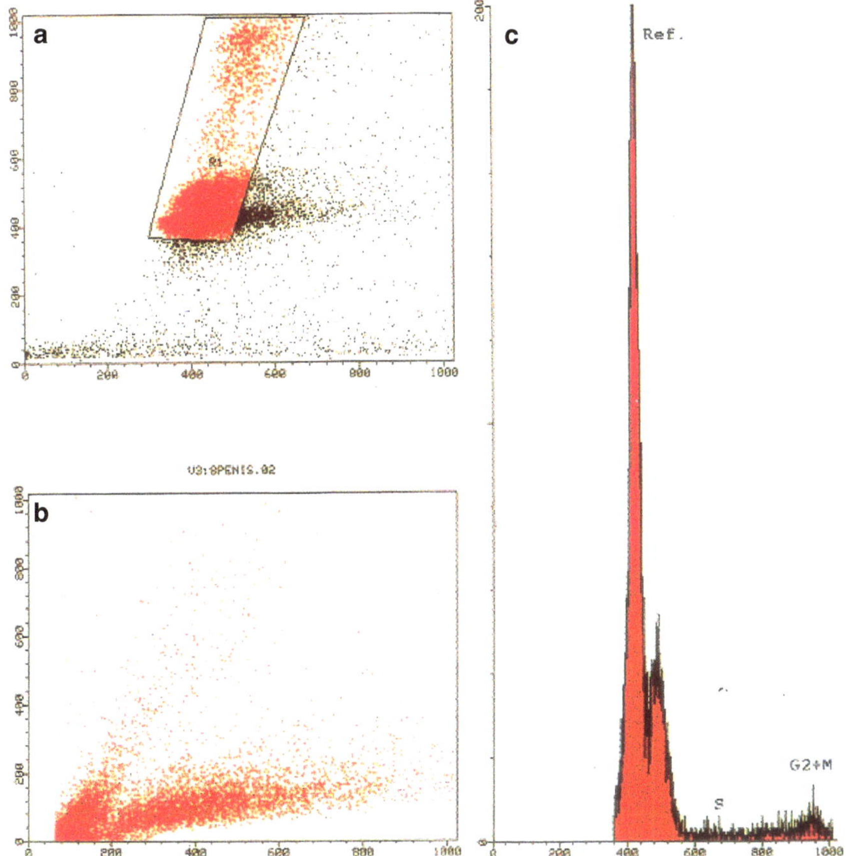

Fig. 4.11 Distribution pattern of nuclear DNA content (aneuploid tumor). (**a**, **b**) Hyperdiploid cell line was identified. (**c**) Singlet nuclear fluorescence intensity showing a hyperdiploid population with DNA index of 1.15 and the diploid reference cells (**c**, From Ornellas et al. [24])

requires different fluorochromes for labeling of DNA that was extracted from a tumor (tumor DNA), and DNA was extracted from one tissue tumor-free (normal DNA). The tumor and normal DNAs compete for hybridization in normal chromosomes, and regions with large chromosomal amplifications or deletions in chromosomes are distinguished by a computer program associated with a fluorescence microscope according to the difference of intensity of labeled tumor and normal DNA which hybridized to normal chromosomes.

DNA samples from 26 SSCP cases were assayed by CGH; six tumors were well-differentiated invasive tumors and the other 20 tumors moderately differentiated. The changes observed were similar to those described in other squamous cell carcinomas, such as oral and nasopharynx. This finding indicates that epidermoid tumors of various organs can be originated from similar genetic alterations. The regions of gene amplification observed most common were 8q24, 16p11-12, 20q11-13, 22q,

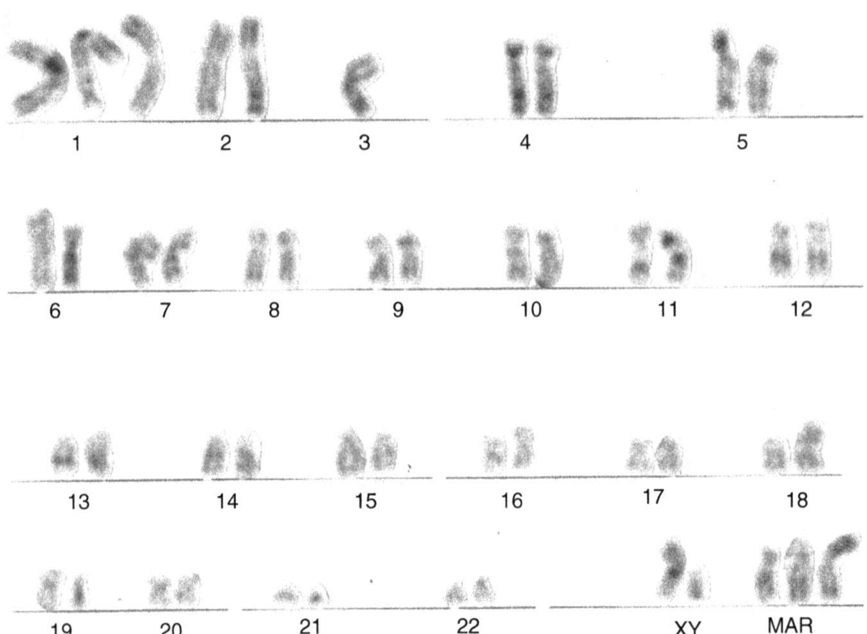

Fig. 4.12 Hyperdiploid moderately differentiated squamous cell carcinoma of the penis with chromosomal alterations. G-banded karyotype showed 49,XY, dup(1)(q21q32), i(1)(q10), 23,add(11)(q23), del(12)(p12),1i(18)(q10),13mar. Primary culture revealed 11 metaphases (From Ornellas et al. [24])

19q13, and 5p15, and the regions with the most frequent deletions were 13q21-22, 4q21-23, and along the X chromosome. In the region 8q24, the proto-oncogene *MYC* that encodes for transcription factor showing a helix-loop-helix leucine zipper protein domain has been mapped. The friendly *MYC* regulates expression of numerous target genes that control key cellular functions, including cell growth and cell cycle progression. *MYC* also has a critical role in DNA replication. Any kind of deregulation on *MYC* leads to constitutive *MYC* activity promotes carcinogenesis.

In 79 cases of SSCP including 11 *in situ* and 68 invasive carcinomas, *MYC* numerical aberrations and c-MYC protein expression were determined and correlated with the clinicopathological parameters and the HPV infection status of the patients [27]. The *MYC* cytogenetic profile was evaluated by fluorescence *in situ* hybridization (FISH) and c-MYC protein by immunohistochemistry (IHC). HPV was detected by polymerase chain reaction amplification (PCR). *MYC* gains were found to increase gradually as penile squamous cell carcinoma progresses from *in situ* to invasive. A significant association between *MYC* gains and tumor progression and poor outcome was demonstrated ($p < 0.05$). These findings were independent of HPV infection. Protein c-MYC expression was increased in samples with HPV infection, probably reflecting direct activation of *MYC*.

Gain in the region 5p15 appears very interesting, because the gene hTERT was mapped on this region. This gene codes for the major protein of the catalytic site of telomerase, the enzyme that stabilizes the telomeres of chromosomes. The stabilization of the end of the chromosomes (telomeres) is critical for promoting immortality. This result can be correlated with the study of analysis of telomerase activity in 51 samples of penile cancer [28]. In addition, gain in region 5p15 was also found in 3/7 men with cutaneous squamous cell carcinoma that were studied by array CGH [29], suggesting that this genetic event could also occur within this histological type.

Tissue and Molecular Alterations

TP53 Tumor Suppressor Gene (p53 Protein)

In an editorial of "Molecule of the Year," p53 was described as: "The molecule p53 is a good guy when it is functioning correctly" [30]. This interpretation suggests that the normal p53 plays a role in controlling cell growth, and when mutated, the surveillance capability of the protein is eliminated and cancer can grow.

When discovered, [31] p53 was just a cellular partner bond to the simian virus 40 large T antigen. After the cloning of the gene *TP53*, p53 was dismissed as an oncogenic protein and recognized as a tumor suppressor that is very frequently mutated in human cancer. Since then more functions for p53 have been revealed [32]. It acts as a transcription factor induced by stress/DNA damage, promoting cell cycle arrest, apoptosis, and senescence, and also regulates cytokines that are required for embryo implantation and metabolic pathways. In addition, p53 promotes oxidative phosphorylation and dampens glycolysis in cells [33] and has a key role in regulating cell growth and autophagy, thereby helping to coordinate the cell's response to nutrient starvation. An altered metabolism can contribute to malignant transformation as cancer cells [34].

Disruption of p53 function is a very common genetic event in many cancers, and there are many ways to cause it. The most common type of mutation causing inactivation of p53 is the missense mutation in the binding domain [35]. However, the SCCP might face another reality due to the common HPV infection [19, 20]. HPV encodes for E6 and E7 proteins that bind to p53 and pRb, respectively, leading to uncontrolled cell division and reduced apoptosis. In this situation, in spite of gene *TP53* being intact, p53 is blocked by E6.

One study [36] with Chinese patients analyzed p53 accumulation by immunohistochemistry in a series of 42 primary penile carcinomas (seven verrucous carcinomas, 14 well-differentiated, 15 moderately differentiated, and six poorly differentiated squamous cell carcinomas) using the p53 protein-specific mouse monoclonal antibody on paraffin sections. The mutant p53 protein frequently accumulates within the cell and can be viewed on fixed tissues by immunohistochemistry with the application of specific antibodies. However, the determination of specific mutations must be detected by DNA sequencing. The p53 protein was detected in 40 % (17 cases) of the tumors. The p53 staining was not observed in six cases of penile warts nor in seven cases of verrucous carcinomas. Positive p53 staining was identified only in the less differentiated tumor cells in the periphery of the tumor cell nests in all the cases. The noninvasive dysplastic epithelium next to the tumors could also be positive for p53 protein. Furthermore, 100 % of the human papillomavirus (HPV)-positive cases showed positive p53 staining. The authors concluded that p53 accumulation is present in penile squamous cell carcinomas and adjacent noninvasive tumor cells. In agreement, another immunohistochemistry study identified the accumulation of p53 in two cases of HPV-positive (6 or 11) invasive carcinoma [37]. One of the cases carried a mutation in *TP53* revealed by DNA sequencing. In contrast, another study did not detect the accumulation of p53 in 25 cases of carcinoma *in situ* [38]. Therefore, according to these reports, it seems that mutant p53 could play a role in the progression of malignancy into invasion, but this remains controversial. Biopsies of penile lesions were obtained for diagnostic purposes from 13 with 1 to 3 therapy-resistant genital warts or intraepithelial neoplasias. In addition, 4 archival specimens of SSCP were obtained. In the specimens, presence of HPV DNA was assayed by *in situ* hybridization and PCR analysis, and p53 accumulation was determined by immunohistochemistry. At the molecular level mutations in the DNA binding domain (exons 4–8) of *TP53* were assayed in gel by single-strand conformation polymorphism (SSCP) after amplification by polymerase chain reaction (PCR). Band shifts were sequenced to detect possible mutations [39]. No correlation between p53 accumulation and HPV status was found. No mutations in the binding domain of *TP53* were found in any of the lesions. The authors concluded that accumulation of p53 did not indicate existence of *TP53* mutation in male genital warts, premalignant lesions, or malignant squamous cell carcinomas.

The accumulation of p53 and p21 (another tumor suppressor protein) in 49 SSCP cases was investigated by immunohistochemistry [40]. The accumulation of p21 and p53 was noted in 40 and 89 %, respectively, of the 47 patients with primary penile carcinoma with squamous differentiation. Positive p21 and p53 expression was also seen in two cases of Paget disease. Staining for p21 was often weak and was found in the suprabasal region of carcinomas with squamous differentiation, while p53 expression was seen in the basal region of squamous cell carcinomas. Preinvasive lesions also showed p21 and p53 expression. An inverse correlation between p53 and p21 expression (p53(+)/p21(−) or p53(−)/p21(+)) was noted in half of the squamous cell carcinomas, 4 of 5 verrucous carcinomas, 2 of 3 basaloid squamous cell carcinomas, and 1 spindle-cell carcinoma. The other cases did not show this correlation. Therefore, p21 and p53 expression seems to be independent in SCCP. The relationship between expression-positive/expression-negative p53 and p21 did not show a direct correlation with histological subtypes and staging. However, a strong association between positivity for HPV16 and p21 was found.

Alterations in p53 protein were also identified in 22 of 63 (35 %) patients with epidermoid tumors and invasive penile stage pT2-4 N1-3 MX [41]. The presence or absence of p53 in the nucleus has been correlated in primary lesions and nodal metastasis in 20 patients. Of these 20 patients (90 %), 18 agreed on the levels of p53 expression in primary lesions and nodal metastasis. Two patients have only p53 expression in nodal metastasis.

The impact of p53 as a prognostic marker was investigated in 82 SSCP patients undergoing penile amputation and bilateral inguinal lymphadenectomy [2]. Immunoreactivity of p53 was studied with other clinicopathological parameters, and HPV DNA was detected by PCR using generic primers. Nuclear accumulation of p53 was detected in 34 of 82 samples (41.5 %). Clinical lymph node N stage, lymphatic and venous embolization by neoplastic cells, and p53 positivity were significantly associated with lymph node metastasis. Multivariate analysis revealed that only lymphatic embolization and p53 positivity were independent factors for lymph node metastasis. Patients with negative p53 had significantly better 5- and 10-year overall survival than those in whom tumors stained positive for p53. When tumors were p53 positive and HPV DNA positive, overall survival was worse.

The prognostic significance of p53, Ki-67, E-cadherin, and Matrix metalloproteases-9 (MMP-9) was evaluated in SSCP tumors of 73 Chinese patients who have penile amputation and regional lymphadenectomy [42]. The expression of molecular markers was determined by immunohistochemistry. By multivariate analysis, tumor embolization and the expression of p53 were independent predictors of metastasis. In stage T1 tumors, high expression of p53 was significantly associated with metastasis and poor survival.

Telomerase Activity

A telomere is the "cap" at the end of chromosomes. It is composed of repetitive DNA sequences and specialized proteins that protect the end of the chromosome from degradation of genes near the ends of chromosomes. The loss of telomeric DNA sequences that occur in each cell division rules the process of cell aging or senescence. Very short telomeres trigger the cell death process, so that they act as a "molecular clock" that determines the lifetime of a cell. Cell immortalization depends on stopping telomeric DNA degradation by the reactivation of telomerase that adds DNA sequence repeats ("TTAGGG" in all vertebrates) to the 3' end of DNA strands in the telomere.

Telomerase, a ribonucleoprotein enzyme, carries its own RNA molecule, which is used as a template for elongating telomeres, which are shortened after each replication cycle. The activity mode of telomerase resembles the activity of the reverse transcriptase enzyme of the retrovirus. The existence of a compensatory mechanism for telomere shortening was first predicted by biologist Alexey Olovnikov in 1973 [43] who also suggested the telomere hypothesis of aging and the telomere's connections to cancer. Telomerase was discovered by Carol W. Greider and Elizabeth Blackburn in 1984 in the ciliate *Tetrahymena* [44]. In humans, telomerase activity usually is detected during embryogenesis, in germ cells, stem cells, and B and T lymphocytes.

Telomerase activity was measured in 48 samples of SSCP and three penile verrucous carcinomas [28] by the Telomeric Repeat Amplification Protocol (TRAP), a PCR-based assay with fluorescence label. In some patients, it was also possible to measure the activity of telomerase in the region adjacent to the tumor, either skin or corpus cavernous, which were free of tumor cells according to histopathological analysis. Among the specimens of invasive carcinomas, 41/48 (85.4 %) showed positive telomerase activity, and three samples of verrucous carcinoma were also positive. The results of adjacent tissues were more surprising; 9/11 (81.8 %) of the adjacent skin samples and 8/10 (80 %) of corpus cavernous adjacent samples also were positive for telomerase activity. As controls, five samples of skin and corpus cavernous of prostate cancer patients were tested negative for telomerase activity. These results indicated that telomerase was reactivated in normal tissues or adjacent tissues of SCCP. This could be happening due to angiogenesis/invasion or inflammation next to the tumor. The original TRAP assay [45] used radioactivity labeling for the detection of amplified telomeric DNA sequences that were previously polymerized by a telomerase extract from the tissues. In addition, the activity of telomerase was detected in other case, a 46-year-old man with a penile giant condyloma acuminatum [46]. This information may be valuable for evaluating the degree of malignancy of giant condyloma acuminatum and in obtaining a differential diagnosis between the benign and malignant cases.

Bax and Bcl-2 Apoptotic Proteins

Apoptosis or programmed cell death is a physiological mechanism, characterized by specific morphological and biochemical changes such as cell shrinkage, chromatin condensation, protein cleavage, DNA breakdown, and phagocytosis. Biochemical events lead to characteristic cell changes (morphology) and death. Many proteins have been identified to play a role in apoptosis.

Bcl-2 family consists of approximately 15 members, some of which are antiapoptotic while others are proapoptotic. The first Bcl-2 gene was identified because of its involvement in B-cell malignancies, and it is located on chromosome segment 18q21.3; Bcl-2 stands for B-cell lymphoma/leukemia-2 gene [47]. The Bcl-2 family of proteins can be identified by the presence of the domains BH1 to BH4. Most antiapoptotic members contain, at least, the BH1 and BH2 domains, while the proapoptotic Bcl-2 family members have the four BH domains.

Expression of two members of Bcl-2 family (the antiapoptotic Bcl-2 and the proapoptotic Bax) was analyzed in 16 SCCP (tumor-free adjacent skin tissue and corpus cavernous) comparing with five controls (skin and corpus cavernous) using Western blot (a technique for identifying a particular protein using antibodies after electrophoretic separation in a gel and transfer to a membrane). It was observed that the proteins Bcl-2 and Bax showed a clear homogeneous expression pattern in normal skin and corpus cavernous; Bcl-2 expression was higher than Bax's. However, Bcl-2 and Bax were completely imbalanced when the tumor, adjacent either skin or corpus cavernous, was compared in the same way. This means that the adjacent tissues are at least under the influence of the tumor. The Bcl-2/Bax results are in agreement with the results of the analysis of telomerase activity [28].

Oncogenes

Alterations in the cellular growing signaling pathways downstream of growth receptors caused by oncogenes are one of the most common events in various cancers. This, in part, is because these receptors control two major signaling pathways (RAS and PI3K pathways). RAS is a family of related proteins with GTPase activity, which are involved in transmitting signals within cells (cellular signal transduction). When *RAS* activity is under control, cell growth and division occur normally. Mutations in RAS that prevents GTP hydrolysis, let ras protein on permanently, resulting in overactivity that can ultimately lead to cancer. *RAS* is the most common oncogene in human cancer and was the first to be discovered in the human genome in the early 1980s [48].

Mutations in *RAS* leading to overexpression are found in 20–25 % of all human tumors and up to 90 % in certain types of cancer. Yet, only one study was published reporting mutations of *RAS* family members in 28 SSCP cases [49]. In this study, single-stranded conformational and direct DNA sequencing were performed to evaluate mutations in *HRAS, KRAS, and NRAS*. In addition, mutations in *PIK3CA, PTEN*, and *BRAF* oncogenes were also evaluated. Considering all oncogenes that were surveyed, missense mutations were found in 11 of the 28 penile cancer samples (39 %), including 1 (3 %) mutation in *KRAS* (G12S) and 2 (7 %) mutations in *HRAS* (G12S and a Q61L). *HRAS* and *KRAS* mutations were found in larger and more advanced tumors. In addition, 8 (29 %) mutations (E542K or E545K) were identified in the *PIK3CA*. The mutations in *RAS* and *PIK3CA* were mutually exclusive, suggesting that deregulation of either the phosphatidylinositol 3-kinase or ras pathway would be sufficient for the development and progression of penile carcinoma.

Genes Silenced by DNA Methylation

Regulation of gene expression includes a wide range of mechanisms acting at either the transcriptional initiation, or at mRNA level, or at protein posttranslational modification. At transcriptional level, epigenetic changes such as DNA methylation at the promoter act to silence gene expression. Gene promoter hypermethylation plays a major role in cancer through transcriptional silencing of critical tumor suppressor genes.

In general, the studies that have searched for DNA methylation of tumor suppressor genes in SSCP also addressed other questions related to gene expression control (in special HPV infection), reflecting the complexity of this issue. However, all of them applied the methylation-specific PCR (MSP) method for assaying. In this reaction, the DNA is modified by sodium bisulfite, converting all unmethylated cytosines to uracil. But those cytosines that are methylated (5-methylcytosine) are resistant to this modification and remain as cytosine. Primers for subsequent amplification can be designed to distinguish methylated from unmethylated DNA in bisulfite-modified DNA, taking advantage of the sequence differences resulting from bisulfite modification. MSP requires only small quantities of DNA and is sensitive to 0.1 % methylated alleles of a given CpG island locus [50].

Two publications from the same group [51, 52] analyzed DNA methylation status of several gene promoters. A total of 26 SSCP tumors from Japanese men were assayed for HPV, *TP53* alterations, and methylation promoter regions [50]. HPV DNA was detected in 3/26 patients (11.5 %). Overexpression of p53 was observed in 13/26 patients (50 %), and *TP53* mutations were detected in 4 /26 patients (15.4 %). The frequencies of methylation in the promoter gene regions were as follows: *DAPK*, 26.9 % (7/26); *FHIT*, 88.4 % (23/26); *MGMT*, 19.2 % (5/26); *p14*, 3.8 % (1/26); *p16*, 23.1 % (6/26); *RAR-beta*, 23.1 % (6/26); *RASSF1A*, 11.5 % (3/26); and *RUNX3*, 42.3 % (11/26). *FHIT* gene promoter methylation was the highest, suggesting that it plays an important role in the pathogenesis of SSCP. Absence of Fhit protein expression was associated with promoter hypermethylation [52]. *FHIT* has a role in the regulation of apoptosis and the cell cycle, which may be lost upon promoter hypermethylation.

The HPV types, the methylation status in the promoter region of thrombospondin-1 (*TSP-1*), RAS association domain family 1A (*RASSF1-A*), and *p16* genes and expression of TSP-1, CD31, p16, and p53 proteins were analyzed by reverse line blot, methylation-specific polymerase chain reaction, and immunohistochemistry, respectively, in 24 SSCP [53]. As results, HPV infection was detected in 11 of 24 cases (46 %), and *TSP-1*, *RASSF1-A*, and *p16* genes were hypermethylated in 46, 42, and 38 % of the tumors, respectively. *TSP-1* hypermethylation was associated with unfavorable histological grade (grade 3; $p=0.033$), vascular invasion ($p=0.023$), weak expression of TSP-1 protein ($p=0.041$), and shorter overall survival ($p=0.04$). TSP-1 expression was not associated with microvessel density. However, *RASSF1-A* hypermethylation was more frequent in T1 tumors ($P=0.01$), and *p16* hypermethylation was not associated with any of the tested variables except for absence of p16 expression ($p=0.022$).

A study was performed on 53 SSCP to gain more insight into the mechanisms that may be involved in disruption of the p16^{INK4A}/cyclin D/Rb pathway that functions as cell cycle regulatory proteins [54]. To that end, human papillomavirus (HPV) presence, *p16* expression and promoter methylation, and expression of the BMI-1 polycomb gene product were studied. Only 9/53 carcinomas (17 %) revealed positivity with methylation-specific primers. The frequency of *p16* promoter methylation was higher in HPV DNA-negative tumors (21 %) than in HPV-positive cases (10 %). Overall data indicated that p16/cyclin D/Rb pathway could become disrupted by either HPV E7 or by methylation of the *p16* promoter or by overexpression of the BMI-1 polycomb gene product.

At Metastasis

Metastasis is a multiple step process by which cancer cells spread to other parts of the body. This can happen when cancer cells invade nearby normal tissue, or when they reach the lymphatic system and the bloodstream to spread to other parts of the body. The starting point for metastasis is when cancer cells break away from the primary tumor and attach to and degrade proteins that make up the surrounding extracellular matrix (ECM), which separates the tumor from adjoining tissues. By degrading these proteins, cancer cells are able to breach the ECM and escape. In addition to that, angiogenesis stimulates the growth of new blood vessels to obtain a blood supply. A blood supply is needed to obtain the oxygen and nutrients necessary for continued tumor growth. Some gene products that are implicated in the basis of metastasis have been studied in SSCP.

E-cadherins are cell adhesion molecules that are expressed in normal epithelia. Downregulation of E-cadherins is involved in the mechanism of metastasis, allowing cancer cells to detach from primary site. Matrix metalloproteases (MMPs) are enzymes that degrade type IV collagen in the basal membrane and are involved in the invasion mechanism. An increase in expression of MMPs is expected in the process of metastasis. E-cadherin and MMP-2 and MMP-9 were assayed by immunohistochemistry in SSCP tumors from 125 Brazilian patients [55]. Several parameters (age, race, disease evolution time, venereal background, clinical and pathological stage, tumor thickness, differentiation grade, venous and lymphatic embolization, koilocytosis, type of invasion, lymph node metastases, and survival) were assessed. On univariate analysis, lower E-cadherin immunoreactivity was associated with a greater risk of lymph node metastases, while higher MMP-9 immunoreactivity was considered an independent risk factor for disease recurrence. Another study has concluded that the less differentiated tumors are associated with the overexpression of MMPs [56]. In addition, lower E-cadherin immunoreactivity was reported in 45 % of SSCP Chinese cases and has been correlated with a greater risk of lymph node metastasis [42].

Prostaglandin E2 (PGE_2) plays a role in invasiveness and metastasis. The synthesis of PGE_2 from arachidonic acid requires the action of two isoenzymes in sequence. Cyclooxygenase (COX-1 and COX-2) catalyzes the synthesis of PGH2, which is converted, in turn, by microsomal prostaglandin E synthase (mPGES-1) to PGE2. In general, COX-1 is constitutively expressed and COX-2 is only expressed following induction by cytokines, growth factors, oncogenes, and tumor promoters. An investigation about COX-2 or mPGES-1 expression was performed in 7 *in situ* carcinomas and in 6 SSCP tumors [57]. Immunohistochemistry and Western blotting were used to evaluate the expression of COX-2 and mPGES-1 in benign and malignant lesions including metastases to lymph nodes. The expression of intratumoral PGE_2 was quantified by enzyme immunoassay. Reverse transcription PCR was used to determine the expression of each of the four known receptors (EP(1–4)) for PGE_2. Because HPV has been linked to the development of SSC, COX-2 overexpression was measured in SSCP in an HPV16 transgenic mouse. Immunohistochemistry demonstrated increased expression of COX-2 and mPGES-1 in dysplasia, *in situ* carcinoma, invasive SCC, and metastases to lymph nodes. Immunoblot analysis confirmed that COX-2 and mPGES-1 were consistently overexpressed in SSCP. PGE_2 and all four of the PGE_2 receptor subtypes were detected in each of the tumor samples. Elevated levels of COX-2 were also detected in SCC arising in an HPV16 transgenic mouse. Although limited in a number of cases, this study has shown the importance of COX-2 and mPGES-1 upregulation in SSCP.

Ki-67, a Proliferation Marker

Ki-67 is a nuclear protein encoded by *MKI67* gene. This protein is considered as a cellular marker for proliferation and was associated with ribosomal RNA transcription [58]. The fact that the Ki-67 protein is present during all active phases of the cell cycle (G1, S, G2, and mitosis), but is absent from resting cells (G0), makes it an excellent marker for determining the so-called growth fraction of a given cell population [59]. Ki-67 expression seems to be tissue type dependent based on studies performed by immunohistochemistry. Ki-67 expression was found higher in basaloid carcinomas and lower in verrucous carcinomas in study assaying the expression of DNA topoisomerase I and II (Topo I and II) to pursue the possibility of future chemotherapy regimens for SCCP [60]. Additionally, lower expression of Ki-67 (as well as *p16*) could differentiate penile verrucous carcinoma from usual type squamous cell carcinoma. Probably, the lower Ki-67 expression is reflecting the slow-growing nature of verrucous tumors [61].

The prognostic significance of Ki-67 index has been investigated by immunohistochemistry. In a study with 44 SSCP tumors, the mean Ki-67 labeling index indicated an association with advanced local tumor stage, nodal metastasis, and clinical disease progression, but the difference between tumors with and without metastasis did not reach statistical significance [62]. Ki-67 was evaluated (in combination with other molecular makers – p53, E-cadherin, and MMP-9) as the presence of lymph node metastasis and survival in 73 Chinese SSCP tumors. High expression of Ki-67 was found in 26/73 (36 %) of the tumors. No significant difference was observed in inguinal metastases or in the 3-year survival rates between patients with low and high Ki-67 expression [61].

However, a different result was obtained when Ki-67 expression (also known as MIB-1) was evaluated in combination with another proliferation marker (proliferating cell nuclear antigen – PCNA) in 125 SSCP tumors [63]. In a univariate analysis, lower Ki-67 expression, the presence of lymphovascular permeation, clinically positive lymph nodes, tumor thickness greater than 5 mm, and infiltration of cavernous bodies were correlated with lymph node metastasis. However, the independent factors for lymph node metastasis risk were Ki-67 and PCNA, lymphovascular permeation, and clinical nodal stage. Independent variables for disease-free survival were urethra infiltration and the presence of lymph node metastasis. For death risk evaluation, the independent variables were age, lymph node metastasis, and clinical stage. In agreement, another study showed positive correlation between high Ki-67 expression and metastasis [64]. Four of 28 patients who were tested showed a weak Ki-67 expression, without displaying lymph node metastasis. Among 17 patients showing an intermediate Ki-67 index, eight exhibited metastases, while in all seven patients with a strong expression of Ki-67 lymph node metastases were found.

The median Ki-67 expression in metastatic lesions was significantly different (50.3 %) from tumors without lymph node metastasis (31.8 %) ($p=0.024$). Furthermore, a correlation between presence of HPV DNA and strong Ki-67 expression was found ($p=0.009$).

The expressions of Ki-67 and cyclin D1 were investigated [65] in 21 SSCP tissues and in premalignant lesions of the penis (7 lichen sclerosus, 5 condyloma acuminatum, and 2 erythroplasia of Queyrat) and correlated with clinicopathological parameters and patient survival. Cyclin D plays an important role in regulating the progression of cells through the G1 phase of the cell cycle. Cyclin D1 overexpression was found in 13/21 SSCP (61.9 %) and in one case of erythroplasia of Queyrat. Strong reactivity for Ki-67 was found in 16 (76.2 %) SSCP, 3 condyloma acuminatum, and 1 case of erythroplasia of Queyrat. A tendency for an association between cyclin D1 expression and tumor differentiation ($p=0.07$) but not the level of tumor invasion ($p=0.50$) was found. The Ki-67 expression was notably increased with the advance of tumor grade, but the difference did not reach a statistically significant level ($p=0.46$). A slight tendency towards a relationship between Ki-67 and cyclin D1 protein expression was observed ($p=0.32$). Two patients relapsed and one died from the disease over a median follow-up period of 4.6 years (range 0.1–10.3 years). Ki-67 and cyclin D1 overexpression were in parallel, supporting the concept that cyclin D1 serves as a cell cycle activator.

PCNA, Proliferation Cell Nuclear Antigen

PCNA is a protein found in the nucleus of cells and is a cofactor of DNA polymerase delta. PCNA is important for both DNA synthesis and DNA repair because it shows further exonuclease activity. Since the exonuclease activity is proofreading, it is expected to play a significant role in the maintenance of the fidelity of mammalian DNA replication. Due to its properties, PCNA was originally identified as an antigen that is expressed in the nuclei of cells during the DNA synthesis phase of the cell cycle (S) [66]. PCNA antigen is, therefore, a marker of proliferation that competes with Ki-67.

PCNA expression was assayed by immunohistochemistry [67] and compares to biological aggressiveness (stage and grade) of 50 SSCP tumors from patients who underwent surgical penile amputation (total or partial). Fifteen of them required associated inguinal lymphadenectomy due to suspicion of lymph node metastasis. A diffuse and strong pattern of staining (high level) was found in 18/34 well-differentiated, 10/12 moderately differentiated, and 4/4 undifferentiated tumors. All tumors with metastasis were strong staining, including 4/18 well-differentiated and 4/10 moderately differentiated tumors exhibiting such pattern of staining. There was a positive relation between the strong staining of PCNA and the tumor staging ($p=0.003$), but not with grading ($p=0.06$). The authors argued that PCNA seemed to be an independent marker to guide medical management. Two years later, a complementary paper was published [68] that included data on p53. In this comparison p53 "won" as a prognostic marker. In a univariate analysis, PCNA staining showed association only with nodal metastasis ($p=0.04$), while p53 staining exhibited correlation with tumor pT stage ($p=0.0005$), grade ($p=0.02$), lymphatic spread ($p=0.02$), and cause-specific survival ($p=0.003$). Multivariate analysis showed that p53 immunoreactivity was the only factor with prognostic significance for disease progression and cause-specific survival. Tumor pT stage, grade, and PCNA staining have no significance for nodal metastases and cause-specific death.

The comparison of the prognostic value of PCNA and Ki-67 [63] revealed that there was a correlation between the expression of both and the presence of lymph node metastasis. However, PCNA and Ki-67 immunohistochemical expression did not have a relationship with survival and death risk.

Circulating Proteins Markers

Proteomics is the large-scale study of proteins and is associated traditionally with displaying a large number of proteins from a given cell line or organism. Curiously, there is no strict linear relationship between genes and the protein complement or "proteome" of a cell. Proteomics is complementary to genomics, because it focuses on the gene products, which are the active agents in cells.

There are two strategies for finding protein biomarkers in tissues or in biological fluids. Several possible biomarkers have been identified using a gel-based approach in bidimensional electrophoresis (with and without stable isotopic labeling) and mass spectrometry. However, since this approach is very laborious and time-consuming, a new method has been developed to solve this problem. ClinProt matrix-assisted laser desorption/ionization time-of-flight (MALDI-TOF), which is based on affinity bead-based prefractionation of proteome, has recently emerged to fill in this gap. This method is fast and quite suitable for the following step that is the accurate mass determination by mass spectrometry (MS) [69]. ClinProt MALDI-TOF uses different chemical chromatographic surfaces on an outer layer of magnetic beads (such as Cu or cation coated) to selectively purify certain subsets of proteins, allowing unbound impurities to be removed by washing with buffers. Proteins bound to the magnetic beads are then eluted, diluted, and directly analyzed. Bioinformatics algorithms are used to align and integrate hundreds of mass data points from large numbers of samples, helping the resolution of complex mixtures. This is especially important for plasma proteomics, because plasma contains high abundance proteins (e.g., albumin, immunoglobulins) that could mask the presence of the secreted tumor protein markers which are found more diluted.

With the application of a ClinProt MALDI-TOF platform, proteins from plasma of 36 healthy subjects (controls) were compared to 25 plasmas from patients with SCCP [70]. The peptides were enriched by super-paramagnetic microparticles functionalized with a hydrophobic C8 coating, separating peptides and proteins according to their hydrophobicity. A cluster of two peptides was able to discriminate patients from control subjects. Cross-validation analysis using the whole casuistic showed 62.5 and 86.76 % sensitivity and specificity, respectively. The cluster also showed very high sensitivity (100 %) and specificity (97 %) for SCCP patients that died due to the disease. Furthermore, patients with lymph node involvement presented sensitivity and specificity of 80 and 97 %, respectively.

The two peptides were identified by an MALDI-TOF-TOF as fragments of C3 and C4a/b complement proteins. The conclusion was that fragments C3 and C4 a/b are less expressed in comparison with healthy subjects as the disease progresses. This finding is very promising in comparison to a previously described circulating SSCP marker, TA-4 antigen, also known as SSC antigen [71]. This antigen was originally isolated from patients showing squamous cell carcinoma of the uterine cervix, and later it was shown [59] that TA-4 values were elevated in serum of metastatic SSCP patients. However, TA-4 has shown limited value in the primary prediction of occult lymph node metastases because its levels increased significantly only after massive lymph node involvement or metastatic disease had occurred [72].

Summary

Pathological factors with a known prognostic value, other than lymph node metastasis, are tumor thickness, grade, histological type, lymphovascular embolization, and stage.

Oncoviruses such as human papillomavirus (HPV) and Epstein-Barr virus (EBV) can help to cause penile cancers. HPV encodes for E6 and E7 proteins that are able to bind to two important tumor suppressor proteins, p53 and pRB, respectively, inactivating them.

In penile cancer, the rarity of karyotype description is due to technical difficulties related to the low mitotic index, contamination of primary cultures, and the occurrence of large areas of necrosis in the tumor. The frequency of DNA aneuploidy showed correlation with histological type of invasive squamous cell carcinoma of the penis.

A significant association between *MYC* gains and tumor progression and poor outcome was demonstrated. These findings were independent of HPV infection. Protein c-MYC expression was increased in samples with HPV infection, probably reflecting direct activation of *MYC*.

The prognostic significance of p53, Ki-67, PCNA, E-cadherin, and Matrix metalloproteases-9 (MMP-9) was evaluated in SCCP tumors. Tumor embolization and the expression of p53 are independent predictors of metastasis. The comparison of the prognostic value of PCNA and Ki-67 revealed that there was a correlation between the expression of both and the presence of lymph node metastasis.

Among the specimens of invasive carcinomas, 85.4 % showed positive telomerase activity. In some patients it was also possible to measure the activity of telomerase in the region adjacent to the tumor, which was free of tumor cells according to histopathological analysis. These results indicated that telomerase was reactivated either in normal tissues or adjacent tissues of SCCP.

Bcl-2 and Bax were completely imbalanced when the tumor, adjacent either skin or corpus cavernous, was compared in the same way. This means that the adjacent tissues are at least under the influence of the tumor.

The mutations in *RAS* and *PIK3CA* were mutually exclusive, suggesting that deregulation of either the phosphatidylinositol 3-kinase or ras pathway would be sufficient for the development and progression of penile carcinoma.

Fragments of C3 and C4a/b complement proteins are less expressed in plasma of SCCP patients in comparison with healthy subjects as the disease progresses.

TA-4 antigen, also known as SCC antigen, was elevated in serum of metastatic SCCP patients. However, this antigen has shown limited value in the primary prediction of occult lymph node metastases.

References

1. Ornellas AA, Nóbrega BLB, Chin EWK, Wisnescky A, Silva PCB, Schwindt ABS. Prognostic factors in invasive squamous cell carcinoma of the penis: analysis of 196 patients treated in Brazilian National Cancer Institute. J Urol. 2008;180:1354–9.
2. Lopes A, Bezerra AL, Pinto CA, Serrano SV, de Mello CA, Villa LL. p53 as a new prognostic factor for lymph node metastasis in penile carcinoma: analysis of 82 patients treated with amputation and bilateral lymphadenectomy. J Urol. 2002;168:81–6.
3. Soria JC, Fizazi K, Piron D, Kramar A, Geraulet A, Haie-Meder C, et al. Squamous cell carcinoma of the penis: multivariate analysis of prognostic factors and natural history in a monocentric study with a conservative policy. Ann Oncol. 1997;8:1089–98.
4. Velazquez EF, Amin MB, Epstein JI, Grignon DJ, Humphrey PA, Pettaway CA, Renshaw AA, Reuter VE, Srigley JR, Cubilla AL. Protocol for the examination of specimens from patients with carcinoma of the penis. Arch Pathol Lab Med. 2010;134:923–9.
5. Ornellas AA, Chin EWK, Nóbrega BLB, Wisnescky A, Koifman N, Quirino R. Surgical treatment of invasive squamous cell carcinoma of the penis: Brazilian National Cancer Institute long-term experience. J Surg Oncol. 2008;97:487–95.
6. Ferrándiz PC, de Torres I, García PV. Penile squamous cell carcinoma. Actas Dermosifiliogr. 2012;103(6):478–87.
7. Mosconi AM, Roila F, Gatta G, Theodore C. Cancer of the penis. Crit Rev Oncol Hematol. 2005;53(2):165–77.
8. Guimarães GC, Cunha IW, Soares FA, Lopes A, Torres J, Chaux A, Velazquez EF, Ayala G, Cubilla AL. Penile squamous cell carcinoma clinicopathological features, nodal metastasis and outcome in 333 cases. J Urol. 2009;182(2):528–34.
9. Chaux A, Reuter V, Lezcano C, Velazquez EF, Torres J, Cubilla AL. Comparison of morphologic features and outcome of resected recurrent and nonrecurrent squamous cell carcinoma of the penis: a study of 81 cases. Am J Surg Pathol. 2010;33(9):1299–306.
10. Cubilla AL, Lloveras B, Alemany L, Alejo M, Vidal A, Kasamatsu E, Clavero O, Alvarado-Cabrero I, Lynch C, Velasco-Alonso J, Ferrera A, Chaux A, Klaustermeier J, Quint W, de Sanjosé S, Muñoz N, Bosch FX. Basaloid squamous cell carcinoma of the penis with papillary features: a clinicopathologic study of 12 cases. Am J Surg Pathol. 2012;36(6):869–75.
11. Velasquez EF, Melamed J, Barrreto JF, Aguero F, Cubilla AL. Sarcomatoid carcinoma of the penis: a clinico-patholocical study of 14 cases. Am J Surg Pathol. 2005;29(9):1152–8.
12. Lont AP, Gallee MPW, Snijders P, Horenblas S. Sarcomatoid squamous cell carcinoma of the penis: a clinical and pathological study of 5 cases. J Urol. 2004;172(3):932–5.

13. Bezerra AL, Lopes A, Landman G, Alencar GN, Torloni H, Villa LL. Clinicopathologic features and human papillomavirus dna prevalence of warty and squamous cell carcinoma of the penis. Am J Surg Pathol. 2001;25(5):673–8.
14. Chuanyu S, Ke X, Jie Z, Guowei X, Zujun F, Qiang D. Surgical treatment for 11 cases of penile verrucous carcinoma. Ann Dermatol. 2011;23(3):346–9.
15. Secretan B, Straif K, Baan R, Grosse Y, El Ghissassi F, Bouvard V, Benbrahim-Tallaa L, Guha N, Freeman C, Galichet L, Cogliano V, WHO International Agency for Research on Cancer Monograph Working Group. A review of human carcinogens–Part E: tobacco, areca nut, alcohol, coal smoke, and salted fish. Lancet Oncol. 2009;10(11):1033–4.
16. Straif K, Benbrahim-Tallaa L, Baan R, Grosse Y, Secretan B, El Ghissassi F, Bouvard V, Guha N, Freeman C, Galichet L, Cogliano V, WHO International Agency for Research on Cancer Monograph Working Group. A review of human carcinogens–part C: metals, arsenic, dusts, and fibres. Lancet Oncol. 2009;10(5):453–4.
17. El Ghissassi F, Baan R, Straif K, Grosse Y, Secretan B, Bouvard V, Benbrahim-Tallaa L, Guha N, Freeman C, Galichet L, Cogliano V, WHO International Agency for Research on Cancer Monograph Working Group. A review of human carcinogens–part D: radiation. Lancet Oncol. 2009;10(8):751–2.
18. Baan R, Grosse Y, Straif K, Secretan B, El Ghissassi F, Bouvard V, Benbrahim-Tallaa L, Guha N, Freeman C, Galichet L, Cogliano V, WHO International Agency for Research on Cancer Monograph Working Group. A review of human carcinogens–Part F: chemical agents and related occupations. Lancet Oncol. 2009;10(12):1143–4.
19. Scheiner MA, Campos MM, Ornellas AA, Chin EW, Ornellas MH, Andrada-Serpa MJ. Human papillomavirus and penile cancers in Rio de Janeiro, Brazil: HPV typing and clinical features. Int Braz J Urol. 2008;34:467–74.
20. Afonso LA, Moyses N, Alves G, Ornellas AA, Passos MR, Oliveira Ldo H, Cavalcanti SM. Prevalence of human papillomavirus and Epstein-Barr virus DNA in penile cancer cases from Brazil. Mem Inst Oswaldo Cruz. 2012;107(1):18–23.
21. Buitrago-Pérez A, Garaulet G, Vázquez-Carballo A, Paramio JM, García-Escudero R. Molecular signature of HPV-induced carcinogenesis: pRb, p53 and gene expression profiling. Curr Genomics. 2009;10(1):26–34.
22. Xiao S, Feng XL, Shi YH, Liu QZ, Li P. Cytogenetic abnormalities in a squamous cell carcinoma of the penis. Cancer Genet Cytogenet. 1992;64(2):139–41.
23. Ornellas AA, Ornellas MH, Simões F, Soares R, Campos MM, Harab RC, Silva MLM. Cytogenetic analysis of an invasive, poorly differentiated squamous cell carcinoma of the penis. Cancer Genet Cytogenet. 1998;101:78–80.
24. Ornellas AA, Ornellas MH, Otero L, Simões F, Campos MM, Harab RC, Silva MLM. Karyotypic findings in two cases of moderately differentiated squamous cell carcinoma of the penis. Cancer Genet Cytogenet. 1999;115:77–9.
25. Ornellas AA, Campos MM, Ornellas MH, Wisnescky A, Koifman N, Harab RC. Cancer du pénis: étude dela ploïdie par cytométrie de flux chez 90 patients. Progrès Urol. 2000; 10:72–7.
26. Alves G, Heller A, Fiedler W, Campos MM, Claussen U, Ornellas AA, Liehr T. Genetic imbalances in 26 penile SSC cases. Genes Chromosomes Cancer. 2001;31(1):48–53.
27. Masferrer E, Ferrándiz-Pulido C, Lloveras B, Masferrer-Niubò M, Espinet B, Salido M, Rodríguez-Rivera M, Alemany L, Placer J, Gelabert A, Servitje O, García-Patos V, Pujol RM, Toll A. MYC copy number gains are associated with poor outcome in penile squamous cell carcinoma. J Urol. 2012;188(5):1965–71.
28. Alves G, Fiedler W, Guenther E, Nascimento P, Campos MM, Ornellas AA. Determination of telomerase activity in squamous cell carcinoma of the penis. Int J Oncol. 2001;18(1):67–70.
29. Salgado R, Toll A, Espinet B, González-Roca E, Barranco CL, Serrano S, Solé F, Pujol RM. Analysis of cytogenetic abnormalities in squamous cell carcinoma by array comparative genomic hybridization. Actas Dermosifiliogr. 2008;99(3):199–206.
30. Koshland Jr DE. Molecule of the year. Science. 1993;262(5142):1953.

31. Lane DP, Crawford LV. T antigen is bound to a host protein in SV40-transformed cells. Nature. 1979;278(5701):261–3.
32. Levine AJ, Oren M. The first 30 years of p53: growing ever more complex. Nat Rev Cancer. 2009;9(10):749–58.
33. Vazquez A, Liu J, Zhou Y, Oltvai Z. Catabolic efficiency of aerobic glycolysis: the Warburg effect revisited. BMC Syst Biol. 2010;4:58. doi:10.1186/1752-0509-4-58. PMC 2880972. PMID 20459610.
34. Vousden KH, Ryan KM. p53 and metabolism. Nat Rev Cancer. 2009;9(10):691–700.
35. Petitjean A, Mathe E, Kato S, Ishioka C, Tavtigian SV, Hainaut P, Olivier M. Impact of mutant p53 functional properties on TP53 mutation patterns and tumor phenotype: lessons from recent developments in the IARC TP53 database. Hum Mutat. 2007;28(6):622–9.
36. Lam KY, Chan AC, Chan KW, Leung ML, Srivastava G. Expression of p53 and its relationship with human papillomavirus in penile carcinomas. Eur J Surg Oncol. 1995;21:613–6.
37. Pilotti S, Donghi R, D'Amato L, et al. HPV detection and p53 alteration in squamous cell verrucous malignancies of the lower genital tract. Diagn Mol Pathol. 1993;2:248–56.
38. Ranki A, Lassus J, Niemi KM. Relation of p53 tumor suppressor protein expression to human papillomavirus (HPV) DNA and to cellular atypia in male genital warts and in premalignant lesions. Acta Derm Venereol. 1995;75:180–6.
39. Castren K, Vahakangas K, Heikkinen E, Ranki A. Absence of p53 mutations in benign and pre-malignant male genital lesions with over-expressed p53 protein. Int J Cancer. 1998;77:674–8.
40. Lam KY, Chan KW. Molecular pathology and clinicopathologic features of penile tumors: with special reference to analyses of p21 and p53 expression and unusual histologic features. Arch Pathol Lab Med. 1999;123:895–904.
41. Seigne JD, Ornellas AA, Faria P. Altered expression of the retinoblastoma (Rb) and P53 tumor suppressor genes in squamous cell carcinoma of the penis. J Urol. 1997;157(suppl):46.
42. Zhu Y, Zhou XY, Yao XD, Dai B, Ye DW. The prognostic significance of p53, Ki-67, epithelial cadherin and matrix metalloproteinase-9 in penile squamous cell carcinoma treated with surgery. BJU Int. 2007;100(1):204–8.
43. Olovnikov AM. A theory of marginotomy. The incomplete copying of template margin in enzymic synthesis of polynucleotides and biological significance of the phenomenon. J Theor Biol. 1973;41(1):181–90.
44. Greider CW, Blackburn EH. Identification of a specific telomere terminal transferase activity in Tetrahymena extracts. Cell. 1985;43(2 Pt 1):405–13.
45. Kim NW, Piatyszek MA, Prowse KR, Harley CB, West MD, Ho PL, Coviello GM, Wright WE, Weinrich SL, Shay JW. Specific association of human telomerase activity with immortal cells and cancer. Science. 1994;266(5193):2011–5.
46. Ikeda R, Kobayashi Y, Shiroma K, Suzuki K, Ueda Y. Telomerase activity in giant condyloma acuminatum. Urol Int. 2000;65(4):220–3.
47. Tsujimoto Y, Cossman J, Jaffe E, Croce CM. Involvement of the bcl-2 gene in human follicular lymphoma. Science. 1985;228(4706):1440–3.
48. Malumbres M, Barbacid M. RAS oncogenes: the first 30 years. Nat Rev Cancer. 2003; 3(6):459–65.
49. Andersson P, Kolaric A, Windahl T, Kirrander P, Söderkvist P, Karlsson MG. PIK3CA, HRAS and KRAS gene mutations in human penile cancer. J Urol. 2008;179:2030–4.
50. Herman JG, Graff JR, Myöhänen S, Nelkin BD, Baylin SB. Methylation-specific PCR: a novel PCR assay for methylation status of CpG islands. Proc Natl Acad Sci U S A. 1996; 93(18):9821–6.
51. Yanagawa N, Osakabe M, Hayashi M, Tamura G, Motoyama T. Detection of HPV-DNA, p53 alterations, and methylation in penile squamous cell carcinoma in Japanese men. Pathol Int. 2008;58(8):477–82.
52. Yanagawa N, Osakabe M, Hayashi M, Tamura G, Motoyama T. Frequent epigenetic silencing of the FHIT gene in penile squamous cell carcinomas. Virchows Arch. 2008;452(4):377–82.

53. Guerrero D, Guarch R, Ojer A, Casas JM, Ropero S, Mancha A, Pesce C, Lloveras B, Garcia-Bragado F, Puras A. Hypermethylation of the thrombospondin-1 gene is associated with poor prognosis in penile squamous cell carcinoma. BJU Int. 2008;102(6):747–55.
54. Ferreux E, Lont AP, Horenblas S, Gallee MP, Raaphorst FM, von Knebel Doeberitz M, Meijer CJ, Snijders PJ. Evidence for at least three alternative mechanisms targeting the p16INK4A/cyclin D/Rb pathway in penile carcinoma, one of which is mediated by high-risk human papillomavirus. J Pathol. 2003;201(1):109–18.
55. Campos RS, Lopes A, Guimarães GC, Carvalho AL, Soares FA. E-cadherin, MMP-2, and MMP-9 as prognostic markers in penile cancer: analysis of 125 patients. Urology. 2006; 67(4):797–802.
56. Soares FA, da Cunha IW, Guimarães GC, Nonogaki S, Campos RS, Lopes A. The expression of metaloproteinases-2 and −9 is different according to the patterns of growth and invasion in squamous cell carcinoma of the penis. Virchows Arch. 2006;449(6):637–46.
57. Golijanin D, Tan JY, Kazior A, Cohen EG, Russo P, Dalbagni G, Auborn KJ, Subbaramaiah K, Dannenberg AJ. Cyclooxygenase-2 and microsomal prostaglandin E synthase-1 are overexpressed in squamous cell carcinoma of the penis. Clin Cancer Res. 2004;10(3):1024–31.
58. Bullwinkel J, Baron-Lühr B, Lüdemann A, Wohlenberg C, Gerdes J, Scholzen T. Ki-67 protein is associated with ribosomal RNA transcription in quiescent and proliferating cells. J Cell Physiol. 2006;206(3):624–35.
59. Scholzen T, Gerdes J. The Ki-67 protein: from the known and the unknown. J Cell Physiol. 2000;182(3):311–22.
60. Berney DM, Stankiewicz E, Adlan AM, Kudahetti S, Biedrzycki OJ, Hadway P, Watkin N, Corbishley C. DNA topoisomerase I and II alpha expression in penile carcinomas: assessing potential tumour chemosensitivity. BJU Int. 2008;102(8):1040–4.
61. Stankiewicz E, Kudahetti SC, Prowse DM, Ktori E, Cuzick J, Ambroisine L, Zhang X, Watkin N, Corbishley C, Berney DM. HPV infection and immunochemical detection of cell-cycle markers in verrucous carcinoma of the penis. Mod Pathol. 2009;22(9):1160–8.
62. Berdjis N, Meye A, Nippgen J, Dittert D, Hakenberg O, Baretton GB, Wirth MP. Expression of Ki-67 in squamous cell carcinoma of the penis. BJU Int. 2005;96(1):146–8.
63. Guimarães GC, Leal ML, Campos RS, Zequi Sde C, da Fonseca FP, da Cunha IW, Soares FA, Lopes A. Do proliferating cell nuclear antigen and MIB-1/Ki-67 have prognostic value in penile squamous cell carcinoma? Urology. 2007;70(1):137–42.
64. Protzel C, Knoedel J, Zimmermann U, Woenckhaus C, Poetsch M, Giebel J. Expression of proliferation marker Ki67 correlates to occurrence of metastasis and prognosis, histological subtypes and HPV DNA detection in penile carcinomas. Histol Histopathol. 2007; 22(11):1197–204.
65. Papadopoulos O, Betsi E, Tsakistou G, Frangoulis M, Kouvatseas G, Anagnostakis D, Kouvidou C. Expression of cyclin D1 and Ki-67 in squamous cell carcinoma of the penis. Cancer Res. 2007;27(4B):2167–74.
66. Leonardi E, Girlando S, Serio G, Mauri FA, Perrone G, Scampini S, Dalla Palma P, Barbareschi M. PCNA and Ki67 expression in breast carcinoma: correlations with clinical and biological variables. J Clin Pathol. 1992;45(5):416–9.
67. Martins ACP, Faria SM, Velludo MAL, Cologna AJ, Suaid HJ, Tucci Jr S. Carcinoma of the penis: the value of proliferating cellular antigen (PCNA). Braz J Urol. 2000;26(1):38–42.
68. Martins AC, Faria SM, Cologna AJ, Suaid HJ, Tucci Jr S. Immunoexpression of p53 protein and proliferating cell nuclear antigen in penile carcinoma. J Urol. 2002;167(1):89–92.
69. Cheng AJ, Chen LC, Chien KY, Chen YJ, Chang JT, Wang HM, Liao CT, Chen IH. Oral cancer plasma tumor marker identified with bead-based affinity-fractionated proteomic technology. Clin Chem. 2005;51(12):2236–44.
70. Ornellas P, Ornellas AA, Chinello C, Gianazza E, Mainini V, Cazzaniga M, Pereira DA, Sandim V, Cypriano AS, Koifman L, da Silva PC, Alves G, Magni F. Downregulation of C3 and C4A/B complement factor fragments in plasma from patients with squamous cell carcinoma of the penis. Int Braz J Urol. 2012;38(6):739–49.

71. Wishnow KI, Johnson DE, Fritsche H. Squamous cell carcinoma antigen (TA-4) in penile carcinoma. Urology. 1990;36(4):315–7.
72. Hungerhuber E, Schlenker B, Schneede P, Stief CG, Karl A. Squamous cell carcinoma antigen correlates with tumor burden but lacks prognostic potential for occult lymph node metastases in penile cancer. Urology. 2007;70(5):975–9.

Chapter 5
Prognostic Factors

Joel Slaton

Introduction

Identification and stratification of patients based on risk factors that predict for recurrence and progression of penile cancer are critical for patient and provider understanding of the disease as well as identification of appropriate therapy. Penile cancer is a relatively orderly cancer with cancer spreading from the primary to the superficial inguinal lymph nodes to the deep inguinal lymph nodes, to the pelvic nodes, and then to create distant metastases. Prognostic factors have primarily been studied in two clinical scenarios in penile cancer. First is the identification of the patient with invasive primary cancer at high risk for developing inguinal lymph node metastases. The importance of this aspect is due to the high risk of morbidity in patient undergoing resection or radiation of these lymph nodes. There is substantial data available to predict this risk. Second is among those with inguinal lymph node metastases, predicting cancer-specific survival. This information will be quite significant for identifying patients for neoadjuvant or adjuvant chemotherapy in the future. However, there is a relative paucity of studies regarding prognostic information in this area. This chapter will lay out the currently available information regarding significant individual predictors for penile cancer progression as well as nomograms combining multiple predictors that have been developed.

J. Slaton, MD
Department of Urology, University of Oklahoma Health Science Center,
920 SL Young Blvd, WP 3150, Oklahoma City, OK 73104, USA
e-mail: joel-slaton@ouhsc.edu, jwsuro@hotmail.com

D.J. Culkin (ed.), *Management of Penile Cancer*,
DOI 10.1007/978-1-4939-0461-7_5, © Springer Science+Business Media New York 2014

Table 5.1 TNM staging

A. Primary tumor (T)	
TX	Primary tumor cannot be assessed
T0	No evidence of primary tumor
Tis	Carcinoma in situ
Ta	Noninvasive verrucous carcinoma
T1a	Tumor invades subepithelial connective tissue without lymph vascular invasion and is not poorly differentiated (i.e., grades 3–4)
T1b	Tumor invades subepithelial connective tissue with lymph vascular invasion or is poorly differentiated
T2	Tumor invades corpus spongiosum or cavernosum
T3	Tumor invades urethra
T4	Tumor invades other adjacent structures
B. Regional lymph nodes (N)	
Clinical stage definition	
cNX	Regional lymph nodes cannot be assessed
cN0	No palpable or visibly enlarged inguinal lymph nodes
cN1	Palpable mobile unilateral inguinal lymph node
cN2	Palpable mobile multiple or bilateral inguinal lymph nodes
cN3	Palpable fixed inguinal nodal mass or pelvic lymphadenopathy unilateral or bilateral
Pathological stage definition	
pNX	Regional lymph nodes cannot be assessed
pN0	No regional lymph node metastasis
pN1	Metastasis in a single inguinal lymph node
pN2	Metastases in multiple or bilateral inguinal lymph nodes
pN3	Extranodal extension of lymph node metastasis or pelvic lymph node(s) unilateral or bilateral
C. Distant metastasis (M)	
M0	No distant metastasis
M1	Distant metastasis[a]

Used with the permission of the American Joint Committee on Cancer (AJCC), Chicago, Illinois. The original source for this material is the *AJCC Cancer Staging Manual*, Seventh Edition (2010) published by Springer Science and Business Media LLC, www.springer.com

[a]Lymph node metastasis outside of the true pelvis in addition to visceral or bone sites

Staging

The most basic approach to stratifying patients for risk for progression is to divide them into different staging groups. The most commonly used system is the American Joint Commission on Cancer Staging System (Table 5.1). Tumors are stratified according to the invasiveness of the primary tumor (T stage), clinically enlarged or pathologically positive lymph nodes (N stage), or the presence of distant metastases (including lymph node metastases outside the pelvis). In the most recent update in 2009, patients with invasion below the surface (pT1) were subdivided into T1a, no lymphovascular invasion and well/moderately differentiated, and T1b, presence of lymphovascular invasion or poorly differentiated [1]. T3 now refers to cancer invading into the urethra; invasion into the prostate is now considered stage T4. Nodal

Table 5.2 Anatomic stage/prognostic groups

Stage	T	N	M
0	Tis	N0	M0
	Ta	N0	M0
I	T1a	N0	M0
II	T1b	N0	M0
	T2	N0	M0
	T3	N0	M0
IIIa	T1–3	N1	M0
IIIb	T1–3	N2	M0
IV	T4	Any N	M0
	Any T	N3	M0
	Any T	Any N	M1

Used with the permission of the American Joint Committee on Cancer (AJCC), Chicago, Illinois. The original source for this material is the *AJCC Cancer Staging Manual*, Seventh Edition (2010) published by Springer Science and Business Media LLC, www.springer.com

staging has been divided into clinical and pathological, and there is no longer distinction between superficial and deep inguinal lymph nodes. TNM stages are further grouped into anatomic stage or prognostic groups (Table 5.2) to reflect their risk for progression.

Predicting Positive Inguinal Lymph Nodes

Histological Grade

Tumor grade has long been recognized as providing added value to stage in patients with squamous penile cancer. In 1989, Fraley et al. were one of the earliest investigators who identified a relationship between stage and histological differentiation in the predicting of metastases to the inguinal lymph nodes [2]. They reported that of the 23 cases of carcinoma in situ or well-differentiated disease, only 1 became metastatic, while of the 35 cases of moderately to poorly differentiated disease, 31 metastasized to the groin. Similar data were reported by McDougal in a series of 76 cases, where 82.7 % of the patients with poorly differentiated or invasive tumors had lymph node metastases [3]. As described by a number of studies detailed below, grade often serves as a significant parameter on multivariate analysis of predictors for lymph node metastases.

Recently, Chaux et al. found that comparison of tumor at the time of the primary diagnosis and of recurrence shows that histological subtype and grade were identical in 76 % of the cases and converted to a higher-grade tumor in 24 % of the cases [4]. Eighty percent of patients with high-grade tumors died from penile cancer. In addition, Chaux et al. developed a grading model for penile cancer to determine the influence on nodal metastasis of the various proportions of grades. When histologically evaluating penile carcinomas, they recommended a careful search of areas of grade 3. They concluded that any focus of grade 3 should be sufficient to grade the neoplasm as a high-grade tumor in order to enhance predictability of nodal metastases [5].

Lymphatic Invasion

In a cancer where there is orderly metastasis along lymphatic chains, invasion of the lymphatic system in the primary tumor might be expected to be a strong prognostic factor. Lopes et al. studied prognostic factors in 145 patients with penile cancer treated with penile amputation and lymphadenectomy [6]. The 5-year disease-free and overall survival rates were 45.3 and 54.3 %, respectively. Venous and lymphatic embolizations were the main factors significantly affecting the incidence of lymph node metastasis, which were the main risk factors for recurrence and death, while level of invasion into adjacent structures was not a significant predictor.

Slaton et al. reported on 48 patients treated at the MD Anderson Cancer Center [7]. They found that none of 15 pT1 tumors exhibited lymphovascular invasion or lymph node metastases. Of 33 patients with pT2 or greater tumors, 21 (64 %) had lymphovascular invasion and 18 (55 %) had metastases. Only 4 of 25 patients (15 %) with 50 % or less poorly differentiated cancer in the penile tumor had metastases compared with 14 of 23 patients (61 %) with greater than 50 % poorly differentiated cancer ($p = 0.001$).

When Ficarra et al. analyzed a number of pathological features, they found that only venous embolization, lymphatic embolization, pT stage, and histological grade were independent predictors of lymph node metastases [8]. In addition, in a subgroup analysis performed in cN0 patients, vascular and lymphatic embolizations were shown to be the most powerful predictors of nodal metastasis ($p = 0.01$).

Combining Factors for Risk Group Formation

As noted above, investigators are making efforts to combine various prognostic factors to predict nodal metastases. Solsona et al. first reported an attempt to formally combine stage and grade in an effort to stratify patients by risk factors. In their analysis, patients with pT1G1 disease could be classified as having a low risk of nodal involvement, while those with pT1G2–3 or pT2G1 as having an intermediate risk, and those with pT2 grades 2–3 or greater than stage pT3 as having a high risk [9]. The percentage of nodal metastases in the low-, intermediate-, and high-risk groups were 0, 36.4, and 80 %, respectively. This classification was confirmed in 2001 in 37 patients in whom the percentages of inguinal metastases were 0 % for the low-, 33 % for the intermediate-, and 83 % for the high-risk group [10].

The European Association of Urology (EAU) guidelines suggest a different classification: (a) low risk for those with stage pTis, pTaG1–2, or pT1G1 disease; (b) intermediate risk for those with pT1G2 tumors; and (c) high risk for those with stage pT2 or greater or G3 cancer [11]. The risk of inguinal metastases according to the EAU classification was 4 % for low-risk, 34.8 % for intermediate-risk, and 45.8 % for high-risk patients. Unfortunately, Novara et al. showed that both the Solsona et al. and the EAU risk groups had low prognostic accuracy [12, 13]. These efforts to incorporate grade and lymphovascular embolization laid the groundwork for subdivision of T1 into T1a and T1b in the updated AJCC guidelines.

Generation of Nomograms

Nomograms represent the most contemporary effort to stratify patients by risk factors [14]. Chaux et al. proposed the prognostic index to predict for metastasis of penile cancer including multiple factors associated with depth of invasion (in glans, lamina propria, numerical value of 1; corpus pongiosum, 2; and corpus cavernosum). In foreskin, they were lamina propria, numerical value of 1; dartos, 2; and skin, 3 [15]. A logistic regression model was the basis for the nomogram. The nomogram was validated by (a) calculation of the concordance index to evaluate discrimination and (b) assessment of calibration, grouping patients with respect to their nomogram-predicted probabilities and then comparing the mean of the group with the observed proportion of positive lymph nodes.

Mean follow-up obtained in all patients was of 81 months. The distribution of cases and rate of metastasis according to index scores were 2 (1 case), no metastasis; 3 (17 cases), no metastasis; 4 (35 cases), 20 % of metastasis; 5 (50 cases), 50 % of metastasis; 6 (47 cases), 66 % of metastasis; and 7 (43 cases), 79 % of metastasis. On logistic regression analysis evaluating various pathological factors, prognostic index scores were found as the best predictors of inguinal node metastasis and patients' survival compared to stage and grade.

Ficarra and Kattan developed a formal nomogram to predict nodal involvement [16]. They collected the clinical and pathological data of 175 patients who had undergone surgical therapy for squamous cell carcinoma of the penis from 1980 to 2002 at 11 urological centers in northeastern Italy. A logistic regression model was used to construct the nomogram. Data was integrating from eight clinical and pathological variables (i.e., clinical inguinal lymph node stage, pathological tumor thickness, growth pattern, histological grade, lymphatic and/or venous embolization, corpora cavernosa infiltration, corpus spongiosum, and/or urethral infiltration; Fig. 5.1). The nomogram had excellent concordance index (0.876). However, this nomogram has yet to undergo external validation.

More recently, Zhu et al. report on a group of 110 men with penile cancer and clinically negative lymph nodes from 1990 to 2008 [17]. The final model, presented as a nomogram, included T stage, grade, lymphovascular invasion, and p53 expression (Fig. 5.2). Only lymphovascular invasion showed independent prognostic value

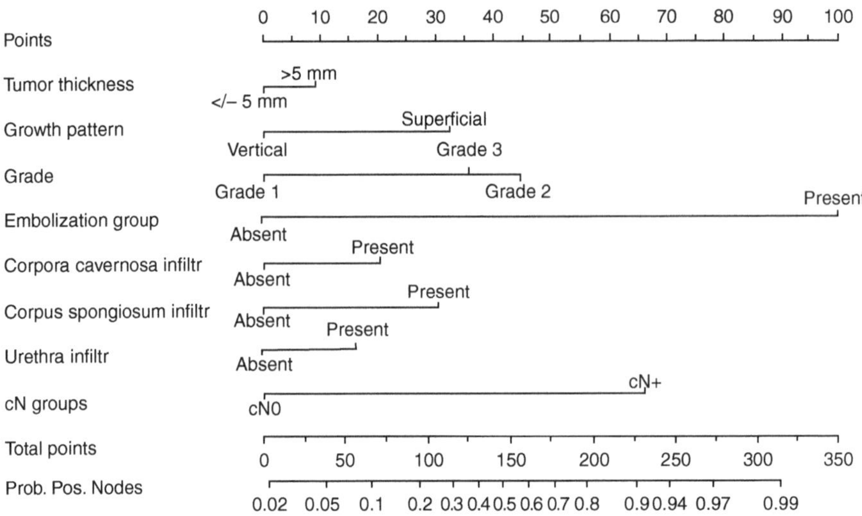

Fig. 5.1 Nomogram predicting probability of pathological lymph node involvement. *Probability positive nodes*, probability of pathologically positive lymph node. *See* Appendix I *for instructions on use* (Reprinted from Ficarra et al. [16], Copyright 2006, with permission from Elsevier)

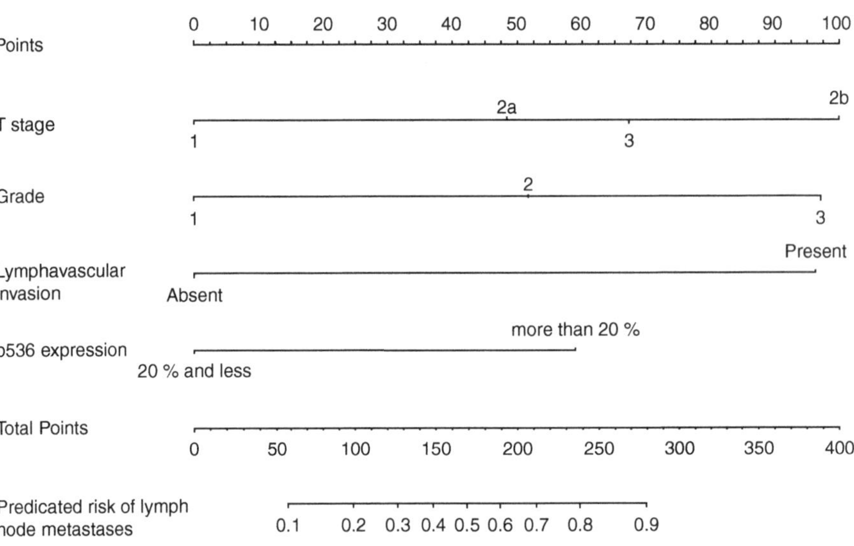

Fig. 5.2 Nomogram predicting lymph node involvement (Reprinted from Zhu et al. [17], with permission from Elsevier)

Table 5.3 Five-year cancer-specific survival stratified by pathological nodal stage

	Pathological nodal stage (%)				
Study	pN0	pN+	pN1	pN2	pN3
Srinivas et al. [18]	85	32	NA	NA	NA
Ornellas et al. [19]	87	29	NA	NA	NA
Pow-Sang et al. [20]	92	NA	80	NA	17
Ravi [21]	95	NA	86	60	0
Kulkarni and Kamat [22]	91	NA	NA	NA	NA
Brkovic et al. [23]	90	NA	80	NA	17
Hegarty et al. [24]	100	NA	100	73	67
Novara et al. [25]	94	29	89	7	0
Pandey et al. [26]	95	51	NA	21	0
Ornellas et al. [27]	96	35	NA	NA	NA
Zhu et al. [28]		NA	87	57	32
Chaux and Cubilla [29]	91	48	NA	NA	NA

Adapted by permission from Macmillan Publishers Ltd Novara et al. [25], copyright 2007

on multivariate analysis ($p=0.024$). The model also showed good calibration (bootstrap-corrected concordance index 0.79). The primary difference between the Kattan and Zhu nomogram was the inclusion of the biomarker, tumor suppression protein p53.

Predicting Cancer-Specific Survival

It has been a challenge to study the prognostic factors for cancer-specific survival in patients with penile carcinoma due to the limited number of patients included in published series.

N Stage

A number of investigators have reported on the value of TNM N stage for predicting survival after lymph node dissection (Table 5.3) [18–29]. For N0 patients, 3–5-year survival ranges from 85 to 100 %, for N1 79 to 100 %, for N2 7 to 73 %, and for N3 0 to 67 %. Zhu et al. studied how changes in the N stage from the 6th edition of the AJCC staging system to the 7th edition impacted survival [28]. In the 7th edition, there is no longer a staging distinction between inguinal superficial and deep lymph nodes, and extranodal extension of regional lymph node metastases is classified as N3 disease. Among a group of 60 patients, using the 6th edition N classification, the 3-year recurrence-free survival rate was 69.8, 48.2, and 33.3 % for the N1, N2, and N3 categories, respectively. However, log rank survival analysis failed to show a statistical difference ($p=0.054$). In the new 7th edition N categories, the 3-year recurrence-free survival rate was 87.5, 57, and 31.8 % in the corresponding N1 to N3 groups. Better survival stratification was observed on analysis ($p < 0.001$). Thus, the new N staging system better reflects the prognosis in patients with penile cancer.

Number of Lymph Nodes and Ratio of Positive to Negative Lymph Nodes

The absolute number of metastatic lymph nodes will impact upon survival. Ravi reported that 5-year survival rate among patients with positive inguinal lymph nodes varied according to the number of positive nodes; 5-year survival rate for those with 1–3 positive nodes was 81 %, while for those with >3 nodes was 50 % [21]. Svatek et al. reported that 8.3 % patients with ≤2 positive lymph nodes died by the last follow-up, while 76 % with >2 metastatic lymph nodes died of metastatic disease. The optimal cutoff for lymph node number is debatable [30]. Zhu et al. found there was no significant difference in the survival rates among patients with 1–3 positive lymph nodes [31]. The survival rate significantly decreased when there were 4 or more metastatic nodes. Leijte et al. validated this finding when a significant difference was observed between 1 and 3 positive inguinal nodes and 4 or greater nodes ($p = 0.029$) [32].

In several neoplasms, investigators have found that lymph node density of positive lymph nodes is a superior predictor for survival compared to the actual number of positive lymph nodes. Svatek et al. reported an estimated 5-year disease-specific survival in patients with lymph node density of 6.7 % or less were significantly better than that in patients with lymph node density greater than 6.7 % (91.2 % vs 23.3 %, $p < 0.001$) [30]. In models comparing lymph node density to known prognostic features, lymph node density remained statistically significant, while the other factors were no longer statistically associated with disease-specific survival. In a series of 73 penile cancer patients, Zhu et al. found that involvement of pelvic lymph nodes correlated with inguinal lymph node density of at least 30 % had 100 % specificity in predicting pelvic nodal disease [31]. Furthermore, this same group demonstrated that lymph node density was a strong predictor for disease-free survival with a concordance index of 0.68. Due to the relatively low number of patients in each study, validation in a larger cohort is needed.

Extracapsular Extension

The incidences of extracapsular extension in node-positive penile cancer patients vary from 15 to 51 % [33]. Analyzing 156 patients with positive inguinal lymph nodes, Graafland et al. found the presence of ECE was correlated with clinical nodal status (13 % cN0 and 66 % in cN+patients) [34]. On multivariate analysis, extracapsular extension and pelvic lymph node involvement remained associated with decreased cancer-specific survival (HR 2.37 and 2.20, respectively).

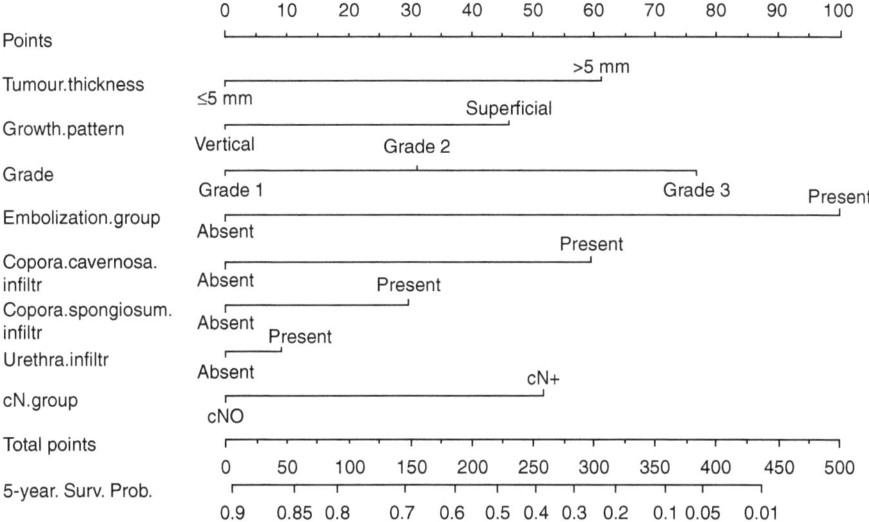

Fig. 5.3 Nomogram predicting 5-year cancer-specific survival according to pathological findings of primary tumor and clinical stage of lymph nodes. *Corpora.cavernosa.infiltr.*, infiltration of corpora cavernosa. *Corpus.spongiosum.infiltr.*, infiltration of corpus spongiosum. *urethra.infiltr.*, infiltration of urethra. *cN.group*, clinical lymph node stage. *5-years. Surv. Prob.*, 5-year cancer-specific survival probabilities. *See* Appendix I *for instructions on use* (Reprinted from Kattan et al. [36], Copyright 2006, with permission from Elsevier)

Several series have demonstrated that extracapsular extension correlates with poor 5-year survival. Pandey found that overall survival rate in patients with extracapsular extension was 9 % compared to 91 % in those without extranodal extension [26]. Both Pandey and Graafland et al. found that extracapsular extension was an independent prognostic factor for 5-year disease-specific survival [26, 34]. Furthermore, Graafland et al. showed that extracapsular extension was of greater prognostic significance than the number of positive lymph nodes. Even among patients receiving neoadjuvant chemotherapy, patients with extracapsular extension in the residual inguinal lymph node tumor had a median overall survival of 10 months compared to greater than 50 months with patients without extracapsular extension [35].

Nomograms

Working with the same dataset of 175 patients used to create their nomogram for predicting the presence of positive lymph nodes, Kattan and Ficarra generated the first model to predict for survival (Fig. 5.3) based upon the pathological findings of the primary tumor after penectomy and on the clinical stage of groin lymph nodes. A second model (Fig. 5.4) incorporated the pathological data of the primary tumor and groin lymph nodes [36]. The concordance for the first model was 0.728 and for the second model 0.747.

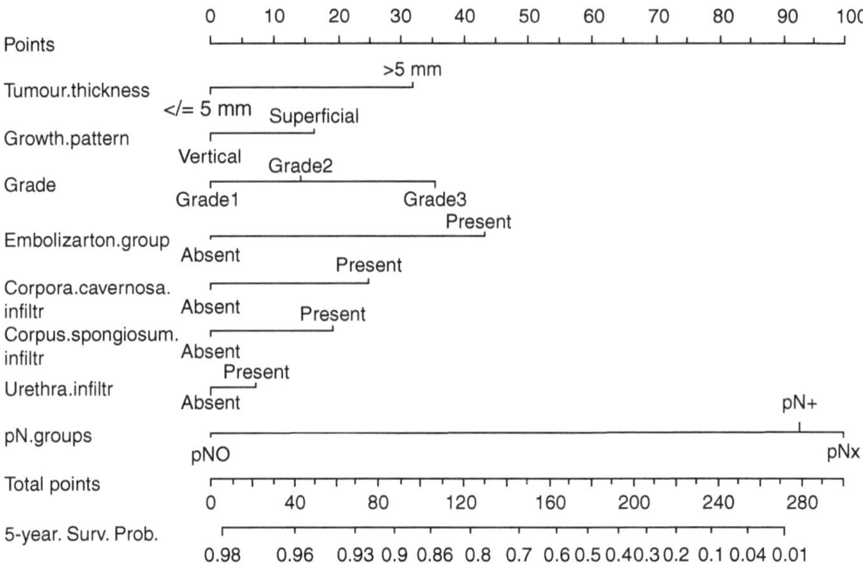

Fig. 5.4 Nomogram predicting 5-year cancer-specific survival according to pathological findings of primary tumor and pathological stage of lymph nodes. *Corpora.cavernosa.infiltr.*, infiltration of corpora cavernosa. *Corpus.spongiosum.infiltr.*, infiltration of corpus spongiosum. *urethra.infiltr.*, infiltration of urethra. *pN.group*, pathological lymph node stage. *5-years. Surv. Prob.*, 5-year cancer-specific survival probabilities. *See* Appendix I *for instructions on use* (Reprinted from Kattan et al. [36], Copyright 2006, with permission from Elsevier)

Some have criticized this Kattan model given its dependence upon several pathological variables (tumor thickness and growth patterns) which are not routinely used in clinical practice. Zini took another approach analyzing the SEER database to identify predictors for survival among 856 patients with penile cancer [37]. The predictors consisted of age, race, SEER stage (localized vs regional vs metastatic), tumor grade, type of surgery (excisional biopsy, partial penectomy, and radical penectomy), and lymph node status (pN0 vs pN1–3 vs pNx). SEER stage and histological grade achieved independent predictor status and qualified for inclusion in the model. The model achieved 73.8 % accuracy for prediction of cancer-specific survival at 5 years after surgery. Unfortunately, the SEER staging system has been supplanted by the TNM system making application of this model to the real world more challenging.

Furthermore, Theuret et al. recently attempted to simplify the process by adding grade to the patients with AJCC stage within the SEER database finding that this combination was the simplest, most accurate cancer-specific mortality prediction strategy after primary tumor excision for penile squamous cell carcinoma [38]. They concluded that this method was more accurate than two previous cancer-specific mortality prediction models. The same authors extended their work to develop the first predictive tool that accounts for conditional survivorship (the concept that long-term cancer survivors have a better prognosis than newly diagnosed individuals) to their model and externally validated it [39].

Summary

Over the past 20 years, substantial efforts have been undertaken to identify and integrate prognostic factors into models that can predict for both inguinal nodal metastases and survival among those with nodal metastases. Nomograms to predict for nodal metastases will allow the provider to carefully select patients for intervention on the lymph nodes while avoiding the potential side effect that such intervention may generate. Furthermore, a clear understanding of the factors which predict for survival will allow for optimal selection of patients for clinical trials testing novel therapeutic strategies to treat metastatic disease. Further integration of biomarkers detailed in Chap. 4 into these nomograms may further enhance their accuracy.

Appendix I

Instructions for Physicians: Locate the tumor thickness on the tumor thickness axis. Draw a line straight upward to the Points axis to determine the number of points received for tumor thickness. Repeat this process for the remaining axes, each time drawing straight upward to the Points axis. Sum the points achieved for each predictor and locate the sum on the Total Points axis. Draw a line straight down to find the 5-year cancer-specific survival of the patient.

Instructions to Patient: "Mr. *X*, if we had 100 men exactly like you, we would expect the predicted percentage from the nomogram to be free of disease-specific death in 5 years, assuming no one died of another cause."

References

1. AJCC. Penis. In: Edge SB, Byrd DR, Compton CC, et al., editors. AJCC cancer staging manual. 7th ed. New York: Springer; 2010. p. 447–55.
2. Fraley EE, Zhang G, Manivel C, Niehans GA. The role of ilioinguinal lymphadenectomy and significance of histological differentiation in treatment of carcinoma of the penis. J Urol. 1989;142(6):1478–82.
3. McDougal WS. Carcinoma of the penis: improved survival by early regional lymphadenectomy based on the histological grade and depth of invasion of the primary lesion. J Urol. 1995;154(4):1364–6.
4. Chaux A, Reuter V, Lezcano C, Velazquez EF, Torres J, Cubilla AL. Comparison of morphologic features and outcome of resected recurrent and nonrecurrent squamous cell carcinoma of the penis: a study of 81 cases. Am J Surg Pathol. 2009;33(9):1299–306.
5. Chaux A, Torres J, Pfannl R, Barreto J, Rodriguez I, Velazquez EF, Cubilla AL. Histologic grade in penile squamous cell carcinoma: visual estimation versus digital measurement of proportions of grades, adverse prognosis with any proportion of grade 3 and correlation of a Gleason-like system with nodal metastasis. Am J Surg Pathol. 2009;33(7):1049–57.
6. Lopes A, Hidalgo GS, Kowalski LP, Torloni H, Rossi BM, Fonseca FP. Prognostic factors in carcinoma of the penis: multivariate analysis of 145 patients treated with amputation and lymphadenectomy. J Urol. 1996;156(5):1637–42.

7. Slaton JW, Morgenstern N, Levy DA, Santos Jr MW, Tamboli P, Ro JY, Ayala AG, Pettaway CA. Tumor stage, vascular invasion and the percentage of poorly differentiated cancer: independent prognosticators for inguinal lymph node metastasis in penile squamous cancer. J Urol. 2001;165(4):1138–42.
8. Ficarra V, Zattoni F, Cunico SC, Galetti TP, Luciani L, Fandella A, Guazzieri S, Maruzzi D, Sava T, Siracusano S, Pilloni S, Tasca A, Martignoni G, Gardiman M, Tardanico R, Zambolin T, Cisternino A, Artibani W, Gruppo Uro-Oncologico del Nord Est (Northeast Uro-Oncological Group) Penile Cancer Project. Lymphatic and vascular embolizations are independent predictive variables of inguinal lymph node involvement in patients with squamous cell carcinoma of the penis: Gruppo Uro-Oncologico del Nord Est (Northeast Uro-Oncological Group) Penile Cancer data base data. Cancer. 2005;103(12):2507–16.
9. Solsona E, Iborra I, Ricós JV, Monrós JL, Dumont R, Casanova J, Calabuig C. Corpus cavernosum invasion and tumor grade in the prediction of lymph node condition in penile carcinoma. Eur Urol. 1992;22(2):115–8.
10. Solsona E, Iborra I, Rubio J, Casanova JL, Ricós JV, Calabuig C. Prospective validation of the association of local tumor stage and grade as a predictive factor for occult lymph node micrometastasis in patients with penile carcinoma and clinically negative inguinal lymph nodes. J Urol. 2001;165(5):1506–9.
11. Solsona E, Algaba F, Horenblas S, Pizzocaro G, Windahl T, European Association of Urology. EAU guidelines on penile cancer. Eur Urol. 2004;46(1):1–8.
12. Novara G, Artibani W, Cunico SC, De Giorgi G, Gardiman M, Martignoni G, Siracusano S, Tardanico R, Zattoni F, Ficarra V, GUONE Penile Cancer Project. How accurately do Solsona and European Association of Urology risk groups predict for risk of lymph node metastases in patients with squamous cell carcinoma of the penis? Urology. 2008;71(2):328–33.
13. Ficarra V, Novara G, Boscolo-Berto R, Artibani W, Kattan MW. How accurate are present risk group assignment tools in penile cancer? World J Urol. 2009;27(2):155–60.
14. Kattan MW. When and how to use informatics tools in caring for urologic patients. Nat Clin Pract Urol. 2005;2(4):183–90.
15. Chaux A, Caballero C, Soares F, Guimarães GC, Cunha IW, Reuter V, Barreto J, Rodríguez I, Cubilla AL. The prognostic index: a useful pathologic guide for prediction of nodal metastases and survival in penile squamous cell carcinoma. Am J Surg Pathol. 2009;33(7):1049–57.
16. Ficarra V, Zattoni F, Artibani W, Fandella A, Martignoni G, Novara G, Galetti TP, Zambolin T, Kattan MW, G.U.O.N.E. Penile Cancer Project Members. Nomogram predictive of pathological inguinal lymph node involvement in patients with squamous cell carcinoma of the penis. J Urol. 2006;175(5):1700–4.
17. Zhu Y, Zhang HL, Yao XD, Zhang SL, Dai B, Shen YJ, Ye DW. Development and evaluation of a nomogram to predict inguinal lymph node metastasis in patients with penile cancer and clinically negative lymph nodes. J Urol. 2010;184(2):539–45.
18. Srinivas V, Morse MJ, Herr HW, Sogani PC, Whitmore Jr WF. Penile cancer: relation of extent of nodal metastasis to survival. J Urol. 1987;137(5):880–2.
19. Ornellas AA, Seixas AL, de Moraes JR. Analyses of 200 lymphadenectomies in patients with penile carcinoma. J Urol. 1991;146(2):330–2.
20. Pow-Sang JE, Benavente V, Pow-Sang JM, Pow-Sang M. Bilateral ilioinguinal lymph node dissection in the management of cancer of the penis. Semin Surg Oncol. 1990; 6(4):241–2.
21. Ravi R. Correlation between the extent of nodal involvement and survival following groin dissection for carcinoma of the penis. Br J Urol. 1993;72(5 Pt 2):817–9.
22. Kulkarni JN, Kamat MR. Prophylactic bilateral groin node dissection versus prophylactic radiotherapy and surveillance in patients with N0 and N1-2A carcinoma of the penis. Eur Urol. 1994;26(2):123–8.
23. Brkovic D, Kälble T, Dörsam J, Pomer S, Lötzerich C, Banafsche R, Riedasch G, Staehler G. Surgical treatment of invasive penile cancer–the Heidelberg experience from 1968 to 1994. Eur Urol. 1997;31(3):339–42.

24. Hegarty PK, Kayes O, Freeman A, Christopher N, Ralph DJ, Minhas S. A prospective study of 100 cases of penile cancer managed according to European Association of Urology guidelines. BJU Int. 2006;98(3):526–31.
25. Novara G, Galfano A, De Marco V, Artibani W, Ficarra V. Prognostic factors in squamous cell carcinoma of the penis. Nat Clin Pract Urol. 2007;4(3):140–6.
26. Pandey D, Mahajan V, Kannan RR. Prognostic factors in node-positive carcinoma of the penis. J Surg Oncol. 2006;93(2):133–8.
27. Ornellas AA, Nóbrega BL, Wei Kin Chin E, Wisnescky A, da Silva PC, de Santos Schwindt AB. Prognostic factors in invasive squamous cell carcinoma of the penis: analysis of 196 patients treated at the Brazilian National Cancer Institute. J Urol. 2008;180(4):1354–9.
28. Zhu Y, Ye DW, Yao XD, Zhang SL, Dai B, Zhang HL. New N staging system of penile cancer provides a better reflection of prognosis. J Urol. 2011;186(2):518–23.
29. Chaux A, Cubilla AL. Stratification systems as prognostic tools for defining risk of lymph node metastasis in penile squamous cell carcinomas. Semin Diagn Pathol. 2012;29(2):83.
30. Svatek RS, Munsell M, Kincaid JM, et al. Association between lymph node density and disease specific survival in patients with penile cancer. J Urol. 2009;182:272.
31. Zhu Y, Ye D-w. Lymph node metastases and prognosis in penile cancer. Chin J Cancer Res. 2012;24(2):90–6.
32. Leijte JA, Gallee M, Antonini N, Horenblas S. Evaluation of current TNM classification of penile carcinoma. J Urol. 2008;180(3):933–8.
33. Zhu Y, Zhang SL, Ye DW, et al. Predicting pelvic lymph node metastases in penile cancer patients: a comparison of computed tomography, Cloquet's node, and disease burden of inguinal lymph nodes. Onkologie. 2008;31:37.
34. Graafland NM, Moonen LM, van Boven HH, et al. Prognostic significance of extranodal extension in patients with pathological node positive penile carcinoma. J Urol. 2010;184:1347.
35. Pagliaro LC, Williams DL, Daliani D, Williams MB, Osai W, Kincaid M, Wen S, Thall PF, Pettaway CA. Neoadjuvant paclitaxel, ifosfamide, and cisplatin chemotherapy for metastatic penile cancer: a phase II study. J Clin Oncol. 2010;28(24):3851–7.
36. Kattan MW, Ficarra V, Artibani W, Cunico SC, Fandella A, Martignoni G, Novara G, Galetti TP, Zattoni F, GUONE Penile Cancer Project Members. Nomogram predictive of cancer specific survival in patients undergoing partial or total amputation for squamous cell carcinoma of the penis. J Urol. 2006;175(6):2103–8.
37. Zini L, Cloutier V, Isbarn H, Perrotte P, Capitanio U, Jeldres C, Shariat SF, Saad F, Arjane P, Duclos A, Lattouf JB, Montorsi F, Karakiewicz PL. A simple and accurate model for prediction of cancer-specific mortality in patients treated with surgery for primary penile squamous cell carcinoma. Clin Cancer Res. 2009;15(3):1013–8.
38. Thuret R, Sun M, Abdollah F, Budaus L, Lughezzani G, Liberman D, Morgan M, Johal R, Jeldres C, Latour M, Shariat SF, Iborra F, Guiter J, Patard JJ, Perrotte P, Karakiewicz PI. Tumor grade improves the prognostic ability of American Joint Committee on Cancer stage in patients with penile carcinoma. J Urol. 2011;185(2):501–7.
39. Thuret R, Sun M, Abdollah F, Schmitges J, Shariat SF, Iborra F, Guiter J, Patard JJ, Perrotte P, Karakiewicz PI. Conditional survival predictions after surgery for patients with penile carcinoma. Cancer. 2011;117(16):3723–30.

Chapter 6
Imaging and Clinical Staging for Penile Cancer

Olivier Bouchot and Jérôme Rigaud

Appropriate diagnosis and evaluation are essential elements for the treatment of squamous cell carcinoma (SCC) of the penis, according to the 2009 TNM classification (Table 6.1). This assessment is even more important in young, sexually active patients in good general health. International guidelines (AUA, EAU) present a number of limitations due to the low incidence of SCC of the penis, the lack of prospective studies, and only a few meta-analyses [33].

The low incidence of penile cancer and the fact that it involves a highly symbolic organ are responsible for (1) poor medical recognition of the diagnosis of SCC of the penis, premalignant lesions, and local and regional staging and (2) delayed diagnosis due to the patient's fears concerning the impact on his sexuality.

Early diagnosis of the primary tumor should allow conservative treatment, particularly for tumors of the glans, and simplify the assessment of inguinal lymph node status.

Imaging and Clinical Staging of the Primary Tumor

The primary tumor can arise anywhere on the penis, but the most common sites are the glans and foreskin. Primary tumors of the body of the penis are rare (<2 %), while secondary tumors, localized in the corpus cavernosum, reflect systemic disease.

The appearance of a tumor of the penis can constitute a warning sign for the patient in the form of induration, increased size, or a papillary or ulcerated lesion. The presence of acquired phimosis may hide a primary tumor that can progress

O. Bouchot, MD, PhD (✉) • J. Rigaud, MD, PhD
Department of Urologic Clinic, University Hospital,
1, Place Ricordeau, BP 1005, Nantes 44093, France
e-mail: obouchot@chu-nantes.fr

D.J. Culkin (ed.), *Management of Penile Cancer*,
DOI 10.1007/978-1-4939-0461-7_6,

Table 6.1 2009 TNM classification

T	*Primary tumor*
TX	Primary tumor cannot be assessed
T0	No evidence of primary tumor
Tis	Carcinoma in situ
Ta	Noninvasive verrucous carcinoma, not associated with destructive invasion
T1	Tumor invades subepithelial connective tissue
T1a	Without lymphovascular invasion and is not poorly differentiated or undifferentiated (T1 G1–2)
T1b	With lymphovascular invasion or poorly differentiated or undifferentiated (T1 G3–4)
T2	Tumor invades corpus spongiosum/corpora cavernosa
T3	Tumor invades urethra
T4	Tumor invades adjacent other structures
N	*Regional lymph nodes*
NX	Regional lymph nodes cannot be assessed
N0	No. palpable gold visibly enlarged inguinal lymph node
N1	Palpable mobile unilateral inguinal lymph node
N2	Palpable mobile multiple or bilateral inguinal lymph nodes
N3	Fixed inguinal nodal mass or pelvic lymphadenopathy unilateral or bilateral
M	*Remote metastases*
M0	No remote metastasis
M1	Remote metastasis

Used with permission from Sobin et al. [42]

unnoticed. Subsequent signs then consist of purulent discharge, urgency, pain, bleeding, or erosion of the tumor through the foreskin.

Physical Examination

During the first consultation, palpation of the penis is essential to locate the primary tumor (glans, foreskin, corpus cavernosum), define the limits of the tumor in relation to other structures (corpus spongiosum, corpus cavernosum, urethra), and determine the size and numbers of tumors and their morphology (flat, papillary, nodular, or ulceration) (Fig. 6.1). This clinical assessment may be distorted by tumor infection and peripheral edema of the tumor or foreskin, suggesting infiltration. The inaccurate clinical staging of the primary tumor has been estimated to concern 26 % of patients, with understaging in 10 % and overstaging in 16 % of cases [15].

The presence of tumor invasion of the corpus cavernosum is a major prognostic factor for survival; in the majority of cases, the presence and extent of inguinal lymph node metastasis contraindicate conservative surgical techniques of the glans.

The 2009 TNM classification, based on clinical signs, is not sufficient for the assessment of prognosis and survival of the patients, as several studies have shown similar survival for stage cT3 or higher compared to stage cT2 [24, 28]. Stage cT3

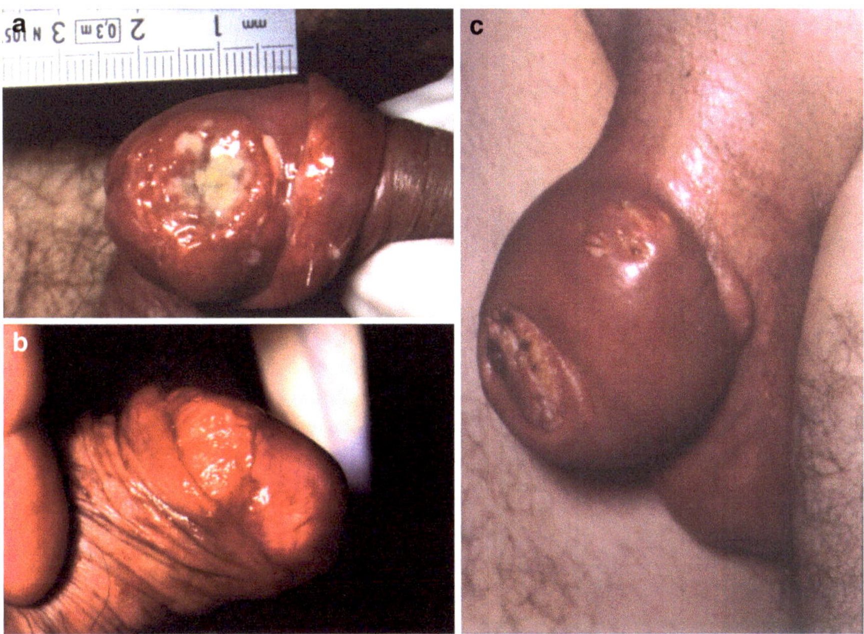

Fig. 6.1 Tumors of the penis. (**a**) Clinical stage T2 limited to the glans. (**b**) Clinical stage T2 with invasion of the corpus cavernosum. (**c**) Clinical stage T3 with invasion of the corpora cavernosum and urethra

corresponds to invasion of the urethra, but the prognosis of the tumors of the glans with invasion of only distal urethra is better than that of tumors with invading the corpus cavernosum.

Penile Ultrasound

7.5 or 10 MHz ultrasound probes are useful for large tumors involving the glans to define the anatomical relations with the corpora cavernosum and urethra [16] but only when these relations cannot be determined on physical examination [29] (Fig. 6.2). Penile ultrasound can demonstrate invasion of the corpora cavernosa and corpus spongiosum, and tunica albuginea infiltration is visualized as interruption of the thin echogenic line of the tunica.

However, this examination is difficult to interpret due to the inflammation and/or infection frequently associated with the primary tumor and in the case of acquired phimosis secondary to large tumors. These tumors may also be hyperechoic and hypoechoic or present mixed echogenicity.

Only one study showed that tumors confined to the glans were often understaged on physical examination, in contrast with tumors invading the body of the penis, and that ultrasound was more reliable than physical examination [1].

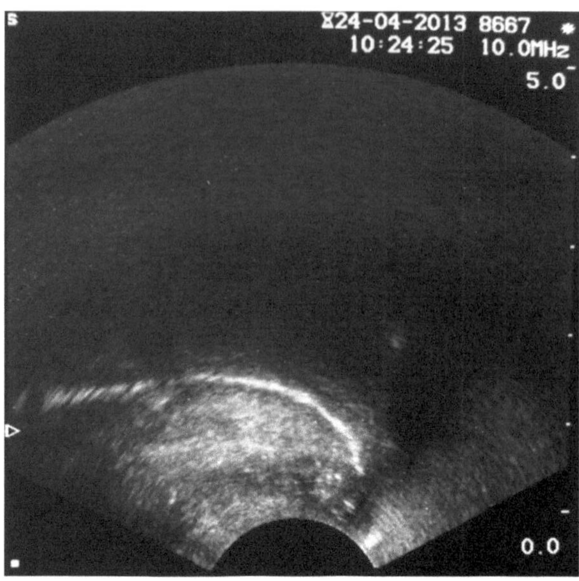

Fig. 6.2 Ultrasound using a 10 MHz probe. Distal tumor of the glans invading the navicular fossa and distal urethra

Penile MRI

Staging of tumors of the glans and foreskin by MRI is designed to demonstrate infiltration of the tunica albuginea of the corpus cavernosum or the urethra (Figs. 6.3 and 6.4). Tumors are hypointense on T1- and T2-weighted sequences and are gadolinium enhanced. The only way to obtain reliable images correlated with the pathological stage is to perform MRI during erection or after intracavernosal injection of 10 μg of prostaglandin E1.

The routine indications for MRI are being extended to improve the selection of patients eligible for penile sparing surgery (local excision, partial or total glansectomy) and brachytherapy [18]. Errors of interpretation are essentially related to tumor infection or secondary to phimosis and the absence of erection.

In tumors of the penile body, MRI is necessary to define tumor margins with respect to the tunica albuginea of the corpora cavernosum and to detect other penile sire sites (Fig. 6.5).

Penile Biopsy

Apart from locally advanced tumors for which the diagnosis is obvious, lesions suspicious of malignancy, involving the glans and/or refractory to treatment, require diagnostic biopsy for histological examination.

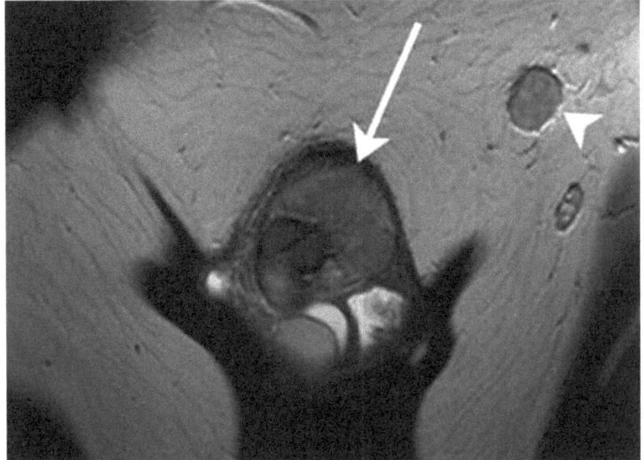

Fig. 6.3 MRI of the penis. Stage T2 tumor of the glans with invasion of the tunica albuginea of corpus cavernosum (*arrow*) and the presence of a left inguinal node (*arrowhead*)

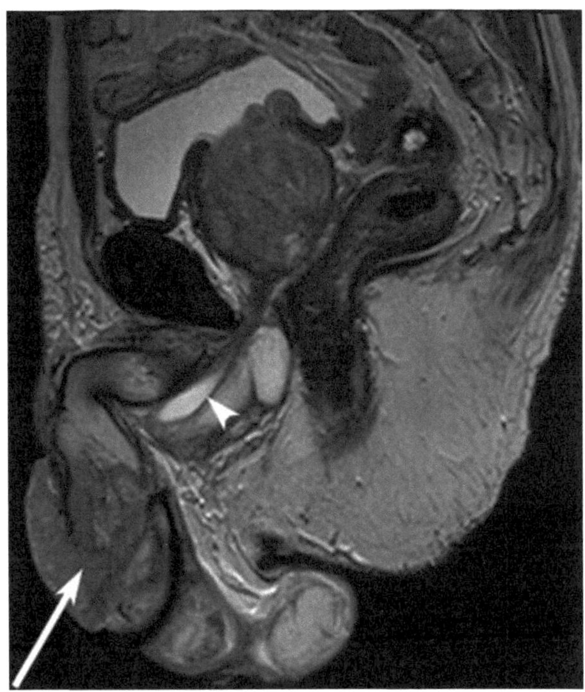

Fig. 6.4 MRI of the penis. Large stage T2 tumor of the glans with extensive invasion of the corpora cavernosa (*arrow*) and urethra (*arrowhead*)

Small superficial biopsies are difficult to analyze [41]. It is preferable to perform a biopsy–excision of the tumor, which provides a maximum of information concerning the histological type, cytological grade, growth patterns, tumor thickness (±3 mm), the presence of lymphatic or vascular embolization, and surgical margins. All this information is useful for treatment and prognosis, especially as tumor subtypes with different prognoses have been recently reported [3].

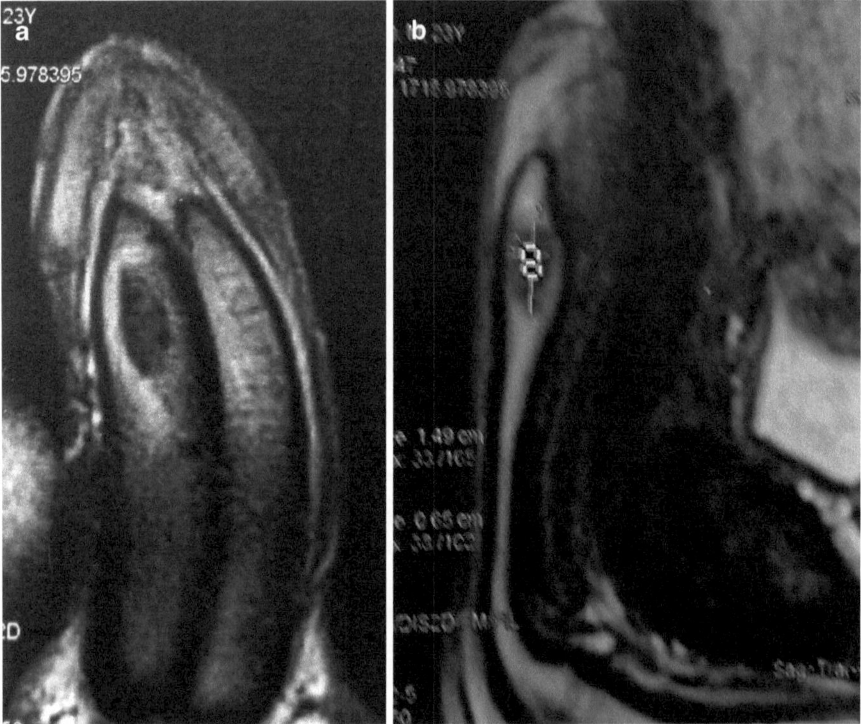

Fig. 6.5 (**a**, **b**) MRI of a primary tumor of the corpus cavernosum without invasion of the tunica albuginea

Imaging and Clinical Staging for Regional Lymph Nodes

Penile cancer essentially spreads via lymphatic dissemination, while vascular dissemination is less common. The first draining lymph nodes are bilateral inguinal lymph nodes [5]. A recent study visualized the lymphatic drainage of penile cancer by single photon emission computed tomography–computed tomography (SPECT-CT), showing that the first inguinal draining node was located in the superior and central quadrants of superficial inguinal lymph nodes, according to Daseler's description, particularly the medial superior quadrant [25]. No direct drainage of the penis to the two inferior quadrants of superficial inguinal lymph nodes and no direct drainage to pelvic lymph nodes were observed [25].

Physical Examination

The presence of palpable superficial inguinal lymph nodes must be determined at the first visit. Palpable inguinal lymph nodes are present in 28–64 % of patients with penile cancer at presentation. Nodal metastases are found in about one-half of these

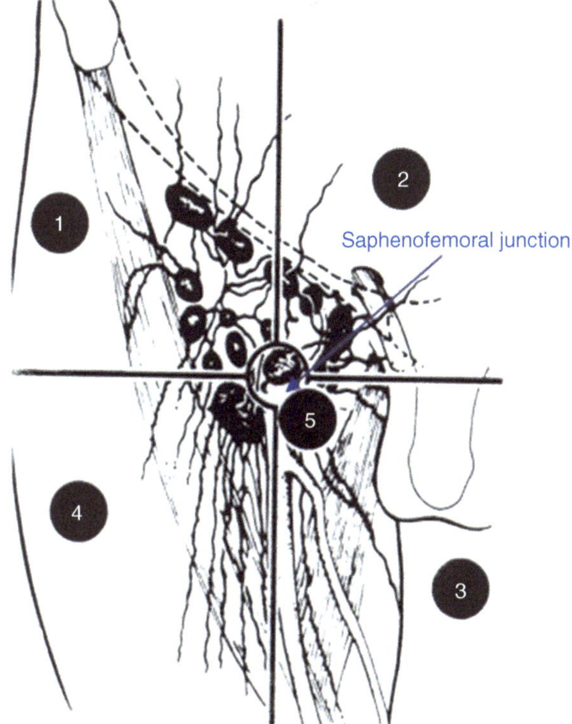

Fig. 6.6 Representation of superficial inguinal lymph node quadrants according to Daseler [5]. The upper quadrants, above the inguinal crease, are zones 1 and 2. Zone 3, next the saphenous arch, represents the central quadrant

cases, while palpable nodes are due to an inflammatory reaction in the remaining cases. About 75 % of patients with palpable inguinal lymph nodes have unilateral invasion, and 25 % have bilateral nodal invasion [8, 14, 17].

The first draining lymph nodes must be thoroughly examined on both sides, with particular attention to the superior quadrants of superficial inguinal lymph nodes. Palpation and ultrasound should therefore both focus on the quadrants above the groin, as the medial superior group lies just lateral to the ipsilateral spermatic cord. The central group, opposite the saphenous arch, is situated in the inguinal crease (Fig. 6.6).

In the presence of palpable lymph nodes, physical examination of the inguinal region should note the following characteristics: number, site (unilateral or bilateral), dimensions, mobility or fixation, relations to other structures (skin, Cooper's ligament), and edema of the penis, scrotum, and/or legs.

Unfortunately, physical examination of inguinal lymph nodes cannot reliably predict the presence of lymph node metastasis, as it has a sensitivity and specificity of 90 and 21 % compared to pathological findings, respectively [15]. Some authors have proposed a course of antibiotics for patients with suspected inflammatory lymph nodes in order to improve the accuracy of physical examination. However, a long course of antibiotic therapy would delay the diagnosis, which would have a negative impact on prognosis. Imaging is useful to distinguish inflammatory and metastatic lymph nodes.

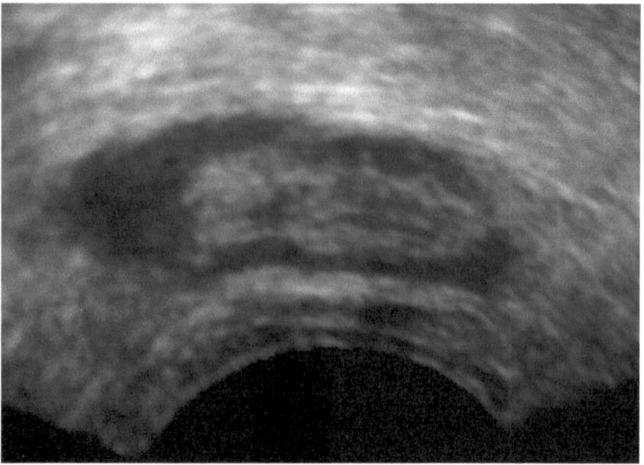

Fig. 6.7 Inguinal ultrasound using a 10 MHz probe. Normal inguinal lymph node homogeneous hypoechoic cortex with intact contours and hyperechoic hilum

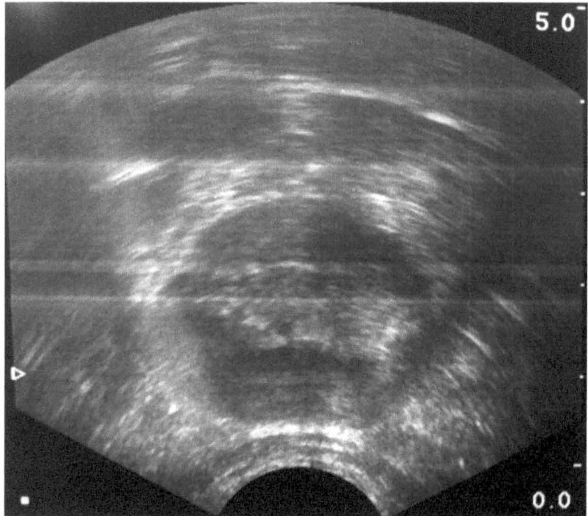

Fig. 6.8 Inguinal ultrasound using a 10 MHz probe. Enlarged node with eccentric cortical hypertrophy suggestive of metastasis

Inguinal Ultrasound Using a 7.5 MHZ or 10 MHz Probe

The role of inguinal ultrasound is to identify metastatic lymph nodes, especially in the superior quadrants and in obese patients in whom physical examination can be particularly difficult.

High-resolution probes allow detailed analysis of inguinal lymph nodes, and features suggestive of tumor invasion include enlarged node, abnormal shape, short-/long-axis ratio <2, eccentric cortical hypertrophy, the absence of echogenic hilum, and hypoechogenicity due to a necrotic zone (Figs. 6.7, 6.8, and 6.9). Pulsed Doppler is also used to demonstrate increased density of the peripheral blood supply of the node [6].

However, ultrasound alone cannot detect micrometastatic inguinal lymph nodes.

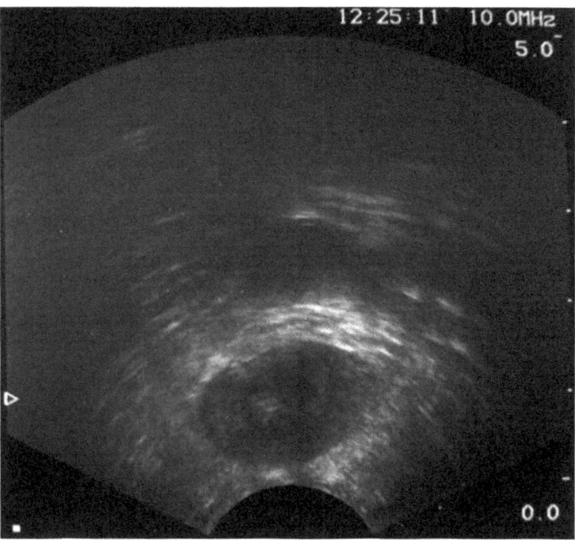

Fig. 6.9 Inguinal ultrasound using a 10 MHz probe. Enlarged node with loss of the hyperechoic hilum suggestive of metastasis

Lymph Node Cytology

Inguinal ultrasound-guided fine-needle aspiration cytology (FNAC) should be systematically performed in patients with clinically palpable lymph nodes and/or abnormal lymph nodes on ultrasound examination, especially in the presence of zones of tumor necrosis. This percutaneous procedure can be performed during physical examination with an intradermal needle (skin–node distance less than 2 cm). The lymph node material obtained is smeared onto a slide, dried, and then sent directly for cytological and/or histological examination.

However, FNAC is only able to detect metastatic inguinal lymph nodes >2 mm in diameter [13, 20]. Ultrasound-guided FNAC is only contributive when positive, as false-negative rates of 29 % have been reported [15, 17, 36]. In the case of negative cytology and suspicious palpable lymph nodes, lymph node aspiration should be repeated after antibiotic therapy [9].

Abdominal and Pelvic CT Scan or MRI

Often performed systematically for all cases of penile tumor, CT scan or MRI is only recommended in the presence of palpable inguinal lymph node (Fig. 6.10) to assess the size, extension (looking for lymph node capsular extension), site, vascular invasion (particularly involving the femoral vein), the presence of pelvic and retroperitoneal lymph nodes, and distant metastases [17].

However, micrometastatic inguinal nodes are rarely demonstrated on CT scan or MRI in patients without palpable lymph nodes [2, 29, 38].

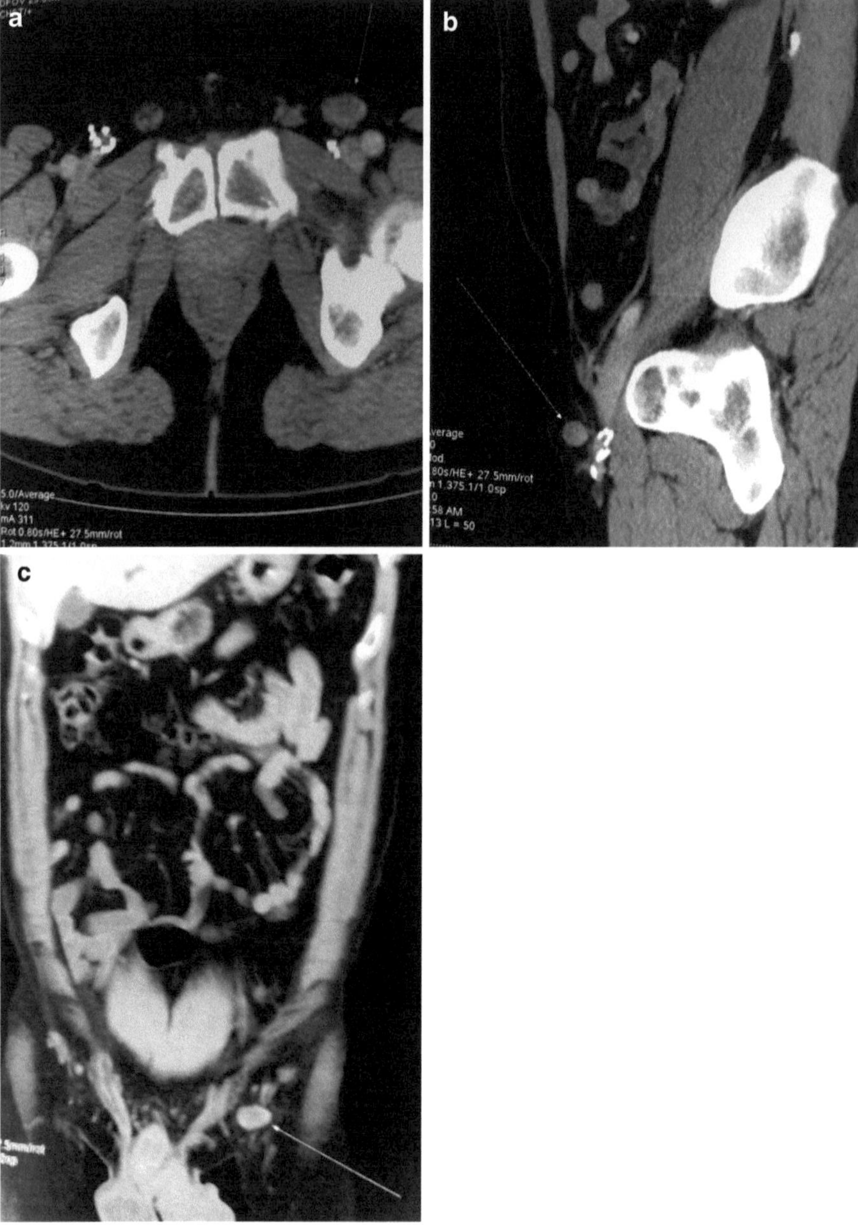

Fig. 6.10 CT scan in a patient with metastatic left inguinal lymph node: (**a**) transversal view, (**b**) view and (**c**) coronal view

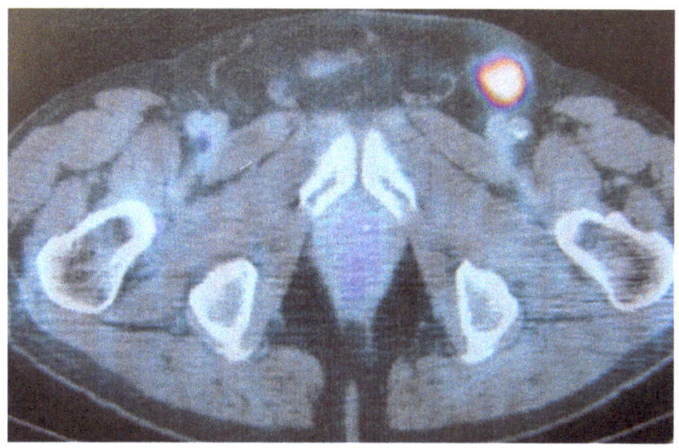

Fig. 6.11 ^{18}F-FDG PET/CT. cN1 patient

The use of lymphotropic nanoparticles coupled with MRI, in a series of seven patients, showed a sensitivity of 100 % and a specificity of 97 % [40]. The mean diameter of the lymph nodes analyzed was 5.4 mm (range: 3–27 mm), and images are interpreted according to node function rather than structure (metastatic nodes do not bind ferumoxtran-10). The smallest metastatic node detected was 3 mm in diameter. This MRI technique is very useful for lymph node staging, but not widely available at the present time.

Positron Emission Tomography/CT (PET/CT)

Fluorine-18-fluorodeoxyglucose PET (18-FDG PET) is widely used for staging and treatment monitoring of a variety of malignancies, with high sensitivity and specificity [19, 30]. PET/CT imaging, by combining anatomical information provided by computed tomography (CT) and functional imaging provided by PET, outperforms PEt alone in terms of the quality of lymph node staging [9]. In 2005, Scher et al showed that 18-FDG PET/CT was a potential tool for diagnosis and staging of penile carcinoma [37].

Several studies have shown a high specificity (>90 %) for cN0 patients but unfortunately a low positive predictive value (between 25 and 37 %), requiring surgical assessment to detect microscopic inguinal lymph node metastases [27, 35, 37, 39].

For patients with palpable inguinal lymph nodes, PET/CT is useful to detect metastatic pelvic lymph nodes and appears promising to assess the exact number of metastatic inguinal lymph nodes (one or multiple) (Figs. 6.11, 6.12, and 6.13). This evaluation has a major impact on the treatment strategy, as the presence of pelvic metastases or more than 2 inguinal metastases constitutes an indication for neoadjuvant chemotherapy. 18-FDG PET/CT is easy to perform, and in view of the improvement of the technique and image quality, this imaging modality should replace CT or MRI for staging of patients with penile cancer, particularly in the presence of palpable inguinal lymph nodes.

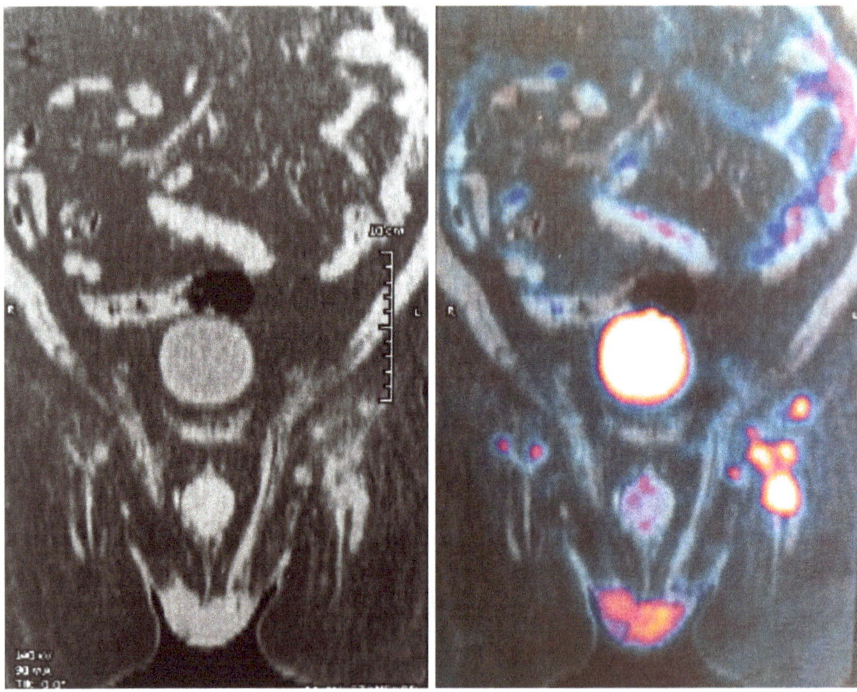

Fig. 6.12 ^{18}F-FDG PET/CT. cN2 patient with at least four metastatic left inguinal lymph nodes

Fig. 6.13 ^{18}F-FDG PET/CT. Increased uptake over left external iliac lymph node

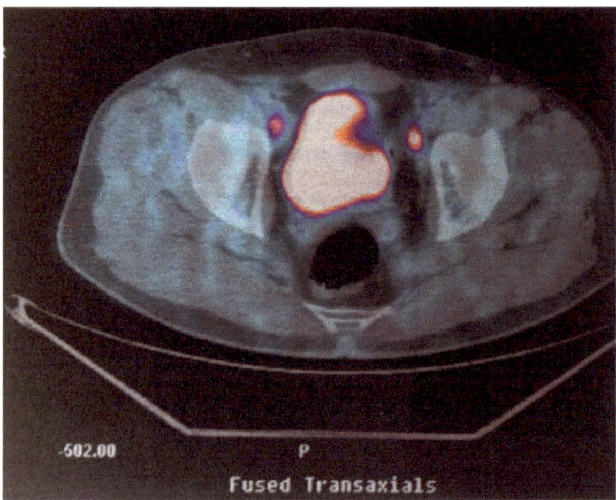

18-FDG PET/CT is also useful to evaluate the response to neoadjuvant chemotherapy in primarily inoperable patients due to locally advanced penile cancer [11].

Lymphoscintigraphy

The imaging technique is performed in the context of sentinel lymph node (SLN) biopsy in patients with a primary tumor ≥T1 G2 without palpable inguinal lymph node (cN0), according to international guidelines [33]. This group of tumors comprises intermediate-risk tumors and tumors at high risk of microscopic inguinal metastases. In the overall population of cN0 patients, the risk of subclinical metastasis is estimated to be between 12 and 20 % [7, 31, 34]. The risk was 4–14 % in the intermediate-risk group and 12–49 % in the high-risk group.

Lymphoscintigraphy is useful to detect the sentinel lymph node, the first draining lymph node. In penile cancer, the SLN is located in the superficial inguinal lymph node group. The Netherlands Cancer Institute team has routinely used dynamic SLN biopsy in patients without clinically palpable inguinal lymph node (cN0) since 1994, by coupling lymphoscintigraphy with ultrasound, intraoperative identification of the SLN by intradermal injection of patent blue dye, and histological examination of serial sections with immunohistochemical staining [23]. Lymphoscintigraphy is performed preoperatively by intradermal injection of technetium 99-labeled nanocolloid around the primary tumor. Dynamic images are acquired at10 min after injection on a coronal view, 30 min, and then 2 h by a dual-head gamma camera [21]. A gamma probe detects the SLN, and patent blue dye is injected at the beginning of the surgical biopsy procedure.

With this sequence, the SLN for penile carcinoma is generally located in the medial superior quadrant of the superficial inguinal lymph nodes in 73 % of cases, in the lateral superior quadrant in 8.7 % of cases, and in the central quadrant in 18.3 % of patients [10, 25].

The dynamic SNL technique is reproducible, as several teams have published equivalent false-negative rates (less than 5 %), lower than those of modified lymphadenectomy techniques, limited to the medial superior quadrant, which do not explore the lateral superior and central quadrants [4, 12, 22, 26]. The SLN biopsy with lymphoscintigraphy is also associated with a low morbidity [32].

Summary

Physical examination is a critical part of the staging assessment of a tumor of the penis. Imaging of the primary tumor is useful if and only if physical examination fails to demonstrate extension to the corpora cavernosum and/or urethra, especially when conservative surgery of the glans is envisaged. Imaging of inguinal lymph nodes is necessary in addition to physical examination for the detection of lymph node metastases (Fig. 6.14).

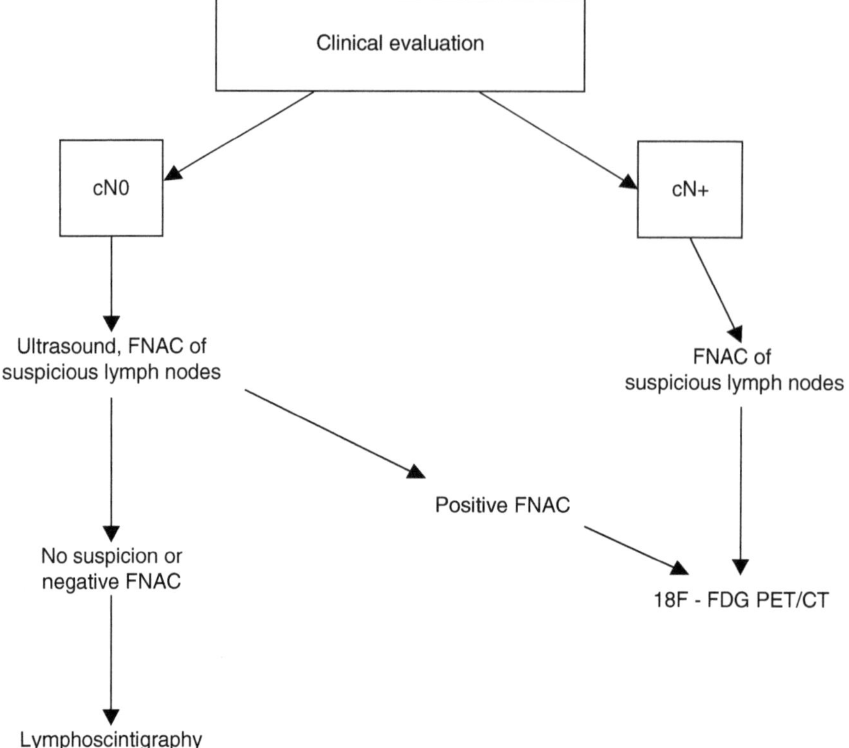

Fig. 6.14 Flow diagram for staging of draining lymph nodes in penile carcinoma

References

1. Agrawal A, Pai D, Ananthakrishnan N, Smile SR, Ratnakar C. Clinical and sonographic findings in carcinoma of the penis. J Clin Ultrasound. 2000;28(8):399–406.
2. Bipat S, Fransen GA, Spijkerboer AM, van der Velden J, Bossuyt PM, Zwinderman AH, Stoker J. Is there a role for magnetic resonance imaging in the evaluation of inguinal lymph node metastases in patients with vulva carcinoma? Gynecol Oncol. 2006;103(3):1001–6.
3. Chaux A, Cubilla AL. Advances in the pathology of penile carcinomas. Hum Pathol. 2012;43(6):771–89.
4. Crawshaw JW, Hadway P, Hoffland D, Bassingham S, Corbishley CM, Smith Y, Pilcher J, Allan R, Watkin NA, Heenan SD. Sentinel lymph node biopsy using dynamic lymphoscintigraphy combined with ultrasound-guided fine needle aspiration in penile carcinoma. Br J Radiol. 2009;82(973):41–8.
5. Daseler EH, Anson BJ, Reimann AF. Radical excision of the inguinal and iliac lymph glands; a study based upon 450 anatomical dissections and upon supportive clinical observations. Surg Gynecol Obstet. 1948;87(6):679–94.
6. Esen G. Ultrasound of superficial lymph nodes. Eur J Radiol. 2006;58(3):345–59.
7. Ficarra V, Zattoni F, Artibani W, Fandella A, Martignoni G, Novara G, Galetti TP, Zambolin T, Kattan MW. Nomogram predictive of pathological inguinal lymph node involvement in patients with squamous cell carcinoma of the penis. J Urol. 2006;175(5):1700–4.
8. Ficarra V, Akduman B, Bouchot O, Palou J, Tobias-Machado M. Prognostic factors in penile cancer. Urology. 2010;76(2 Suppl 1):S66–73.

9. Graafland NM, Leijte JA, Valdes Olmos RA, Hoefnagel CA, Teertstra HJ, Horenblas S. Scanning with 18F-FDG-PET/CT for detection of pelvic nodal involvement in inguinal node-positive penile carcinoma. Eur Urol. 2009;56(2):339–45.
10. Graafland NM, Leijte JA, Valdes Olmos RA, van Boven HH, Nieweg OE, Horenblas S. Repeat dynamic sentinel node biopsy in locally recurrent penile carcinoma. BJU Int. 2010; 105(8):1121–4.
11. Graafland NM, Valdes Olmo RA, Teertstra HJ, Kerst JM, Bergman AM, Horenblas S. (18) F-FDG PET/CT for monitoring induction chemotherapy in patients with primary inoperable penile carcinoma: first clinical results. Eur J Nucl Med Mol Imaging. 2010;37(8):1474–80.
12. Graafland NM, Lam W, Leijte JA, Yap T, Gallee MP, Corbishley C, van Werkhoven E, Watkin N, Horenblas S. Prognostic factors for occult inguinal lymph node involvement in penile carcinoma and assessment of the high-risk EAU subgroup: a two-institution analysis of 342 clinically node-negative patients. Eur Urol. 2010;58(5):742–7.
13. Hadway P, Smith Y, Corbishley C, Heenan S, Watkin NA. Evaluation of dynamic lymphoscintigraphy and sentinel lymph-node biopsy for detecting occult metastases in patients with penile squamous cell carcinoma. BJU Int. 2007;100(3):561–5.
14. Horenblas S, van Tinteren H. Squamous cell carcinoma of the penis. IV. Prognostic factors of survival: analysis of tumor, nodes and metastasis classification system. J Urol. 1994; 151(5):1239–43.
15. Horenblas S, Van Tinteren H, Delemarre JF, Moonen LM, Lustig V, Kroger R. Squamous cell carcinoma of the penis: accuracy of tumor, nodes and metastasis classification system, and role of lymphangiography, computerized tomography scan and fine needle aspiration cytology. J Urol. 1991;146(5):1279–83.
16. Horenblas S, Kroger R, Gallee MP, Newling DW, van Tinteren H. Ultrasound in squamous cell carcinoma of the penis; a useful addition to clinical staging? A comparison of ultrasound with histopathology. Urology. 1994;43(5):702–7.
17. Hughes B, Leijte J, Shabbir M, Watkin N, Horenblas S. Non-invasive and minimally invasive staging of regional lymph nodes in penile cancer. World J Urol. 2008;27(2):197–203.
18. Kayes O, Minhas S, Allen C, Hare C, Freeman A, Ralph D. The role of magnetic resonance imaging in the local staging of penile cancer. Eur Urol. 2007;51(5):1313–8.
19. Kitajima K, Murakami K, Yamasaki E, Fukasawa I, Inaba N, Kaji Y, Sugimura K. Accuracy of 18F-FDG PET/CT in detecting pelvic and paraaortic lymph node metastasis in patients with endometrial cancer. AJR Am J Roentgenol. 2008;190(6):1652–8.
20. Kroon BK, Horenblas S, Deurloo EE, Nieweg OE, Teertstra HJ. Ultrasonography-guided fine-needle aspiration cytology before sentinel node biopsy in patients with penile carcinoma. BJU Int. 2005;95(4):517–21.
21. Kroon BK, Valdes Olmos RA, van Tinteren H, Nieweg OE, Horenblas S. Reproducibility of lymphoscintigraphy for lymphatic mapping in patients with penile carcinoma. J Urol. 2005;174(6):2214–7.
22. Lam W, Alnajjar HM, La-Touche S, Perry M, Sharma D, Corbishley C, Pilcher J, Heenan S, Watkin N. Dynamic sentinel lymph node biopsy in patients with invasive squamous cell carcinoma of the penis: a prospective study of the long-term outcome of 500 inguinal basins assessed at a single institution. Eur Urol. 2013;63(4):657–63.
23. Leijte JA, Kroon BK, Valdes Olmos RA, Nieweg OE, Horenblas S. Reliability and safety of current dynamic sentinel node biopsy for penile carcinoma. Eur Urol. 2007;52(1):170–7.
24. Leijte JA, Gallee M, Antonini N, Horenblas S. Evaluation of current TNM classification of penile carcinoma. J Urol. 2008;180(3):933–8.
25. Leijte JA, Valdes Olmos RA, Nieweg OE, Horenblas S. Anatomical mapping of lymphatic drainage in penile carcinoma with SPECT-CT: implications for the extent of inguinal lymph node dissection. Eur Urol. 2008;54(4):885–90.
26. Leijte JA, Hughes B, Graafland NM, Kroon BK, Olmos RA, Nieweg OE, Corbishley C, Heenan S, Watkin N, Horenblas S. Two-center evaluation of dynamic sentinel node biopsy for squamous cell carcinoma of the penis. J Clin Oncol. 2009;27(20):3325–9.
27. Leijte JA, Graafland NM, Valdes Olmos RA, van Boven HH, Hoefnagel CA, Horenblas S. Prospective evaluation of hybrid 18F-fluorodeoxyglucose positron emission tomography/com-

puted tomography in staging clinically node-negative patients with penile carcinoma. BJU Int. 2009;104(5):640–4.
28. Longpre MJ, Lange PH, Kwon JS, Black PC. Penile carcinoma: lessons learned from vulvar carcinoma. J Urol. 2013;189(1):17–24.
29. Lont AP, Besnard AP, Gallee MP, van Tinteren H, Horenblas S. A comparison of physical examination and imaging in determining the extent of primary penile carcinoma. BJU Int. 2003;91(6):493–5.
30. Nahmias C, Carlson ER, Duncan LD, Blodgett TM, Kennedy J, Long MJ, Carr C, Hubner KF, Townsend DW. Positron emission tomography/computerized tomography (PET/CT) scanning for preoperative staging of patients with oral/head and neck cancer. J Oral Maxillofac Surg. 2007;65(12):2524–35.
31. Ornellas AA, Nobrega BL, Wei Kin Chin E, Wisnescky A, da Silva PC, de Santos Schwindt AB. Prognostic factors in invasive squamous cell carcinoma of the penis: analysis of 196 patients treated at the Brazilian National Cancer Institute. J Urol. 2008;180(4):1354–9.
32. Perdona S, Autorino R, De Sio M, Di Lorenzo G, Gallo L, Damiano R, D'Armiento M, Gallo A. Dynamic sentinel node biopsy in clinically node-negative penile cancer versus radical inguinal lymphadenectomy: a comparative study. Urology. 2005;66(6):1282–6.
33. Pizzocaro G, Algaba F, Horenblas S, Solsona E, Tana S, Van Der Poel H, Watkin NA. EAU penile cancer guidelines 2009. Eur Urol. 2010;57(6):1002–12.
34. Protzel C, Alcaraz A, Horenblas S, Pizzocaro G, Zlotta A, Hakenberg OW. Lymphadenectomy in the surgical management of penile cancer. Eur Urol. 2009;55(5):1075–88.
35. Sadeghi R, Gholami H, Zakavi SR, Kakhki VR, Horenblas S. Accuracy of 18F-FDG PET/CT for diagnosing inguinal lymph node involvement in penile squamous cell carcinoma: systematic review and meta-analysis of the literature. Clin Nucl Med. 2012;37(5):436–41.
36. Scappini P, Piscioli F, Pusiol T, Hofstetter A, Rothenberger K, Luciani L. Penile cancer. Aspiration biopsy cytology for staging. Cancer. 1986;58(7):1526–33.
37. Scher B, Seitz M, Reiser M, Hungerhuber E, Hahn K, Tiling R, Herzog P, Reiser M, Schneede P, Dresel S. 18F-FDG PET/CT for staging of penile cancer. J Nucl Med. 2005;46(9):1460–5.
38. Singh AK, Gonzalez-Torrez P, Kaewlai R, Tabatabaei S, Harisinghani MG. Imaging of penile neoplasm. Semin Ultrasound CT MR. 2007;28(4):287–96.
39. Souillac I, Rigaud J, Ansquer C, Marconnet L, Bouchot O. Prospective evaluation of (18) F-fluorodeoxyglucose positron emission tomography-computerized tomography to assess inguinal lymph node status in invasive squamous cell carcinoma of the penis. J Urol. 2012;187(2):493–7.
40. Tabatabaei S, Harisinghani M, McDougal WS. Regional lymph node staging using lymphotropic nanoparticle enhanced magnetic resonance imaging with ferumoxtran-10 in patients with penile cancer. J Urol. 2005;174(3):923–7.
41. Velazquez EF, Barreto JE, Rodriguez I, Piris A, Cubilla AL. Limitations in the interpretation of biopsies in patients with penile squamous cell carcinoma. Int J Surg Pathol. 2004;12(2):139–46.
42. Sobin LH, Gospodarowicz MK, Wittekind CH, eds. International Union Against Cancer (UICC). TNM classification of malignant tumors. 7th ed. Oxford: Wiley-Blackwell; 2009.

Chapter 7
Diagnosis and Management of Premalignant Penile Lesions

Asheesh Kaul, Catherine M. Corbishley, and Nicholas A. Watkin

Introduction

Premalignant penile lesions are a difficult group of disorders to accurately differentiate from benign dermatoses. There is often a history of self-management or management in non-specialist centres leading to a delay in diagnosis. Early recognition and treatment of these lesions may prevent progression to invasive cancer thereby reducing the need for more traumatic interventions. It is important to note that penile cancer is a relatively rare malignancy affecting approximately 1 in 100,000 men per year in Europe and the USA, with premalignant lesions forming a small proportion of new cases. Therefore, the knowledge base relating to the management of premalignant lesions is often from small series or case reports.

The aim of this chapter is to provide a description of aetiology and clinical features of premalignant penile lesions, present the up-to-date histopathological terminology, and give details of management strategies for these lesions. A summary of the clinical and histopathological classifications of premalignant penile lesions can be seen in Table 7.1.

Aetiology of Premalignant Lesions

There are a number of well-known risk factors for the development of penile cancer and premalignant lesions. These include infection with human papillomaviruses (HPV), lichen sclerosus (LS), the uncircumcised state, phimosis,

A. Kaul, MBBS, BSc, MRCS (✉) • N.A. Watkin, MA, MChir, BM, BCL, FRCS
Department of Urology, St. George's Hospital, Blackshaw Road, London SW17OQT, UK
e-mail: asheeshkaul@msn.com; nick.watkin@nhs.net

C.M. Corbishley, BSc, MB ChB, FRCPath
Department of Cellular Pathology, St George's Healthcare NHS Trust, London, UK

D.J. Culkin (ed.), *Management of Penile Cancer*,
DOI 10.1007/978-1-4939-0461-7_7,

Table 7.1 Clinical and histopathological classification of premalignant penile lesions

	Premalignant lesions	Conditions which may be associated with invasive carcinoma
Clinical	Erythroplasia of Queyrat	Lichen sclerosus
	Bowen's disease	Penile cutaneous horn
	Bowenoid papulosis	
	Cutaneous	
	Verrucous hyperplasia	
Histopathological	Undifferentiated PeIN	
	Differentiated PeIN	

chronic inflammation, immunosuppression and smoking. Apart from HPV and LS, which have been investigated specifically for their role in premalignancy, most factors have only been investigated for their association with invasive malignancy.

Immunosuppression, particularly in the HIV and AIDS population, increases the relative risk of penile cancer (RR, 3.9; 95 % CI, 2.1–6.5), as well as leading to a younger age at presentation [1].

Cigarette smoking has been associated with a four- to fivefold risk of developing invasive penile cancer. This association was found to be dose dependent and independent of coexisting phimosis [2].

The role of circumcision in penile cancer prevention is controversial. A systematic review of male circumcision and penile cancer found a strong protective effect of childhood/adolescent circumcision on invasive penile cancer (odds ratio 0.33) [3]. Four studies in the same systematic review found a strong association between the presence of phimosis and invasive cancer (OR 4.9–37.2). The theory for the relationship between the uncircumcised state and the presence of phimosis with penile cancer is that of chronic inflammation caused by poor hygiene. There is no evidence for a carcinogenic role of smegma [4]; however, it is likely to contribute to chronic inflammation. There is also evidence that circumcision reduces the incidence of HPV and HIV infection, themselves risk factors for penile cancer.

HPV is the most studied risk factor for penile cancer with HPV DNA detected in up to 50 % of tumours, and the most important risk factor for HPV infection is increasing number of sexual partners. Sixty percent are HPV subtype 16 and 13 % subtype 18 [5]. HPV infection is therefore further divided into 'high-risk' subtypes 16 and 18 and the less common 'low-risk' subtypes including 6 and 11. The clinically defined lesions associated with HPV will be discussed in subsequent sections.

Dermatoses such as lichen sclerosus and penile cutaneous horn have an association with penile cancer. Other texts refer to these lesions as premalignant [6]. This is a contentious issue as the lesions in themselves are benign. We subsequently refer to these as lesions associated with in situ disease and invasive SCC.

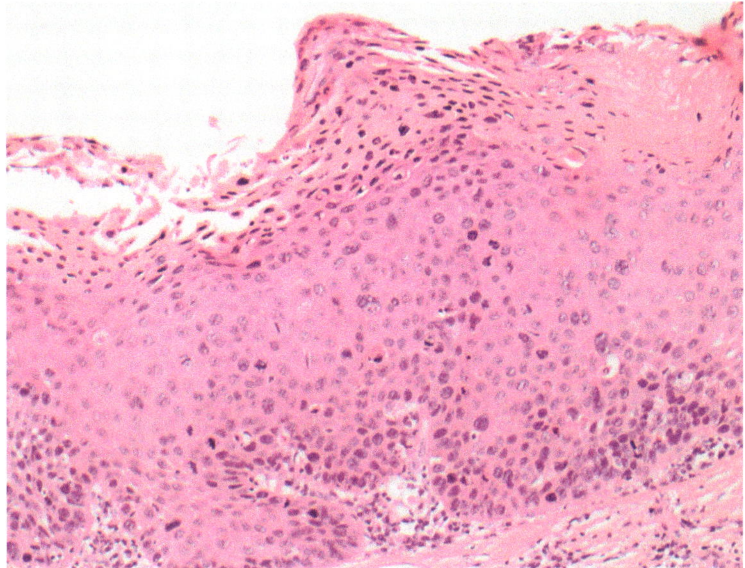

Fig. 7.1 Undifferentiated PeIN

Histopathological Terminology

A number of terms have been used in the histopathological classification of premalignant penile lesions. These include penile intraepithelial neoplasia (PeIN), squamous carcinoma in situ (CIS), high-grade squamous intraepithelial lesion (HSIL) and low-grade squamous intraepithelial lesion (LSIL). In some systems, PeIN was originally graded from I to III (low to high grade).

More recently Velazquez et al. [7] have proposed a simplified system encompassing all these terms and dividing the changes into undifferentiated or differentiated PeIN and have done away with the terms low grade and high grade and with subtyping of PeIN into grades I–III.

Undifferentiated PeIN encompasses squamous carcinoma in situ, severe epithelial dysplasia and the clinically defined mucosal erythroplasia of Queyrat and Bowen's disease of the penile skin. Undifferentiated PeIN is subdivided into basaloid and/or warty subtypes and is frequently associated with HPV 16. Histologically this lesion shows full thickness cytological atypia with lack of differentiation and abnormal mitotic activity (see Fig. 7.1). Undifferentiated PeIN is associated with warty and basaloid invasive carcinomas [8] but may also be seen with usual type squamous carcinoma. Bowenoid papulosis shows the features of warty undifferentiated PeIN and can only be defined clinically.

Differentiated PeIN has only been described and defined more recently. Histologically the atypical squamous cells are confined to the lower layers of the penile squamous epithelium and are usually associated with architectural atypia,

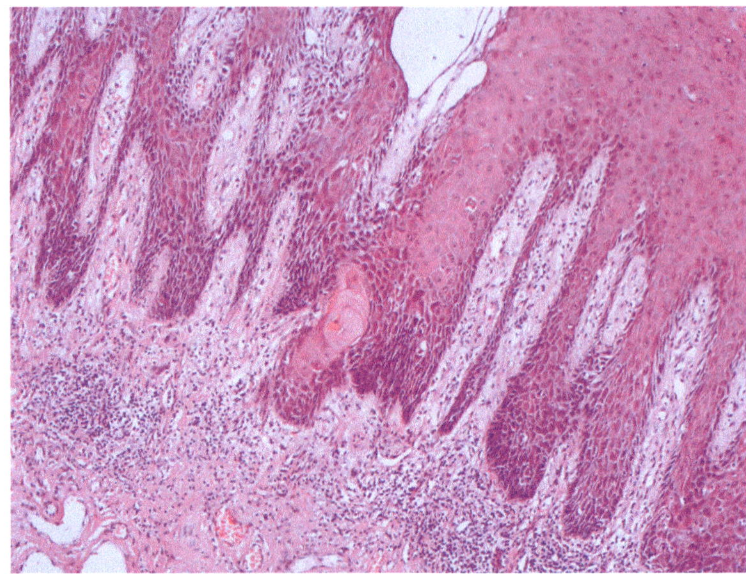

Fig. 7.2 Differentiated PeIN

elongated rete ridges and aberrant intraepithelial keratinisation (see Fig. 7.2). It is often associated with verrucous hyperplasia and lichen sclerosus. It is not associated with high-risk HPV subtypes.

Clinically Defined Premalignant Lesions

Erythroplasia of Queyrat (EQ) (Fig. 7.3)

Erythroplasia of the glans penis was first described by Queyrat in 1911. EQ affects the mucosal surfaces of the penis (glans, inner prepuce or distal urethra) and has a number of clinical presentations. Lesions can vary from patchy erythema to diffuse shiny erythema with or without erosions. EQ can also present as well-demarcated velvety plaques, which can coalesce to form a large contiguous plaque. They are often painless but can be extremely painful with the presence of erosions. Transformation into invasive carcinoma has been reported in up to 33 % of cases [9]. Histopathologically these lesions show undifferentiated PeIN.

Bowen's Disease (BD) (Fig. 7.4)

Bowen's disease is histologically indistinguishable from erythroplasia of Queyrat; however, it involves non-mucosal skin rather than penile mucosa. It usually presents

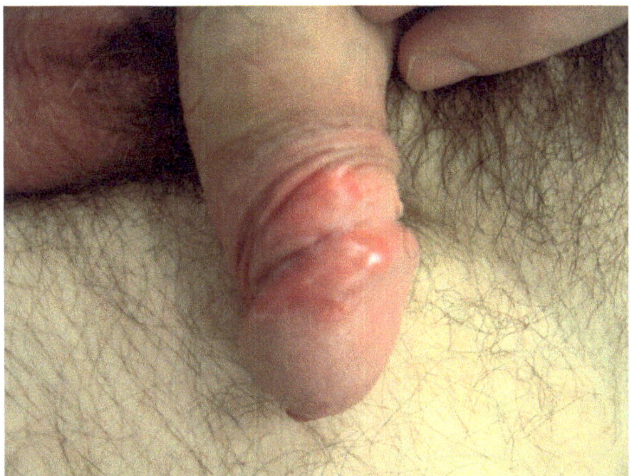

Fig. 7.3 Erythroplasia of Queyrat

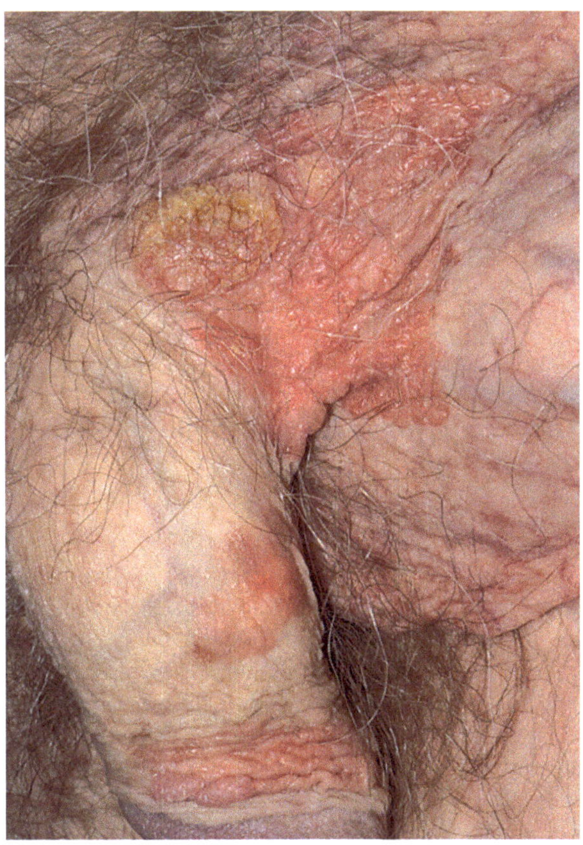

Fig. 7.4 Bowen's disease

as a single well-defined plaque of scaly erythema. The appearances can vary with ulcerated, keratotic or elevated flesh-coloured plaques described. Lesions may even become heavily pigmented and resemble melanoma. Malignant transformation has been reported in 5 % of cases [10].

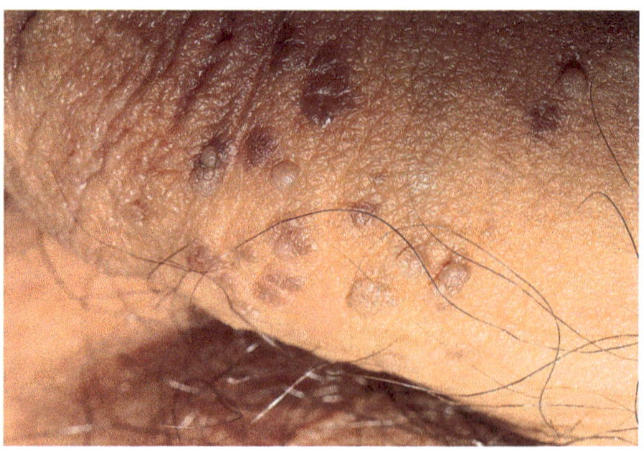

Fig. 7.5 Bowenoid papulosis (Reproduced with permission from Marghoob et al. [35])

Bowenoid Papulosis (BP) (Fig. 7.5)

Bowenoid papulosis occurs mainly in sexually active young men and is strongly associated with HPV subtype 16. It is characterised by pink, velvety papules. The papules are often multiple and can coalesce into plaques. Lesions tend to occur on the penile shaft or mons pubis where they often appear more pigmented. They are less frequently found on the glans or inner prepuce. Lesions can be pruritic but are often asymptomatic. Histologically the lesions show undifferentiated PeIN with warty features. However, it tends to run a more benign course with malignant transformation seen in less than 1 % of cases [11].

Giant Condyloma Accuminatum (Buschke-Lowenstein Tumour) (Fig. 7.6)

Giant condyloma accuminatum (GCA) was first described by Buschke and Lowenstein in 1925. This large, exophytic, cauliflower-like growth results from a confluence of condyloma acuminata, smaller warty growths that can affect any part of the anogenital region. On the penis these lesions tend to be found in the coronal sulcus and frenulum. They have a strong association with HPV 6 and 11. Although GCA was thought originally to be benign, the lesion is now thought to be a type of warty carcinoma, and careful examination of these lesions often shows invasion [12]. Older literature refers to GCA interchangeably as verrucous carcinoma. It is now widely accepted that GCA and verrucous carcinoma are two distinct pathologies due to the well-documented role of HPV in the pathogenesis of GCA, which is not commonly seen with verrucous carcinoma.

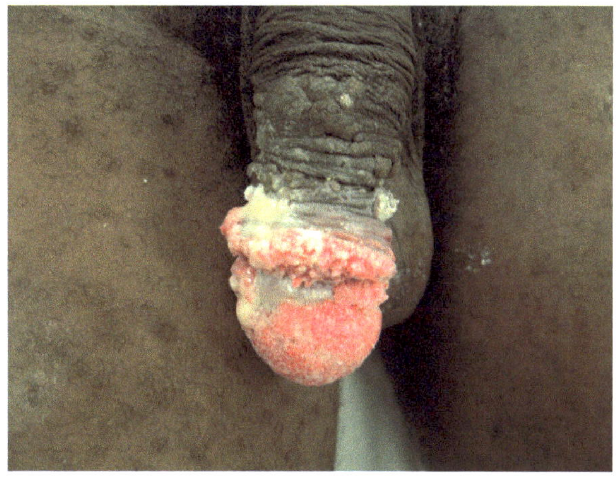

Fig. 7.6 Giant condyloma accuminatum

Verrucous Hyperplasia (Fig. 7.7)

Verrucous hyperplasia appears as thickened pale areas of mucosa without nodularity. Histologically there is epithelial hyperplasia with elongation of broad rete ridges without cytological atypia. It is thought to be a premalignant lesion leading to verrucous carcinoma and should be excised with a narrow margin [13].

Lesions Associated with In Situ Disease and Invasive SCC

Lichen Sclerosus (Fig. 7.8)

Lichen sclerosus (LS) is a chronic inflammatory skin condition of unknown aetiology. Lesions appear as white plaques on the prepuce and glans. The resulting sclerosis can cause phimosis, adherence of the prepuce to the glans, meatal stenosis and urethral strictures.

A number of studies have shown a strong association between LS and penile cancer. Several studies comment on the presence of synchronous penile cancer in LS specimens. Barbagli et al. reviewed the histology of 130 patients with male genital lichen sclerosis and reported the finding of malignant or premalignant lesions in 11 (8.4 %) of the specimens [14]. Nasca et al. reviewed the histology of 86 patients over a 10-year period, finding malignant or premalignant lesions in 5 (5.8 %) of the samples [15]. In the largest series to date, Depasquale et al. identified 12 patients with squamous cell carcinoma from 522 patients (2.3 %) treated for LS over a 14-year period [16]. Seven of these patients had been previously circumcised for LS and later developed SCC, and five had LS in uncircumcised penises. There was no

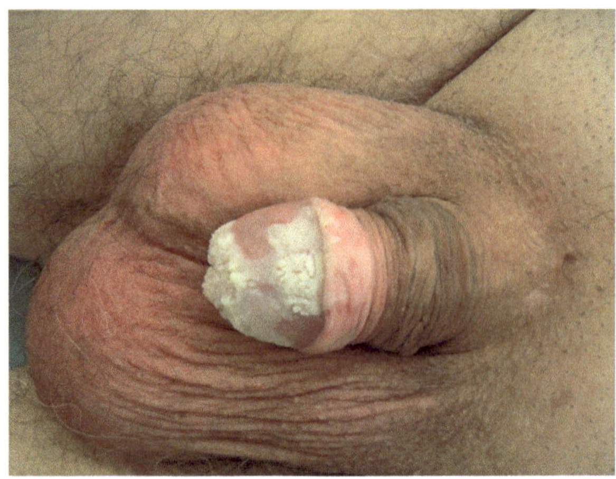

Fig. 7.7 Verrucous hyperplasia

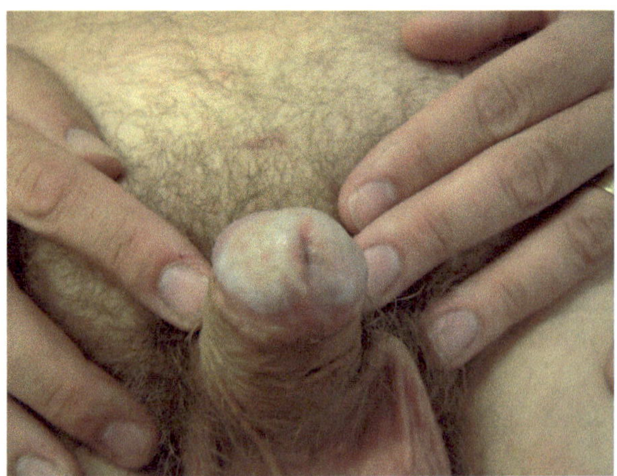

Fig. 7.8 Lichen sclerosus

reference to the inclusion of premalignant lesions in this study, which may account for the rates being lower than those reported in other series. In another smaller series, Campus et al. identified SCC in 2 of 54 patients treated for LS (3.7 %) [17].

There are also a number of studies that report the synchronous finding of LS in the histology of excised malignant and premalignant penile lesions. Velazquez and Cubilla identified synchronous LS in 68 of 207 penile SCC specimens (32.8 %) [18]. Pietrzak et al. identified synchronous LS in 44 of 105 patients with penile SCC or CIS (28 %) [19]. A recent study by Chaux et al. showed the association of LS with differentiated PeIN in 39 of 77 cases (51 %) [20]. Mannweiler investigated the association of LS with 35 patients with differentiated PeIN or HPV and $p16^{INK4a}$ overexpression negative SCC. 26 (74.3 %) of these patients had synchronous LS [21].

Where patients have undergone circumcision for LS, we would advise that the prepuce is always sent for histological analysis to look for differentiated PeIN. Further follow-up depends on the extent of persistent glanular and/or urethral

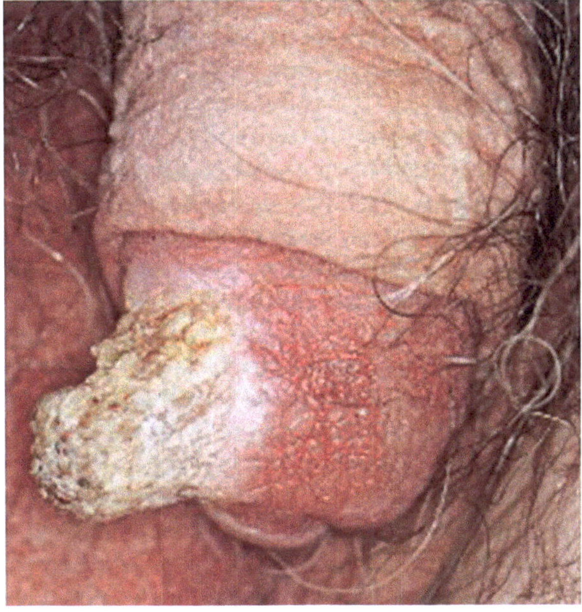

Fig. 7.9 Penile cutaneous horn (Reproduced with permission from Micali et al. [36])

changes. A relatively normal-appearing glans does not require outpatient follow-up, and the patient can be advised to perform regular self-examination. If the glans is particularly inflamed, a period of topical steroid use and follow-up is advised.

Penile Cutaneous Horn (Fig. 7.9)

Penile cutaneous horn describes a conical, protruding, hyperkeratotic mass usually arising from the glans or coronal sulcus. In most cases, there is a history of chronic inflammation and phimosis. The base of the lesion can show dysplastic changes amounting to differentiated PeIN, and these lesions may also be associated with hyperplastic lichen sclerosus.

Diagnosis

Any suspected premalignant lesion of the penis should be biopsied to confirm the diagnosis and rule out invasive disease or other benign penile dermatosis. This should ideally be a full thickness incision of a representative area of the lesion or an excision biopsy if possible. Excision is relatively straightforward with lesions of the prepuce and shaft skin such as Bowen's disease or bowenoid papulosis; however, complete excision of a large area of the glans (EQ) may not be possible due to potential disfigurement. We would advise that these lesions have a generous incision biopsy as they have a tendency to be under staged and architectural subtlety may not be appreciated on a smaller punch biopsy or scraping.

When assessing the penis, we recommend staining the genital skin with a swab soaked in 5 % acetic acid for several minutes before assessment. This elicits a so-called 'aceto-white' reaction of any abnormal epithelium. It must be stated that 'aceto-white' reaction is not specific for premalignancy. Wikström et al. performed acetic acid staining of the penis of 101 men with penile soreness or with female partners known to have genital HPV infection. Ninety one men developed 'aceto-white' reaction and were subsequently biopsied. 18 (20 %) of the biopsies had evidence of PeIN I–III. The majority of 'aceto-white' reaction was due to the HPV-related changes or inflammation [22]. The staining can allow a more precise targeting of any biopsy and may also reveal a more extensive lesion than first appreciated.

We also recommend that all patients with confirmed in situ disease should undergo circumcision if it has not already been performed as part of treatment. This removes a site of potential dysplasia and allows patients and clinicians to examine the glans with ease.

Treatment

Premalignant lesions of the penis, by virtue of their non-invasive nature, are amenable to minimally invasive treatment. Depending on patient factors, the extent of disease and the availability of techniques, a number of treatment modalities can be used. These include topical chemotherapy (5-fluorouracil (5-FU) or 5 % imiquimod), conservative surgery (glans resurfacing or Mohs micrographic techniques) and ablative therapies (laser or cryotherapy). Finally, photodynamic therapy is a relatively new treatment with recent outcome data emerging.

Topical Therapy

Topical therapy with 5-FU is the most common first-line therapy for PeIN. It is best used in immunocompetent patients with focal lesions. There is a lack of consensus on the best treatment regimen for 5-FU. In our practice, we recommend application of cream for 12 h on alternate days for 28 days. Most patients will develop local inflammation and erosion secondary to treatment. This can take up to 4 weeks to heal, at which time the lesion can be reassessed for the results of treatment. In some cases, an allergic reaction can occur leading to a severe dermatitis. The inflammatory processes that inevitably take place during treatment can lead to difficulties with compliance. Topical steroids can be used to help reduce the inflammation; however, it can still take several weeks for affected areas to heal.

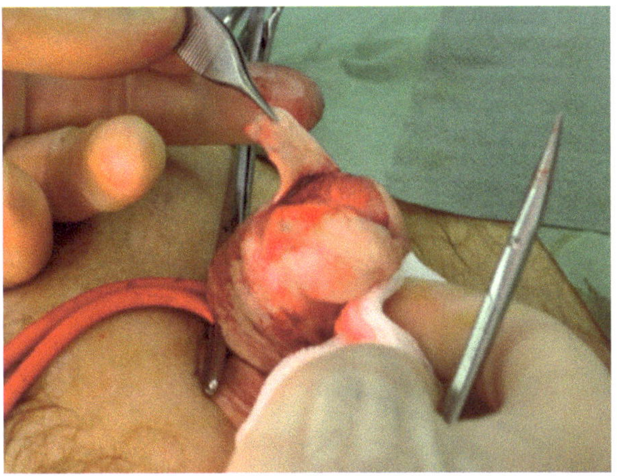

Fig. 7.10 Dissection of the glans epithelium from the corpus spongiosum

In our practice, treatment with 5 % imiquimod is considered second-line therapy when there is no response or only a partial response to 5-FU. However, in some centres it is used as primary treatment. Imiquimod induces cytokine production to produce an innate cell-mediated response to malignant cells. The treatment regimen again varies in the literature. An acceptable regimen would involve application 3–5 days per week for 4–6 weeks. Side effects of inflammation and irritation are similar to those of 5-FU. Most published data on the use of 5 % imiquimod are from case reports or small series. Mahto et al. have performed a review of these studies demonstrating a 70 % rate of complete resolution and 30 % partial resolution with no recurrence up to 12 months [23].

Alnajjar et al. have reported the largest series of topical therapies for PeIN, using 5-FU as first-line therapy and 5 % imiquimod as second-line therapy. Over a 10-year period, 44 out of 86 patients (51 %) with confirmed PeIN received topical therapy. Twenty-five out of 44 (57 %) demonstrated complete response, 6 out of 44 (13.6 %) demonstrated partial response, and 13 out of 44 (29.5 %) demonstrated no response at a mean follow-up of 34 months [24].

Total and Partial Glans Resurfacing

Glans resurfacing can be performed either as primary treatment for biopsy-proven PeIN of the glans or where topical chemotherapy has failed. The procedure can be performed under general or regional anaesthesia. 5 % acetic acid is applied to the glans to highlight abnormal glanular epithelium. Under tourniquet control, a plane is dissected between the sub-epithelial tissue and the corpus spongiosum (see Fig. 7.10). This plane is dissected from the urethral meatus to the coronal sulcus and tissue excised in four quadrants. Once all the glans epithelium and sub-epithelium have been excised, circumcision is performed by a standard sleeve technique. The shaft skin is then approximated proximal to the coronal sulcus with absorbable

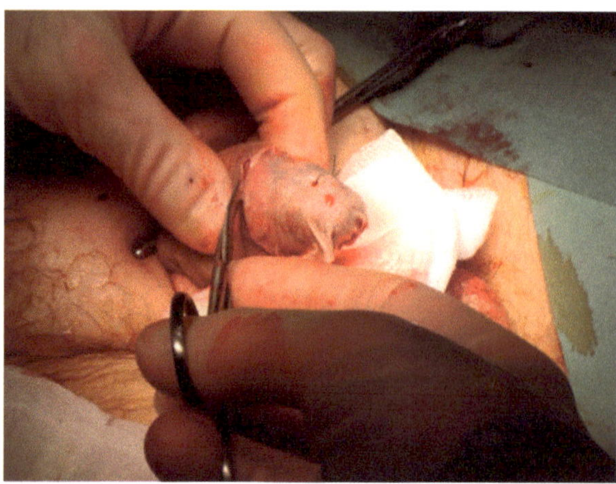

Fig. 7.11 Trimming skin graft and covering the glans

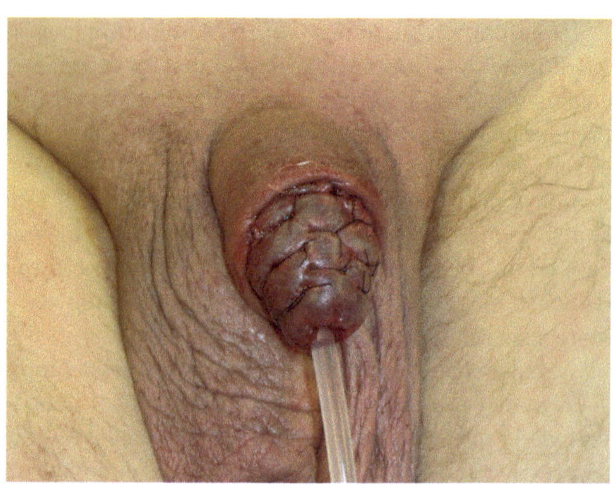

Fig. 7.12 Early post-operative appearance

sutures. Using an air dermatome, a split-thickness skin graft is harvested from the lateral thigh and used to cover the denuded glans (see Fig. 7.11). The graft is sutured directly to the underlying corpus spongiosum and can then be trimmed and sutured to the urethral meatus and shaft skin. A urethral catheter is inserted and a paraffin-covered gauze dressing applied (see Fig. 7.12). The patient remains on strict bed rest for 48 h. The catheter is removed 5 days post-operatively, and the patient discharged with advice to gently dab the graft with saline-soaked gauze to clean daily. The post-operative results can be seen in Fig. 7.13. Hadway et al., in a series of ten patients treated with total glans resurfacing, reported clear resection margins in all cases and no recurrence at a median follow-up of 30 months (7–45 months). Histology of all ten resected samples reported PeIN with no invasive disease [25].

Partial glans resurfacing can be performed when there is a focal area of PeIN affecting <50 % of the glans. Again, we would advocate the use of 5 % acetic acid staining to ensure as complete an excision as possible. The glans epithelium and

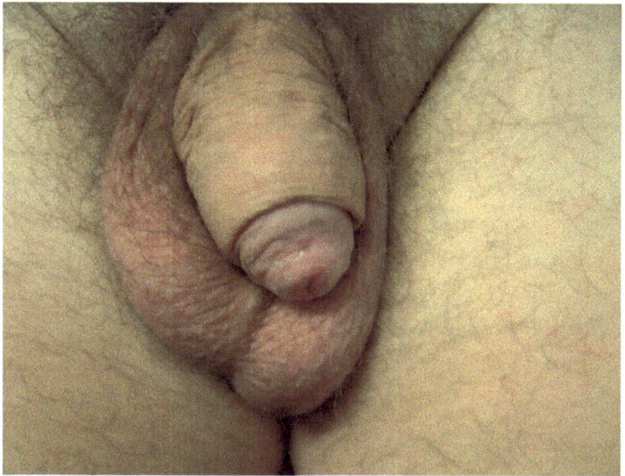

Fig. 7.13 Final appearance after total glans resurfacing

sub-epithelium are excised from the corpus spongiosum leaving a macroscopically clear margin. As with total glans resurfacing, a split-thickness skin graft is applied to the denuded area of the glans and quilted to the underlying corpus spongiosum. Post-operative protocol with regard to bed rest, catheter and sutures is the same as total glans resurfacing.

Shabbir et al. reported on a series of 15 patients with biopsy-proven PeIN treated with partial glans resurfacing. They reported a high rate of positive surgical margins in 10 out of 15 patients (67 %) with a need for further surgery in 6 out of 15 (40 %). This data includes four patients found to have invasive disease (G2 pT1) and two patients with no PeIN on histological examination of the resected samples. Examining the nine patients with PeIN only, six had positive surgical margins. Two described as extensive margin involvement and four described as focal margin involvement. The two patients with extensive margin involvement went on to have total glans resurfacing, and the four patients with focal margin involvement had no evidence of recurrence at a mean follow-up of 23 months. Overall seven of nine patients that underwent partial glans resurfacing for PeIN had no evidence of recurrence at follow-up. The high number of invasive tumours identified highlights the importance of an adequate pretreatment biopsy [26].

Laser Therapy

Two types of laser which either vaporise or coagulate the abnormal tissue have been described for treatment of premalignant lesions. The CO_2 laser, at an energy of 10,600 nm, targets water in the epidermal cells leading to vaporisation of these cells, with minimal penetration to the underlying dermis. Quoted penetration depth is 1–2.5 mm. The laser should be applied to the visualised lesion and surrounding area. The treated area heals by re-epithelialisation from healthy surrounding tissue and takes several weeks. The CO_2 laser can also be used as a scalpel to excise tissue for histological examination. Reported recurrence rates for CO_2 laser alone are 10–26 % [27, 28].

The neodymium (Nd):YAG laser causes protein denaturation and coagulative necrosis. It has a tissue penetration of 3–8 mm. Frimberger et al. reported their 13-year experience with Nd:YAG laser for treating CIS and invasive penile cancers. Their technique consisted of laser coagulation combined with knife excision of the lesion and biopsies of the base. In addition, a 3-mm rim of tissue around the tumour was ablated. This study included 17 patients with CIS. They reported one patient with recurrence at a mean follow-up of 47.6 months (5.6 % recurrence rate) who eventually required a partial penectomy for a G3T1 tumour [29].

Cryotherapy

Cryotherapy typically involves the application of liquid nitrogen to rapidly freeze lesions to temperatures as low as −50 °C. This leads to the destruction of cell membranes and cell death. The evidence for the use of cryotherapy for the treatment of premalignant penile lesions is limited. Hansen et al. compared 5-FU, surgical excision and cryotherapy for the treatment of 299 patients with extra-genital Bowen's disease. Recurrence rate was 9 % for 5-FU, 5.5 % for surgical excision and 13.4 % for cryotherapy [30].

Photodynamic Therapy (PDT)

PDT is a light-sensitive therapy that produces selective cell killing by the production of oxygen-free radicals. A photosensitising agent, which is taken up by malignant cells preferentially, is applied to the lesion and covered for 3 h. The photosensitiser commonly used for premalignant lesions is methylaminolaevulinic acid (MAL). It is activated by exposure to noncoherent light supplied by a PDT lamp. Activation of the photosensitiser leads to the production of oxygen-free radicals, DNA destruction and cell death. The procedure can be performed under local anaesthetic with a circumferential penile ring block. The two most recent studies of MAL-PDT for EQ show markedly different outcomes. Feldmeyer et al. report on 11 cases of EQ treated by MAL-PDT. Only five patients (45 %) showed complete remission at a mean follow-up of 28.3 months [31]. Fai et al. report on 23 cases of EQ treated by MAL-PDT with complete remission in 19 (82.6 %) of patients at a mean follow-up of 18 months [32]. Two other studies show complete response rates of 40 % at a mean follow-up of 35 months [33] and 70 % at a median follow-up of 20 months [34]. All studies reported a high incidence of severe acute pain and inflammation but excellent long-term cosmetic results.

Follow-Up

All premalignant lesions treated with penile-preserving measures should undergo regular clinical review. Again, we apply 5 % acetic acid to the glans to aid assessment. We currently follow European guidelines which recommend follow-up every 3 months for 2 years, followed by 6 monthly visits for a further 3 years after penis-preserving treatment. After 5 years' follow-up, the patient can be discharged with advice on the importance of self-examination.

References

1. Frisch M, Biggar RJ, Engels EA, Goedert JJ, AIDS-Cancer Match Registry Study Group. Association of cancer with AIDS-related immunosuppression in adults. JAMA. 2001; 285(13):1736–45.
2. Hellberg D, Valentin J, Eklund T, Nilsson S. Penile cancer: is there an epidemiological role for smoking and sexual behaviour? Br Med J (Clin Res Ed). 1987;295:1306–8.
3. Larke N, Thomas S, Santos Silva I, Weiss H. Male circumcision and penile cancer: a systematic review and meta-analysis. Cancer Causes Control. 2011;22(8):1097–110.
4. Van Howe RS, Hodges FM. The carcinogenicity of smegma: debunking a myth. J Eur Acad Dermatol Venereol. 2006;20(9):1046–54.
5. Backes DM, Kurman RJ, Pimenta JM, Smith JS. Systematic review of human papillomavirus prevalence in invasive penile cancer. Cancer Causes Control. 2009;20(4):449–57.
6. Pizzocaro G, Algaba F, Horenblas S, Solsona E, Tana S, Van DerPoel H, Watkin NA, European Association of Urology (EAU) Guidelines Group on Penile Cancer. EAU penile cancer guidelines 2009. Eur Urol. 2010;57(6):1002–12.
7. Velazquez EF, Chaux A, Cubilla AL. Histologic classification of penile intraepithelial neoplasia. Semin Diagn Pathol. 2012;29:96–102.
8. Chaux A, Pfannl R, Lloveras B, et al. Distinctive association of p16INK4a overexpression with penile intraepithelial neoplasia depicting warty and/or basaloid features: a study of 141 cases evaluating a new nomenclature. Am J Surg Pathol. 2010;34(3):385–92.
9. Micali G, Innocenzi D, Nasca MR, Musumeci ML, Ferrau F, Greco M. Squamous cell carcinoma of the penis. J Am Acad Dermatol. 1996;35(3 Pt 1):432–51.
10. Lucia MS, Miller GJ. Histopathology of malignant lesions of the penis. Urol Clin North Am. 1992;19(2):227–46.
11. von Krogh G, Horenblas S. Diagnosis and clinical presentation of premalignant lesions of the penis. Scand J Urol Nephrol Suppl. 2000;205:201–14.
12. Cubilla AL, Velazques EF, Reuter VE, Oliva E, Mihm Jr MC, Young RH. Warty (condylomatous) squamous cell carcinoma of the penis: a report of 11 cases and proposed classification of 'verruciform' penile tumors. Am J Surg Pathol. 2000;24(4):505–12.
13. Chaux A, Cubilla AL. Diagnostic problems in precancerous lesions and invasive carcinomas of the penis. Semin Diagn Pathol. 2012;29(2):72–82.
14. Barbagli G, Palminteri E, Mirri F, Guazzoni G, Turini D, Lazzeri M. Penile carcinoma in patients with genital lichen sclerosus: a multicenter survey. J Urol. 2006;175(4): 1359–63.
15. Nasca MR, Innocenzi D, Micali G. Penile cancer among patients with genital lichen sclerosus. J Am Acad Dermatol. 1999;41(6):911–4.
16. Depasquale I, Park AJ, Bracka A. The treatment of balanitis xerotica obliterans. BJU Int. 2000;86(4):459–65.

17. Campus GV, Alia F, Bosincu L. Squamous cell carcinoma and lichen sclerosus et atrophicus of the prepuce. Plast Reconstr Surg. 1992;89(5):962–4.
18. Velazquez EF, Cubilla AL. Lichen sclerosus in 68 patients with squamous cell carcinoma of the penis: frequent atypias and correlation with special carcinoma variants suggests a precancerous role. Am J Surg Pathol. 2003;27:1448–53.
19. Pietrzak P, Hadway P, Corbishley CM, Watkin NA. Is the association between balanitis xerotica obliterans and penile carcinoma underestimated? BJU Int. 2006;98(1):74–6.
20. Chaux A, Velazquez EF, Amin A, et al. Distribution and characterization of subtypes of penile intraepithelial neoplasia and their association with invasive carcinomas: a pathological study of 139 lesions in 121 patients. Hum Pathol. 2012;43(7):1020–7.
21. Mannweiler S, Sygulla S, Beham-Schmid C, Razmara Y, Pummer K, Regauer S. Penile carcinogenesis in a low-incidence area: a clinicopathologic and molecular analysis of 115 invasive carcinomas with special emphasis on chronic inflammatory skin diseases. Am J Surg Pathol. 2011;35(7):998–1006.
22. Wikström A, Hedblad MA, Johansson B, et al. The acetic acid test in evaluation of subclinical genital papillomavirus infection: a comparative study on penoscopy, histopathology, virology and scanning electron microscopy findings. Genitourin Med. 1992;68(2):90–9.
23. Mahto M, Nathan M, O'Mahony C. More than a decade on: review of the use of imiquimod in lower anogenital intraepithelial neoplasia. Int J STD AIDS. 2010;21(1):8–16.
24. Alnajjar HM, Lam W, Bolgeri M, Rees RW, Perry MJ, Watkin NA. Treatment of carcinoma in situ of the glans penis with topical chemotherapy agents. Eur Urol. 2012;62(5):923–8.
25. Hadway P, Corbishley CM, Watkin NA. Total glans resurfacing for premalignant lesions of the penis: initial outcome data. BJU Int. 2006;98(3):532–6.
26. Shabbir M, Muneer A, Kalsi J, Shukla CJ, et al. Glans resurfacing for the treatment of carcinoma in situ of the penis: surgical technique and outcomes. Eur Urol. 2011;59(1):142–7.
27. Porter WM, Francis N, Hawkins D, Dinneen M, Bunker CB. Penile intraepithelial neoplasia: clinical spectrum and treatment of 35 cases. Br J Dermatol. 2002;147:1159–65.
28. Rosemberg SK, Fuller TA. Carbon dioxide rapid superpulsed laser treatment of erythroplasia of Queyrat. Urology. 1980;16:181–2.
29. Frimberger D, Hungerhuber E, Zaak D, Waidelich R, Hofstetter A, Schneede P. Penile carcinoma. Is ND:YAG laser therapy radical enough? J Urol. 2002;168:2418–21.
30. Hansen JP, Drake AL, Walling HW. Bowen's Disease: a four-year retrospective review of epidemiology and treatment at a university center. Dermatol Surg. 2008;34(7):878–83.
31. Feldmeyer L, Krausz-Enderlin V, Töndury B, Hafner J, French LE, Hofbauer GF. Methylaminolaevulinic acid photodynamic therapy in the treatment of erythroplasia of Queyrat. Dermatology. 2011;223(1):52–6.
32. Fai D, Romano I, Cassano N, Vena GA. Methyl-aminolevulinate photodynamic therapy for the treatment of erythroplasia of Queyrat in 23 patients. J Dermatolog Treat. 2012;23(5):330–2.
33. Paoli J, Ternesten Bratel A, Löwhagen GB, Stenquist B, Forslund O, Wennberg AM. Penile intraepithelial neoplasia: results of photodynamic therapy. Acta Derm Venereol. 2006;86(5):418–21.
34. Axcrona K, Brennhovd B, Alfsen GC, Giercksky KE, Warloe T. Photodynamic therapy with methyl aminolevulinate for atypial carcinoma in situ of the penis. Scand J Urol Nephrol. 2007;41(6):507–10.
35. Marghoob A, Sachs D. Skin cancer precursor lesions in atlas of cancer. Current medicine, Inc. Ed. Maurie Markman. Lippincott Williams & Wilkins; 2003:464.
36. Micali G, Nasca MR, Innocenzi D, Schwartz RA. Penile cancer. J Am Acad Dermatol. 2006;54(3):369–91.

Chapter 8
Penile-Sparing Surgery

Nabil K. Bissada and Mohamed H. Kamel

Introduction

Total penectomy has been shown to be devastating for the majority of patients with penile cancer. As a result, penile-sparing surgery for invasive squamous cell carcinoma of the penis emerged as an appealing alternative because of its obvious functional and psychological benefits. As with any conservative cancer surgery, the main challenge is to achieve maximum functional preservation while providing cancer cure comparable to current standard amputations. Penile cancer is most common in the sixth decade of life [1]. Data from the Massachusetts Male Aging Study shows that over 50 % of men in that age group are able to attain an erection sufficient for sexual intercourse [2]. In another study, 68 % of 50 men aged 45–70 years with localized prostate cancer were willing to trade off 10 % survival advantage in order to keep their potency by choosing radiation rather than surgery as their treatment of choice [3]. It is clear that maintaining the ability for sexual intercourse remains important even in the elderly. Fortunately enough, the majority of penile cancers occur in the distal portion of the penis (glans and prepuce) making an organ-sparing surgery an attractive and feasible option [4]. Our goal is to examine how to maximize organ and functional preservation without compromising cancer control.

N.K. Bissada, MD (✉)
Department of Urology, VA Medical Center, Oklahoma University,
920 SL Young Blvd, WP3150, Oklahoma City, OK 73104, USA
e-mail: bissadan@hotmail.com

M.H. Kamel, MD, FACS, FRCS
Department of Urology, University of Arkansas for Medical Sciences,
4301 West Markham, Little Rock, AR 72205, USA
e-mail: mkamel@uams.edu

D.J. Culkin (ed.), *Management of Penile Cancer*,
DOI 10.1007/978-1-4939-0461-7_8,

Indications

Penile-conserving surgery is indicated for noninvasive or invasive squamous cell carcinoma of the penis as long as the cancer can be completely excised with preservation of adequate penile tissue that can improve patient's quality of life.

Advantages of Penile-Sparing Surgery

Maximum penile preservation has obvious functional and psychological advantages. Even when partial penectomy is required, it is better than amputation since the patient may be able to urinate standing and a reasonable percentage of patients are able to have sexual intercourse. Unlike laser treatment, penile-sparing surgery provides tissue for diagnosis. It does not require as much technical expertise and support staff as Mohs micrographic surgery (MMS) and can eradicate cancers that are not eradicated by MMS.

Surgical Techniques

Circumcision

Patients with penile cancer developing in foreskin are typically elderly. The diagnosis should be suspected in the setting of phimosis with bleeding or palpable lump underneath the foreskin. Often, the diagnosis of penile cancer is an incidental finding following routine circumcision for phimosis.

If the penile cancer is small and distal on the preputial skin, circumcision may be adequate as a treatment for the cancer. For the incidentally diagnosed larger and more proximal lesions, more involved surgery such as excision of distal penile skin may be warranted. In all cases, intraoperative careful frozen section examination and final pathological confirmation of all the margins are mandatory.

Penile Cancer in Circumcised Patients

De novo penile cancer developing in circumcision scars is a unique entity [5]. Bissada et al. reported on the characteristics, management, and long-term outcome of these patients. These cancers usually occur after ritual circumcision with extensive scarring. They tend to be of low to moderate grade. Surgical excision whether in the form of local excision, tailored resections, and occasionally up to total penectomy or more extensive surgery appeared to be the only effective treatment. Radiotherapy did not seem to provide cure in that particular group of patients. Node dissection was used selectively based on primary tumor characteristics.

Wedge Resection

Wedge resection or excision of small tumors on the glans or distal penile shaft can be accomplished without difficulty. An essential prerequisite is to perform adequate intraoperative frozen sections from both the base and all the margins to confirm complete excision of all cancer. How much of normal tissue to be excised with the tumor is controversial. However, it is safe to excise the tumor with a relatively small area of normal tissue, provided careful biopsy of all margins is meticulously performed. If the remaining defect is small, primary closure can be attempted using 3-0 synthetic absorbable suture (SAS). More often, the defect can be easily bridged with a flap from perpetual skin. If the patient is circumcised, penile degloving is performed and the freed penile skin can be easily pulled to cover the glandular defect and sutured in place using 3-0 SAS. Alternatively, as well as in rare occasions, when the defect cannot be closed using the aforementioned techniques, a split-thickness skin graft (STSG) is used. (See below)

Glansectomy

The glans is the most common site for squamous cell carcinoma of the penis (48 %). Multifocal or large tumors involving the glans penis are best managed by glansectomy. The technique of glansectomy is simple and the steps are outlined below:

1. Circumferential coronal incision is made.
2. Dissection deep to Buck's fascia (Fig. 8.1).
3. Control of dorsal venous complex.
4. Dissection between urethra and corporal bodies without dividing the urethra.
5. Dissection between the glans and tips of corpora cavernosa.
6. The glans is attached only on the urethra that is divided (Fig. 8.2).
7. Division of the urethra (Fig. 8.3).
8. Adequate frozen sections are sent from the distal tunica.
9. Urethra is spatulated.

Methods of covering the exposed tips of corpora cavernosa following glansectomy:

1. Penile skin advancement: Perhaps, that is the easiest method for covering the exposed corpora. Penile skin is degloved and the penile skin is advanced to be sutured to the edges of the spatulated urethra.
2. Urethral advancement with spatulation: Following glansectomy, a plane of dissection is developed sharply between the urethra and the 2 corpora. Every attempt is made when doing that dissection not to button hole the urethra which is particularly thin dorsally. The urethra is spatulated and advanced over the tips of the corpora and sutured to the penile skin giving an appearance similar to the lost glans (Figs. 8.4, 8.5, 8.6, and 8.7). Patient undergoing glansectomy should

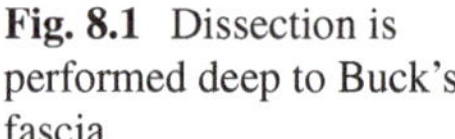

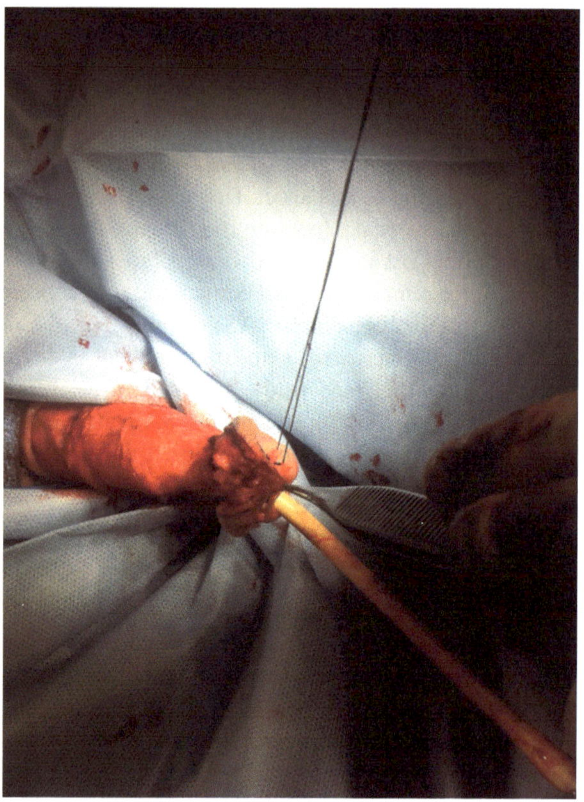

Fig. 8.1 Dissection is performed deep to Buck's fascia

be warned that sometimes their female partners may complain of increased pain during sexual intercourse following that surgery. This is because the cushion effect of the flaccid glans during normal erection is lost.

3. Split-thickness skin graft (STSG): The technique of performing an STSG can be easily performed by most urologists. However, if the surgeon is not adequately trained in STSG, plastic surgeon help should be requested. The donor site selected is typically the inner (non-hairy) aspect of the thigh (Figs. 8.8 and 8.9). Experience has shown that the graft should be taken 30 % larger than the recipient site since it tends to contract after transplanting [6]. Following harvesting, the graft is applied with quilting sutures of 3-0 SAS to immobilize it in place (Fig. 8.12). A key to the success of this type of defect coverage is the dressing that should keep the graft stable (together with the quilting sutures). This allows for improved graft take. Split-thickness skin graft can be used to cover defects on the glans penis or shaft (Figs. 8.10, 8.11, and 8.12). We don't normally use full-thickness skin graft because of poor cosmetic outcome in the penis and poor recipient site intake [7].

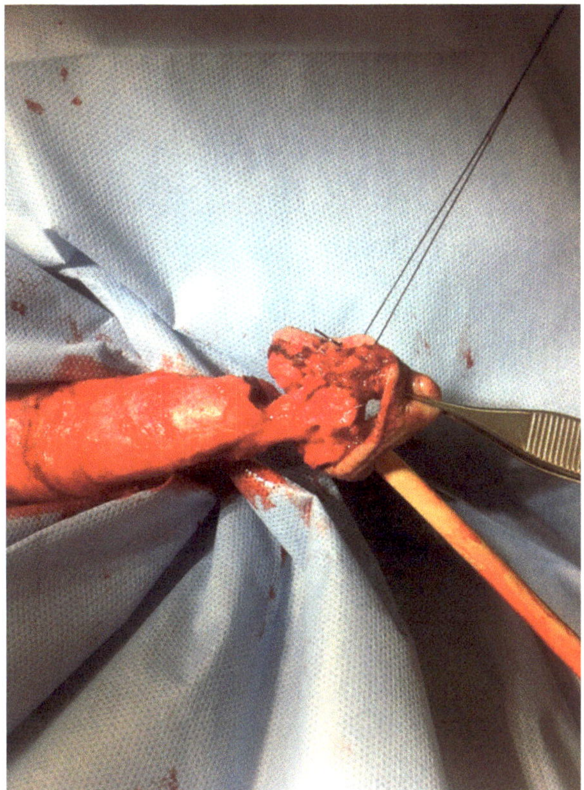

Fig. 8.2 The dorsal venous complex is divided. Glans is hanging on the urethra

Oncological and Functional Outcome of Glansectomy

Smith et al. reported their experience with 72 patients treated by glansectomy and STSG for T1/T2 penile cancer. In that report, the mean follow-up was 27 months. The local recurrence rate was 4 % and only two patients required early re-excision due to positive margin in the permanent specimen [8]. The functional outcome was reported to be adequate in terms of voiding and sexual function. However, it may be associated with increased discomfort of the female partner during intercourse due to loss of the cushion effect of the tumescent glans [9].

Partial Penectomy

Partial penectomy is considered the most aggressive form of penis-conserving surgery. It is indicated for tumors on the glans and extending onto the distal shaft or

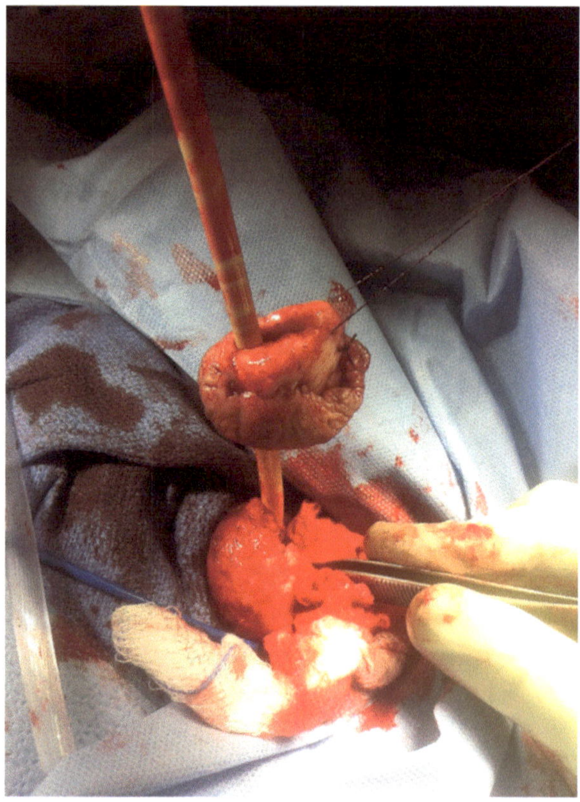

Fig. 8.3 The urethra is divided and glans penis is freed

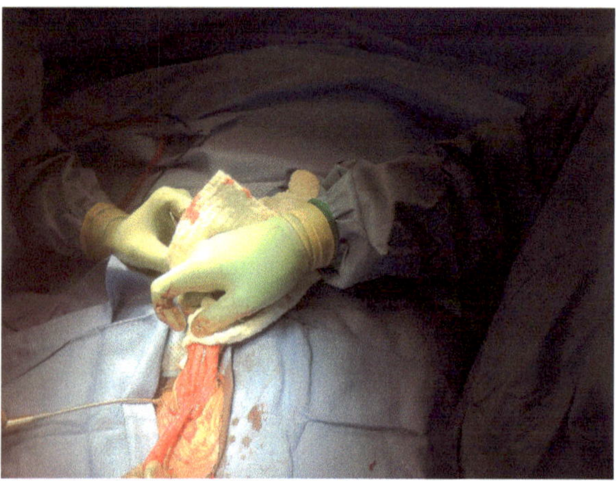

Fig. 8.4 Urethra is mobilized off the corpora cavernosa

tumors of the distal shaft of the penis. The main goal of that surgery is to eradicate the penile cancer while maintaining adequate remaining penile length sufficient for urinating in a standing position and possibly able to attain sexual intercourse. Usually a penile stump of 2–3 cm is enough to achieve that. If that cannot be

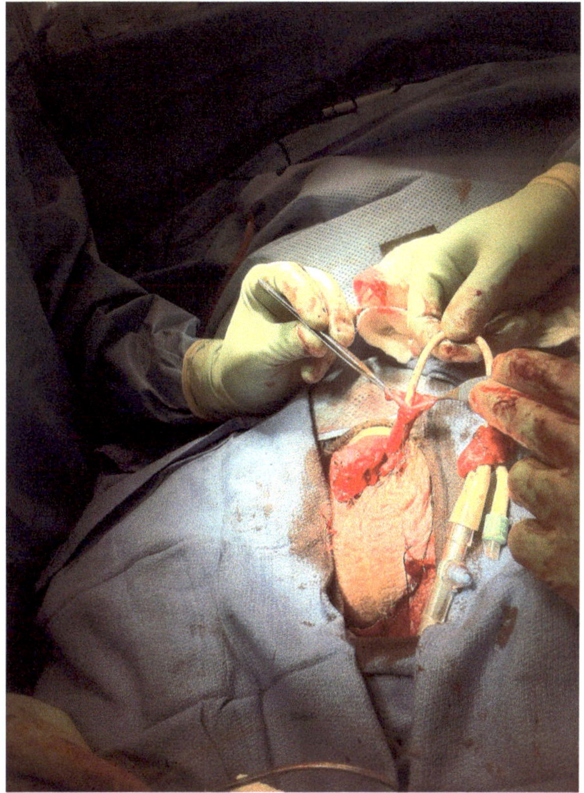

Fig. 8.5 Urethra is spatulated

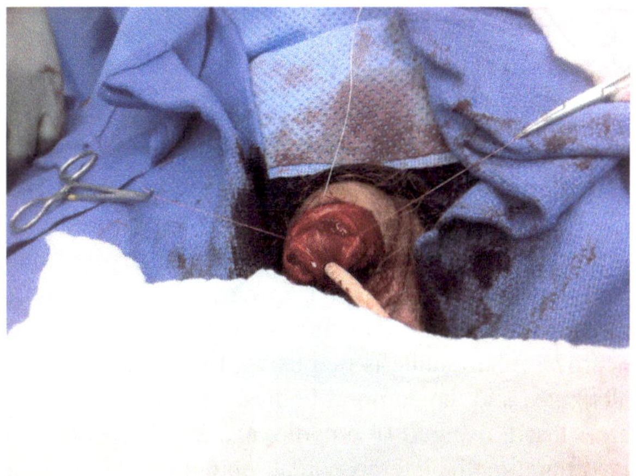

Fig. 8.6 Eversion of the spatulated urethra on the corpora cavernosa

achieved at the time of partial penectomy, total penectomy with perineal urethrostomy is advised. Patients undergoing partial penectomy should be counseled about the risks of urethral meatus stenosis (6 %) and urine spraying during micturition that may necessitate sitting down when urinating [10].

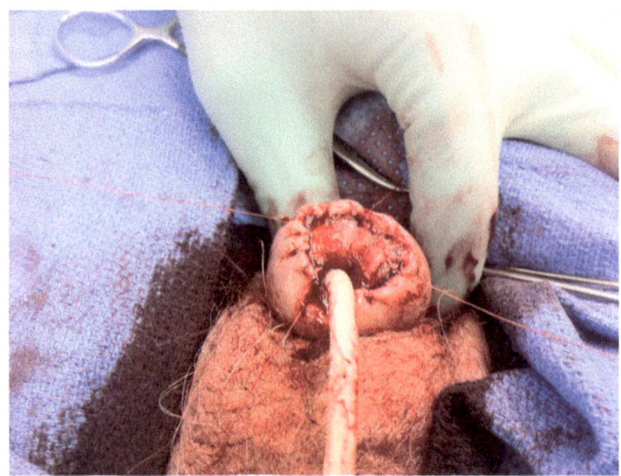

Fig. 8.7 Urethra is sutured to penile skin

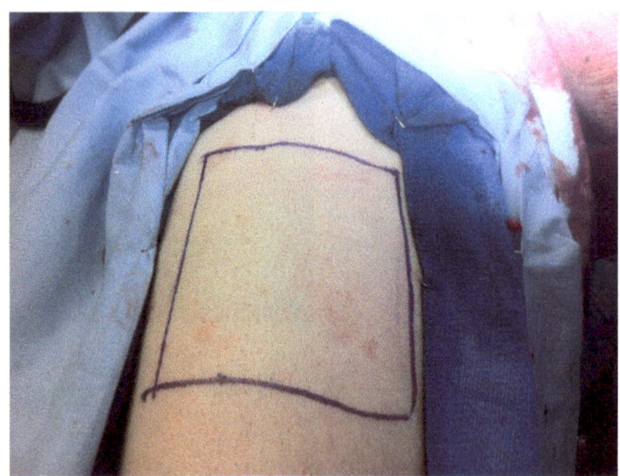

Fig. 8.8 Typical site for donor STSG on the medial aspect of the thigh

Technique of Partial Penectomy

A tourniquet is applied at the base of penis to reduce the blood loss during the surgery. A dorsal skin incision is made 1 cm proximal to the penile tumor and slanting forwards on the side. The incision is deepened deep to Buck's fascia and the dorsal neurovascular bundle is tied using 3-0 SAS. A scalpel is used to divide the tunica albuginea and the corporal bodies. The cut ends of the transected corporal bodies are closed using 2-0 polydioxanone (PDS) in a horizontal mattress fashion incorporating the intercorporeal septum.

The urethra is dissected off the corpora and divided to get an extra 1.5 cm distal to the divided corpora. The urethra is spatulated ventrally. The penile skin is advanced and anastomosed to the spatulated ends of the urethra using 3-0 synthetic absorbable suture (SAS).

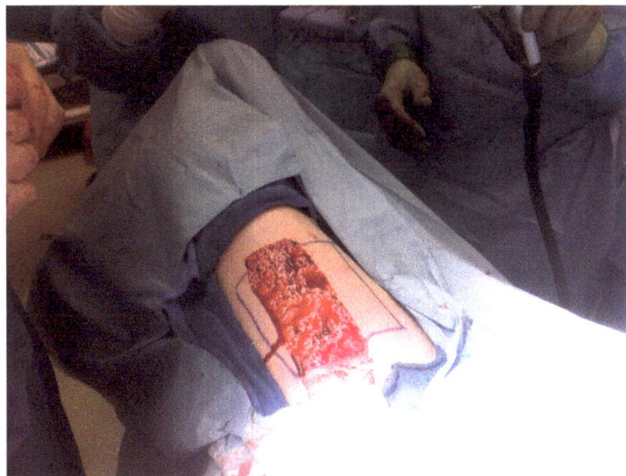

Fig. 8.9 Donor site on the thigh after harvesting

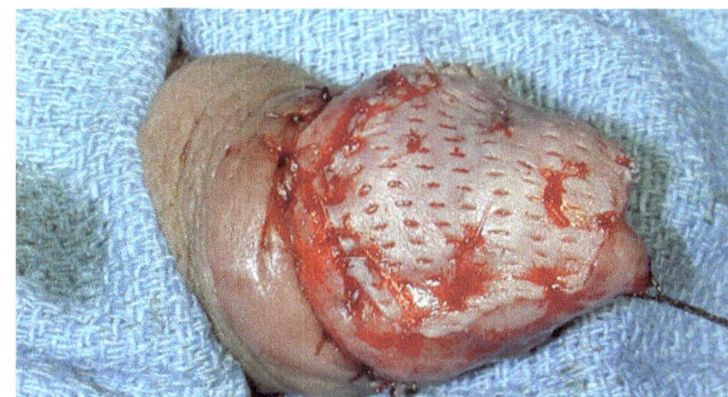

Fig. 8.10 Quilting sutures to fix the graft to the exposed tips of the corpora cavernosa

Margin Controversy in Partial Penectomy

Classic teaching when performing partial penectomy is to divide the penile shaft 2 cm proximal to the tumor. However, this requirement has been questioned. Bissada et al. studied 26 patients who had tailored excisions with median follow-up of 360 months. Margins were determined by an adequate negative frozen section. Local recurrence rate was 7.7 % [6]. Agrawal et al. studied 64 partial/total penectomy specimens examined histologically for microscopic tumor extension beyond visible tumor extension by using 5 mm sections. The authors found that the maximum microscopic tumor extension beyond visible growth was 5 mm for G1/G2 and 10 mm for G3. No skip lesions were identified [11]. Minhas et al. studied 51 patients treated with glansectomy or wide local excision with mean F/U 26 months. Margins were 0–10 mm in 48 % in the study patients and were less than 2 cm in 98 %. Local recurrence rate was noted in only 4 %. These studies demonstrate that a margin of 2 cm is not required as long as an intraoperative frozen section was negative [12]. Final pathological confirmation should be obviously included.

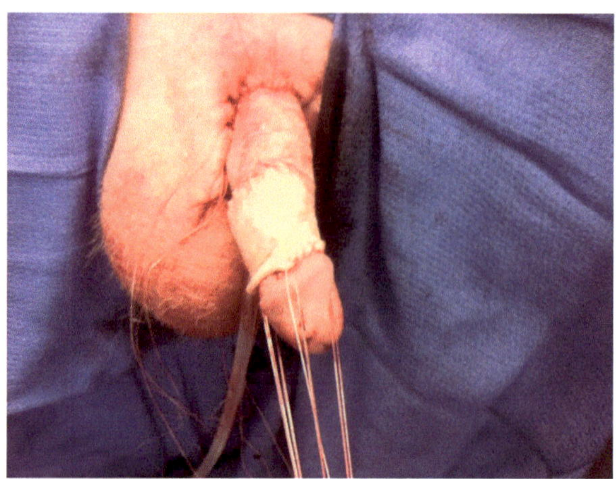

Fig. 8.11 STSG applied on the penile shaft

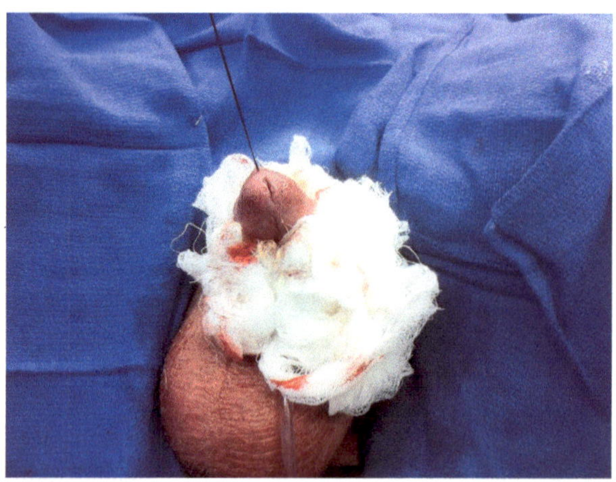

Fig. 8.12 Dressing applied and fixed by tying the long ends of sutures as shown in Fig. 8.11

Techniques to lengthen the penile stump after partial penectomy:

1. Division of suspensory ligaments of the penis
2. Mobilization of corpora proximally from pubic arch
3. V-Y plasty at the penopubic junction
4. Z-plasty at the penoscrotal junction

Oncological and functional outcome of partial penectomy:

Reported local recurrence rate was 0–8 % [10]. Most patients void sitting to prevent spraying. Sexual function is preserved in 20 % of patients [13].

Urethra-Sparing Total Penectomy

Urethra-sparing total penectomy is occasionally feasible when cancer involves the dorsum of the penis with clearly uninvolved ventral aspect and urethra.

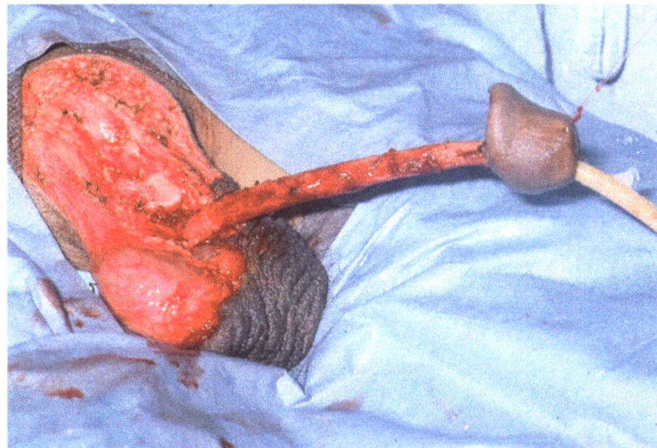

Fig. 8.13 Complete excision of the 2 corpora with urethral sparing. Glans does not survive with this technique

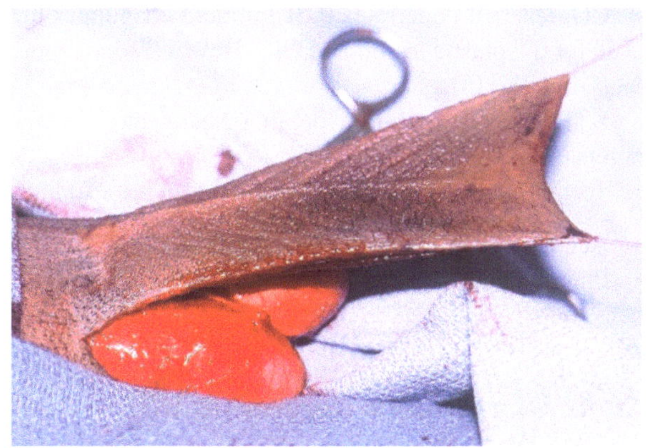

Fig. 8.14 Creation of scrotal flaps

Technique: A urethral catheter is inserted. A small ventral transverse incision proximal to the glans is performed. A vertical ventral midline incision is performed. The urethra is dissected off the 2 corpora down to the penoscrotal junction. A vertical elliptical incision is performed at the pubic area and excision of the 2 corpora is done in a standard fashion. Perineal urethrotomy is created in a standard fashion.

Penile reconstruction after urethra-sparing total penectomy: In patients who previously underwent a urethra-sparing penectomy, the urethra is included in the reconstructed penis to provide a meatal location at the tip of the penis without the added risks of standard urethral reconstruction [14] (Figs. 8.13, 8.14, and 8.15).

Laser Techniques

Laser in general is most suited for Tis or small T1 tumors or small T2 in a patient who refuses more aggressive surgery.

Nd:YAG laser: Most commonly used laser. Penetrates 3–6 mm and coagulates up to 5 mm vessel.

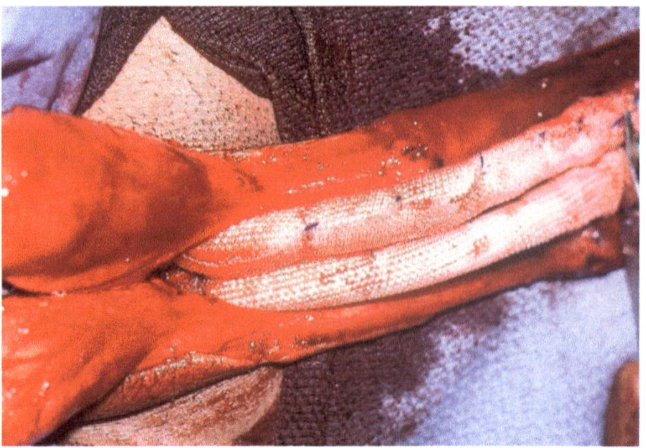

Fig. 8.15 Insertion of semirigid penile implant wrapped into GORE-TEX mesh

CO_2 laser: It penetrates 0.01 mm and coagulates up to 0.5 mm vessel. It can be used for dysplastic lesion and CIS. However, one report shows local recurrence was 33 % in CIS [15].

KTP laser: Penetration depth in between CO_2 and Nd:YAG laser and better hemostasis than CO_2.

Techniques to improve tumor detection prior to laser include:

- Acetic acid application to the penis
- Photodynamic therapy

Mohs Micrographic Surgery (MMS)

This involves removing the skin cancer by excising thin layers of tissue and examining them microscopically. Initial reports by Mohs were encouraging. He reported 5 years cure rate that was dependent on tumor size, <1 cm: 100 %, 1–2 cm: 83 %, 2–3 cm: 75 %, >3 cm: 50 % [16]. However, more contemporary reports show an overall high recurrence rate of 32 % at 5 years' follow-up [17]. We had to perform current techniques to eradicate tumors in several patients who have failed MMS.

Management of Inguinal Lymph Nodes: That follows the same rules as after total/partial penectomy and is discussed in a different chapter in this book.

Summary

Organ preservation for penile cancer surgery is indicated whenever it is feasible to attain complete cancer excision and maintain adequate penile length for forwarded directed urinary stream. Any technique used must adhere to the basics of adequate cancer control. Adequate use of biopsies to confirm that no residual cancer remains is mandatory.

There is a role for laser surgery in small penile cancer in appropriately selected patients. More contemporary literature shows that Mohs micrographic surgery may be associated with a high local recurrence rate on long-term follow-up.

Before performing the surgery, adequate knowledge of the different techniques to cover the resulting defect of cancer excision is imperative. The surgeon should be capable of and ready to perform skin advancement, urethral advancement, or split-thickness skin graft if and as needed.

In this chapter, the evidence for the appropriate use of a tailored approach to the management of penile cancer with the aim of organ preservation while ensuring complete eradication of all malignant tissue yields superior functional and psychological outcomes without compromising oncological control.

References

1. de Kernion JB, Tynberg P, Persky L, Fegen JP. Proceedings: Carcinoma of the penis. Cancer. 1973;32(5):1256–62.
2. Johannes CB, Araujo AB, Feldman HA, Derby CA, Kleinman KP, McKinlay JB. Incidence of erectile dysfunction in men 40 to 69 years old: longitudinal results from the Massachusetts male aging study. J Urol. 2000;163(2):460–3.
3. Singer PA, Tasch ES, Stocking C, Rubin S, Siegler M, Weichselbaum R. Sex or survival: tradeoffs between quality and quantity of life. J Clin Oncol. 1991;9:328–34.
4. Burgers JK, Badalament RA, Drago JR. Penile cancer. Clinical presentation, diagnosis, and staging. Urol Clin North Am. 1992;19(2):247–56.
5. Seyam RM, Bissada NK, Mokhtar AA, Mourad WA, Aslam M, Elkum N, et al. Outcome of penile cancer in circumcised men. J Urol. 2006;175(2):557–61; discussion 561.
6. Bissada NK. Conservative extirpative treatment of cancer of the penis. Urol Clin North Am. 1992;19(2):283–90.
7. Bissada NK, Yakout HH, Fahmy WE, Gayed MS, Touijer AK, Greene GF, et al. Multi-institutional long-term experience with conservative surgery for invasive penile carcinoma. J Urol. 2003;169(2):500–2.
8. Smith Y, Hadway P, Biedrzycki O, Perry MJ, Corbishley C, Watkin NA. Reconstructive surgery for invasive squamous carcinoma of the glans penis. Eur Urol. 2007;52(4):1179–85. Epub 2007 Feb 20.
9. Hatzichristou DG, Tzortzis V, Hatzimouratidis K, Apostolidis A, Moysidis K, Panteliou S. Protective role of the glans penis during coitus. Int J Impot Res. 2003;15(5):337–42.
10. Horenblas S, van Tinteren H, Delemarre JF, Boon TA, Moonen LM, Lustig V. Squamous cell carcinoma of the penis. II. Treatment of the primary tumor. J Urol. 1992;147(6):1533–8.
11. Agrawal A, Pai D, Ananthakrishnan N, Smile SR, Ratnakar C. The histological extent of the local spread of carcinoma of the penis and its therapeutic implications. BJU Int. 2000;85(3):299–301.
12. Minhas S, Kayes O, Hegarty P, Kumar P, Freeman A, Ralph D. What surgical resection margins are required to achieve oncological control in men with primary penile cancer? BJU Int. 2005;96(7):1040–3.
13. Mazza ON, Cheliz GM. Glanuloplasty with scrotal flap for partial penectomy. J Urol. 2001;166(3):887–9.
14. Bissada NK. Penile reconstruction after total penectomy or urethra-sparing total penectomy. J Urol. 1987;137(6):1173–5.
15. van Bezooijen BP, Horenblas S, Meinhardt W, Newling DW. Laser therapy for carcinoma in situ of the penis. J Urol. 2001;166(5):1670–1.

16. Mohs FE, Snow SN, Larson PO. Mohs micrographic surgery for penile tumors. Urol Clin North Am. 1992;19(2):291–304.
17. Shindel AW, Mann MW, Lev RY, Sengelmann R, Petersen J, Hruza GJ, et al. Mohs micrographic surgery for penile cancer: management and long-term followup. J Urol. 2007;178(5):1980–5. Epub 2007 Sep 17.

Chapter 9
Analysis of Contemporary Treatment of Penile Cancer at the Netherlands Cancer Institute

Rosa S. Djajadiningrat, Erik van Werkhoven, and Simon Horenblas

Introduction

The low incidence of penile cancer poses a challenge for the clinicians as many aspects in the management are based on a limited amount of scientific evidence. Until a few decades ago, most evidence was derived from retrospective, single-institutional analyses with limited number of patients. During the last decades, however, there has been a shift towards centralization of penile cancer care in the Netherlands and the United Kingdom with collaboration among large centers. This has resulted in improved knowledge and changes in the diagnosis and treatment of penile cancer.

Historically, the primary tumor has been treated by some form of amputation. Management of the regional lymph nodes varied from observation to prophylactic inguinal lymph node dissection (iLND) in clinically node-negative patients (cN0) and therapeutic iLND in patients with regional metastases. The last decades treatment has shifted to penile-sparing approaches [1–3], risk-adapted iLND [4], and dynamic sentinel node biopsy (DSNB) instead of prophylactic iLND in patients with non-palpable inguinal lymph nodes (cN0) [5]. In 1994, DSNB was introduced at our institute for cN0 patients [6]. First, analysis showed improved survival in patients staged by DSNB compared to those followed by close surveillance [7]. Furthermore, while adjuvant radiotherapy is part of our treatment protocol for years, additional induction chemotherapy has been introduced recently in selected patients with locally advanced penile disease [3, 8]. Thus, in theory, contemporary prognosis and survival may have improved in SCCp. On the other hand, less

R.S. Djajadiningrat, MD (✉) • S. Horenblas, MD, PhD, FEBU
Department of Urology, Netherlands Cancer Institute,
Plesmanlaan 121, Amsterdam, 1066CX, The Netherlands
e-mail: r.djajadiningrat@nki.nl; s.horenblas@nki.nl

E. van Werkhoven, MSc
Biometrics, Netherlands Cancer Institute,
Amsterdam, The Netherlands

D.J. Culkin (ed.), *Management of Penile Cancer*,
DOI 10.1007/978-1-4939-0461-7_9,

invasive surgery could lead to more locoregional recurrences and subsequent decreased survival. Following is an analysis of contemporary treatment results at our institute.

Current Treatment of Primary Tumor

Carcinoma in situ (Tis) and the majority of T1 and T2 tumors smaller than 2–3 cm are treated with penile-preserving strategies, such as laser, local excision, and glans resurfacing [1]. More recently, glans resection with or without reconstruction was introduced for (recurrent) tumors confined to the glans [1, 9]. All abovementioned surgeries are considered penile sparing. In general, patients with larger T2 tumors and all T3–T4 tumors are treated with partial or total penile amputation. Local recurrent tumors are treated by penis preservation if the recurrent tumor stage is T1–T2 or amputation for the larger tumors.

Current Treatment of Regional Lymph Nodes

Surgery remains the treatment of choice in patients with metastatic disease in the groins. Cure can be attained in approximately 80 % of patients who have one or two involved inguinal nodes without extranodal extension.

Dynamic Sentinel Node Biopsy (DSNB)

Sentinel lymph node biopsy is a fairly new technique in medical practice that is becoming the standard of care for regional lymph node staging of many solid tumors. Sentinel lymph node biopsy is the preferred method of lymph node staging in melanoma and breast cancer [10]. This technique is based on the hypothesis of stepwise distribution of malignant cells in the lymphatic system. The absence of tumor cells in the first lymph node(s) in the lymphatic drainage of the tumor indicates the absence of further spread in regional lymph node basin(s). The best definition of a sentinel node is probably that of Morton: "the first lymph node that receives afferent drainage from a primary tumor" [11]. It is important to realize that there is individual variation in the location of the sentinel node. Moreover, although the location is usually in the area traditionally known as the regional lymph node basin, aberrant locations can be seen in a minority of patients. Also more than one sentinel node can be present. All these variations can only be found if one combines all the preoperative information from the lymphoscintigraphy with the findings during surgery.

Since 1994, DSNB has been performed at the authors' institution to stage cN0 patients [5].

In 2001, several procedural changes were made, including preoperative ultrasound of the groins, administration of a reinjection if no nodes were visualized on lymphoscintigraphy, and intraoperative palpation of the wound at the end of the procedure, and finally, histopathological analysis was expanded with serial sectioning and immunohistochemistry [5]. Only in patients with a tumor-positive sentinel node is a completing ipsilateral iLND performed as described before [12]. This procedure has been included in the 2009 European Association of Urology guidelines on penile cancer [4].

Lymphadenectomy

Ipsilateral radical inguinal lymphadenectomy is indicated when tumor-bearing lymph nodes are found with DSNB, FNAC, or excision biopsy. Previous studies have suggested that the likelihood of bilateral inguinal involvement is related to the number of involved nodes in the unilateral resected inguinal specimen [13, 14]. With two or more metastases, the probability of occult lateral involvement is 30 %, and this may warrant an early contralateral inguinal lymphadenectomy. Currently, ultrasound-guided FNAC and DSNB are used to solve this problem in the authors' institute in those patients presenting with unilateral positive nodes. Patients with contralateral groins with tumor-negative sentinel nodes are kept under close surveillance.

If histopathology reveals >2 positive inguinal nodes and/or extranodal extension in the removed inguinal specimen, a subsequent ipsilateral pelvic lymphadenectomy and adjuvant ipsilateral inguinal radiotherapy followed. In patients with tumor-positive pelvic nodes, ipsilateral irradiation to the pelvic region is administered. In general, radiotherapy dose is 50 Gy. Induction chemotherapy is given in locally advanced and/or inoperable regional disease without evidence of distant metastasis [15]. Patients presenting with or progressed to inoperable advanced disease received chemo- and/or radiotherapy for palliation only, together with best supporting care.

Pelvic Lymphadenectomy

Approximately 20–30 % of all patients with positive inguinal nodes harbor tumor-positive pelvic nodes [13, 16, 17]. Although patients with pelvic lymph node involvement are considered to have a poor outcome, pelvic lymphadenectomy can be curative in some patients, particularly patients with occult pelvic metastases benefit. Several studies have shown that the likelihood of pelvic nodal involvement is related to the number of positive nodes in the inguinal specimen and presence of nodal extension [13, 16–22]. At the authors' institute, a pelvic dissection is considered unnecessary in patients with one intranodal inguinal metastasis. In all other patients with two or more inguinal nodes involved or extranodal extension, an ipsilateral pelvic lymphadenectomy is performed. Contralateral pelvic lymphadenectomy is not recommended, since there is no evidence that cross over from groin to the contralateral pelvic area does occur [14, 16, 17]. Therefore, contralateral pelvic lymphadenectomy is not recommended in patients with unilateral nodal involvement. Patients with preoperative evidence of pelvic metastases are unlikely to be cured by surgery alone and are candidates for neoadjuvant chemotherapy before undergoing surgery.

Disease-Specific Survival

Patients

We evaluated all recorded data of 1,000 patients with penile cancer presented at our institute from 1956 until February 2012. Detailed information on patient characteristics, tumor characteristics at presentation, treatment, and follow-up have been registered in our consecutive penile SCC database. Because no adequate analysis was possible with missing grade of differentiation, pT, and pN stage, 36 patients were excluded from the study because of lack of pathology. The majority of these patients were treated with primary radiotherapy in the early years. Twenty patients were excluded who refused treatment or died before they were treated. Thus, in total 56 patients were excluded, leaving 944 patients eligible for analysis. All were treated with surgical resection of the penile tumor.

Staging

All tumors were (re)staged by clinical and pathological stage according to the 2009 TNM classification [4] (Table 9.1). Pathological node status was based on histopathology, obtained either by sentinel node biopsy or lymph node dissection. Patients subjected to close surveillance of the regional lymph nodes, without pathological examination, were staged either pN0 if there was no evidence of lymph node involvement 2 years after primary treatment or pN1, pN2, or pN3 if there was. Patients were staged pNx if treatment of the groins consisted of radiotherapy only or if patients were subjected to close surveillance and had less than 2 years of follow-up or died of another cause within 2 years after primary treatment.

Until 2008, all histopathology was revised by a single experienced uropathologist. Since then, all histopathological examinations were not revised but reported by experienced uropathologists. Grade was assigned as well, moderately or poorly differentiated based on the amount of undifferentiated cells within the tumor on histopathological examination according to Broders [23]. Lymphovascular invasion was defined as the presence of embolic tumor cells in thin-walled vessel-like structures using routinely stained sections. Finally, extranodal extension (ENE) was defined as extension of tumor through the lymph node capsule into the perinodal fibrous adipose tissue.

Table 9.1 2009 TNM classification of penile cancer

Clinical classification		
T	*Primary tumor*	
	TX	Primary tumor cannot be assessed
	T0	No evidence of primary tumor
	Tis	Carcinoma in situ
	Ta	Noninvasive verrucous carcinoma, not associated with destructive invasion
	T1	Tumor invades subepithelial connective tissue
	T1a	Tumor invades subepithelial connective tissue without lymphovascular invasion and is not poorly differentiated or undifferentiated (T1G1–2)
	T1b	Tumor invades subepithelial connective tissue with lymphovascular invasion or is poorly differentiated or undifferentiated (T1G3–4)
	T2	Tumor invades corpus spongiosum/corpora cavernosa
	T3	Tumor invades urethra
	T4	Tumor invades adjacent structures
N	*Regional lymph nodes*	
	NX	Regional lymph nodes cannot be assessed
	N0	No palpable or visibly enlarged inguinal lymph node
	N1	Palpable mobile unilateral inguinal lymph node
	N2	Palpable mobile multiple or bilateral inguinal lymph nodes
	N3	Fixed inguinal nodal mass or pelvic lymphadenopathy, unilateral or bilateral
M	*Distant metastasis*	
	M0	No distant metastasis
	M1	Distant metastasis
Pathological classification		
The pT categories correspond to the T categories. The pN categories are based upon biopsy or surgical excision		
pN	*Regional lymph nodes*	
	pNx	Regional lymph nodes cannot be assessed
	pN0	No regional lymph nodes metastasis
	pN1	Intranodal metastasis
	pN2	Metastasis in multiple or bilateral inguinal lymph nodes
	pN3	Metastasis in pelvic lymph node(s), unilateral or bilateral or extranodal extension of regional lymph node metastasis
pM	*Distant metastasis*	
	pM0	No distant metastasis
	pM1	Distant metastasis
G	*Histopathological grading*	
	Gx	Grade of differentiation cannot be assessed
	G1	Well differentiated
	G2	Moderately differentiated
	G3–4	Poorly differentiated or undifferentiated

Used with permission from Sobin et al. [38]

Patient Follow-Up

Since 1988, the follow-up has been standardized at our institute. This involves physical examination of the penis and groins at the outpatient clinic every 2 months during the first 2 years, at 3-month intervals in the third year, and 6-month intervals thereafter. Imaging with ultrasound and CT was done on indication. Patients were discharged from follow-up after 10 years without evidence of disease. The follow-up scheme was altered after analysis of recurrence patterns and consists now of a more risk-adapted follow-up scheme [24].

Management of Penile Cancer Over Time

We divided patients into four cohorts according to the introduction of changes in treatment.

Cohort 1: 1956–1987

The first cohort consisted of patients documented from 1956. Until 1988, a wait-and-see policy was applied to patients presenting with cN0 groins. Patients who first presented with clinically node-positive patients (cN+) or patients who developed clinical apparent metastatic disease during follow-up underwent an ipsilateral iLND.

Cohort 2: 1988–1993

In 1988, standardized management and follow-up was introduced based on an analysis of treatment results [14, 22, 25, 26]. Also a risk-adapted approach was a standard of care in patients presenting with cN0 groins. In general, elective bilateral iLND was introduced for cN0 patients considered to be at high risk (≥T2G3) for lymphatic invasion. The second cohort consisted of patients diagnosed between January 1988 and January 1994.

Cohort 3: 1994–2000

In 1994, DSNB was introduced for patients presenting with cN0 groins. Patients diagnosed between January 1994 and December 2000 were included in the third cohort.

Cohort 4: 2001–2012

In 2001, several modifications were applied to the DSNB procedure as described earlier [27], thereby increasing its sensitivity [5]. Since 2004, DSNB is also performed for all patients with ≥T1b tumors.

Furthermore, glans resection and resurfacing became more standardized in selected patients. Therefore, the fourth cohort consisted of patients diagnosed with SCCp after 2001.

Patient Characteristics

The median observed follow-up duration of the 944 patients was 64 months. The four cohorts consisted of 97, 55, 164, and 628 patients, respectively. Table 9.2 shows patient characteristics at presentation. No significant age differences were found between the cohorts (p value = 0.3427). During the study period, significantly more patients appeared to have poorer differentiated tumors (G3) (p value = 0.0373).

All patients with pTa (n = 4) and pTis tumors (n = 70) were staged cN0 and either pNx or pN0. The number of patients who had distant metastasis at first presentation was limited and remained limited during the study period (overall 11 of 944, 1 %).

All four Ta and 61 of 70 patients with pTis tumors were alive at last date of follow-up. The remaining 9 patients with pTis tumors died due to a non-cancer cause. Contrary, all 11 patients with distant metastasis died of disease within 9 months (range 0.9–8.2).

To improve prognostic stratification of the different T and N category, these 85 patients (pTa = 4, pTis = 70, distant metastasis = 11) were excluded for further analysis.

Penile Surgery Over Time

Overall, 53 % of patients were treated with penile-preserving surgery, while 47 % of patients had undergone a (partial) amputation. Time was a significant predictor for the probability of amputation (p value = 0.0049) and was nonlinear (p value = 0.06).

Table 9.2 Patient characteristics

	Cohort 1 1956–1987	Cohort 2 1988–1993	Cohort 3 1994–2000	Cohort 4 2001–2012	Total
Number of patients	97	55	164	628	944
Median follow-up (months)	135 (2–399)	161 (2–268)	107 (5–207)	49 (1–127)	64 (1–399)
Median age at diagnosis (range)	65 (30–94)	62 (36–89)	62 (21–92)	65 (23–96)	64 (21–96)
pT stage					
pTis	1 (1 %)	9 (16 %)	13 (8 %)	47 (7 %)	70 (7 %)
pTa	0 (0 %)	0 (0 %)	1 (1 %)	3 (0 %)	4 (0 %)
pT1a	30 (31 %)	17 (31 %)	39 (24 %)	161 (26 %)	247 (26 %)
pT1b	14 (14 %)	4 (4 %)	12 (7 %)	45 (7 %)	75 (8 %)
pT2	47 (48 %)	25 (45 %)	89 (54 %)	319 (51 %)	480 (51 %)
pT3	4 (4 %)	0 (0 %)	7 (4 %)	46 (7 %)	57 (6 %)
pT4	1 (1 %)	0 (0 %)	3 (2 %)	7 (1 %)	11 (1 %)
Grade of differentiation					
CIS	1 (1 %)	9 (16 %)	13 (8 %)	47 (7 %)	70 (7 %)
G1 – well	41 (42 %)	22 (40 %)	54 (33 %)	188 (30 %)	305 (32 %)
G2 – intermediate	43 (45 %)	19 (35 %)	69 (42 %)	248 (39 %)	379 (40 %)
G3 – poor	10 (10 %)	5 (9 %)	27 (17 %)	123 (20 %)	165 (17 %)
Missing	2 (2 %)	0 (0 %)	1 (0 %)	22 (4 %)	25 (4 %)

(continued)

Table 9.2 (continued)

	Cohort 1 1956–1987	Cohort 2 1988–1993	Cohort 3 1994–2000	Cohort 4 2001–2012	Total
Kind of penile surgery[a]					
pT1–2					
Penis preserving[b]	39 (41 %)	19 (41 %)	86 (60 %)	297 (52 %)	441 (51 %)
(Partial) amputation	52 (54 %)	27 (59 %)	51 (35 %)	226 (39 %)	356 (42 %)
pT3–4					
Penis preserving	1 (1 %)	0 (0 %)	1 (1 %)	8 (1 %)	10 (1 %)
(Partial) amputation	4 (4 %)	0(0 %)	6 (4 %)	42 (7 %)	52 (6 %)
cN stage					
cN0	60 (62 %)	47 (85 %)	140 (85 %)	489 (78 %)	736 (78 %)
cN+	37 (38 %)	8 (15 %)	24 (15 %)	139 (22 %)	208 (22 %)
cN1	18	5	11	78	112
cN2	15	3	10	27	55
cN3	4	0	3	34	41
pN stage					
pN0	49 (51 %)	29 (53 %)	111 (68 %)	402 (64 %)	591 (63 %)
pN+	34 (35 %)	21 (38 %)	50 (30 %)	195 (31 %)	300 (31 %)
pN1	3	0	13	64	80
pN2	4	7	5	40	56
pN3	27	14	32	91	164
pNx	14 (14 %)	5 (9 %)	3 (2 %)	31 (5 %)	53 (6 %)
ENE status in pN+					
No	8 (24 %)	9 (43 %)	22 (44 %)	114 (58 %)	153 (51 %)
Yes	19 (56 %)	11 (52 %)	27 (54 %)	77 (40 %)	134 (45 %)
Unknown	7 (20 %)	1 (5 %)	1 (2 %)	4 (2 %)	13 (4 %)
Distant metastasis					
No	97 (100 %)	55 (100 %)	158 (96 %)	623 (99 %)	933 (99 %)
Yes	0 (0 %)	0 (0 %)	6 (4 %)	5 (1 %)	11 (1 %)

[a]Only for patients with T1–2 and T3–4 tumors
[b]Penile-conserving surgery includes laser, local excision, glans resection, or a combination of these methods

The estimated effect is shown in Fig. 9.1. The odds ratio for pT3–4 compared to pT1–2 was 6.65 (95 %–CI: 3.32–13.31, p value < 0.001). The number of penile-preserving operations increased significantly over the years, but after 2000 a slight decrease was seen. This could not be explained by the increasing number of pT3–4 tumors.

Five-year DSS of all patients was 81 %; this was 83 % for patients with a pT1–2 tumor and 63 % for patients with a pT3–4 tumor. When adjusting for relevant covariables such as grade of differentiation, pathological T stage, N stage, lympho-vascular invasion, resection margins, and year of diagnosis, patients treated with (partial) amputation showed no significant differences in survival compared with patients treated with penis-preserving therapies.

This shows that penile-preserving therapies were indeed increasingly used over time in our cohort. Furthermore, it underscores the safety of the use of penile-preserving therapies, since no differences in CSS were observed in patients treated

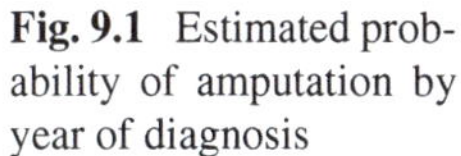

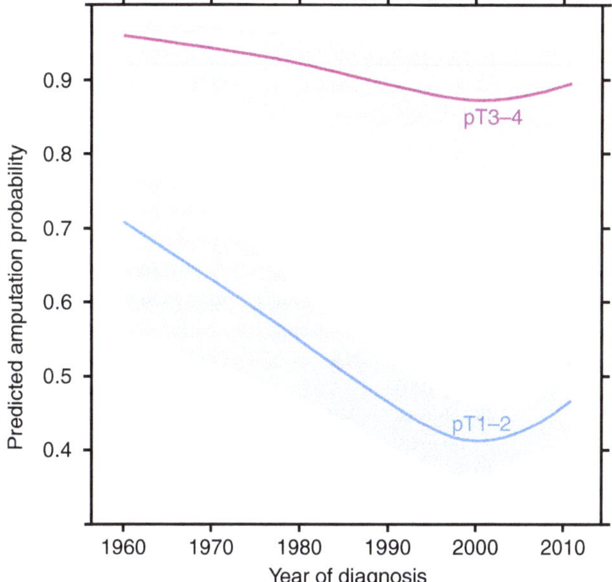

Fig. 9.1 Estimated probability of amputation by year of diagnosis

with penile-preserving therapies than in patients treated with (partial) amputation. Thus, penile-preserving therapies are increasingly used without jeopardizing survival.

This was also shown in another study, where short-term cancer control rates were excellent. In this study, it was concluded that with careful patient selection and meticulous follow-up, most patients with invasive penile carcinoma can undergo penile-preserving surgery [28]. About 80 % of penile carcinomas occur distally, involving the glans, coronal sulcus, or prepuce, and are potentially amenable to organ-preserving surgery [29].

Cancer-Specific Survival of All Patients with Invasive Tumors

The estimated 5-year CSS of all 859 patients with primary invasive tumors (≥T1a) was 81 % (95 % CI: 78–84 %). The estimated 5-year overall survival was 66 % (95 % CI: 63–70 %).

A statistically significant CSS difference was found for all cN0 and cN+ patients and between all pN0 and pN+ categories: cN0 90 % versus cN+ 54 % ($p<0.001$) and pN0 97 % versus pN+ 56 % ($p<0.001$), respectively (Table 9.3).

Cancer-Specific Survival of cN Categories

Contemporary CSS of cN categories is shown in Fig. 9.2. Focusing on the cN0 category, improved CSS was found for cN0 in contemporary series ($p<0.044$) (Fig. 9.3).

Table 9.3 Five-year cancer-specific survival estimates with 95 % confidence intervals

Patients	1956–1987	1988–1993	1994–2000	2001–2012	Overall	p value
cN0	85 % (76–95)	78 %	89 % (84–95)	92 % (88–95)	90 % (87–92)	0.044[a]
cN+	56 % (41–76)	8 subjects, 0 events	51 % (32–83)	51 % (42–62)	54 % (47–62)	0.2
cN1	68 % (47–98)	5 subjects, 0 events	75 % (50–100)	62 % (51–76)	66 % (57–77)	0.32
cN2	48 % (26–85)	3 subjects, 0 events	29 % (9–92)	39 % (22–67)	43 % (30–61)	0.48
cN3	25 % (5–100)	NA	3 out of 3	34 % (19–60)	32 % (18–55)	0.16
pN0	48 subjects, no events	94 % (84–100)	98 % (95–100)	96 % (94–98)	97 % (95–98)	0.47
pN+	40 % (26–61)	75 % (58–97)	57 % (43–74)	57 % (49–66)	56 % (50–63)	0.05[b]
pN1	3 subjects, 0 events	NA	91 % (75–100)	80 % (69–93)	83 % (74–93)	0.48
pN2	50 % (19–100)	83 % (58–100)	60 % (29–100)	66 % (51–87)	66 % (54–82)	0.52
pN3	31 % (17–57)	71 % (51–99)	40 % (25–65)	37 % (27–52)	40 % (32–50)	0.17
pNx	67 % (43–100)	5 subjects, 1 event	3 subjects, 1 event	25 % (5–100)	43 % (22–83)	0.87

[a]Statistically significant
[b]Borderline significant

The 5-year CSS was 91 % after 1994, the year DSNB was introduced, versus 82 % (1956–1993) ($p=0.021$). This difference in CSS since the introduction of DSNB remained, when adjusting for pT stage and grade in a Cox proportional hazard model (HR 2.46, $p=0.01$). In a second model, where cN0 patients in whom a DSNB was performed were compared to cN0 patients without DSNB, 5-year CSS was better for the DSNB group after adjusting for the same covariables (HR 2.63, $p=0.01$).

This is most probably due to the detection of microscopic disease by DSNB resulting in early treatment. This survival difference underscores our initial report [7] and remains after longer follow-up. Thus, men with SCCp benefit from surgical resection of microscopic non-palpable disease when compared to iLND after metastasis becomes clinically apparent [7, 30]. This also attests to the safety of the DSNB procedure as the survival figures in pN+ patients appear better than series that advocate primary iLND in all patients considered to be at risk for lymph node metastases [21].

Contrary to cN0 patients, contemporary survival of patients staged as cN1, cN2, and cN3 appears to be similar with previous cohorts. These figures probably reflect the limits of curative potential of contemporary management of such cN+ patients. New strategies are necessary to improve the outcome of these patients. Surgery alone is curative in a proportion of patients, while other patients could benefit from

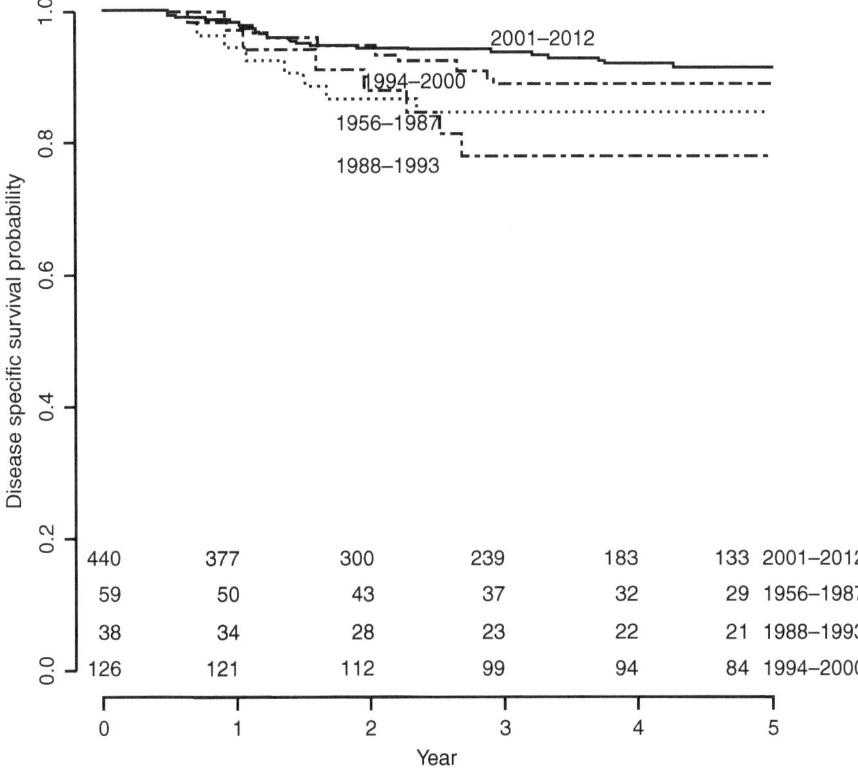

Fig. 9.2 cN0 category CSS curves of the different cohorts (Log rank $p=0.044$). 1956–1987: 85 % (76–95); 1988–1993: 78 % (65–94); 1994–2000: 89 % (84–95); 2001–2012: 92 % (88–95)

adjuvant treatment. More research is needed to distinguish groups of patients with more or less risk for recurrence. Also, nodal involvement is still underestimated with conventional radiologic imaging. This accounts especially for patients with pelvic lymph node involvement [31]. Seventy percent or more of the patients with pelvic lymphadenopathy are not identified preoperatively with CT and thus are understaged. The use of ^{18}F-FDG-PET/CT in recognizing pelvic nodal involvement seems promising in patients with proven inguinal involvement [32], although its value in detecting clinically non-palpable inguinal node is low [33].

Cancer-Specific Survival of pN Categories

Contemporary 5-year CSS according to the different pN categories was 96, 80, 66, and 37 %, respectively ($p<0.001$) (Fig. 9.4).

Differences in 5-year CSS of all pN+ patients between the cohorts were borderline significant. Changes in 5-year CSS for the different pN categories between the cohorts were not significant at all. An overview of the different 5-year CSS estimates of the different cohorts is provided in Table 9.3.

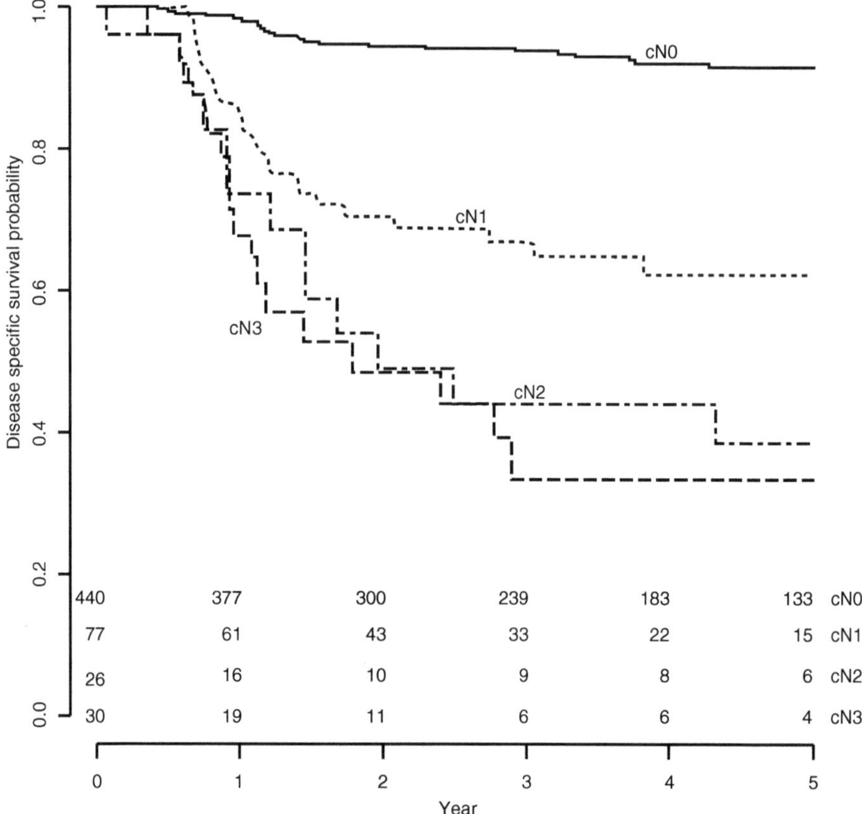

Fig. 9.3 Contemporary cN category CSS curves (Log rank $p<0.0001$). cN0: 92 % (88–95); cN1: 62 % (51–76); cN2: 39 % (22–76); cN3: 34% (19–60)

Results of Cox proportional hazards model in all pN+ patients showed that ENE was associated with worse 5-year CSS than pN+ patients without ENE, when correcting for grade, pT stage, and diagnosis before or after 1994 (HR 3.05, $p<0.0001$).

The current pN staging did have discriminating value in survival between all different pN stages in the contemporary cohort (Fig. 9.4). This underscores the improvement in N staging since the introduction of the recent TNM classification [34, 35].

Role of N Stage

These data show that contemporary 5-year CSS in clinically cN0 patients with SCCp has improved over the years (Fig. 9.2). cN0 patients treated after 1994 showed improved CSS compared to those treated between 1956 and 1994 when adjusted for pT category and grade of differentiation.

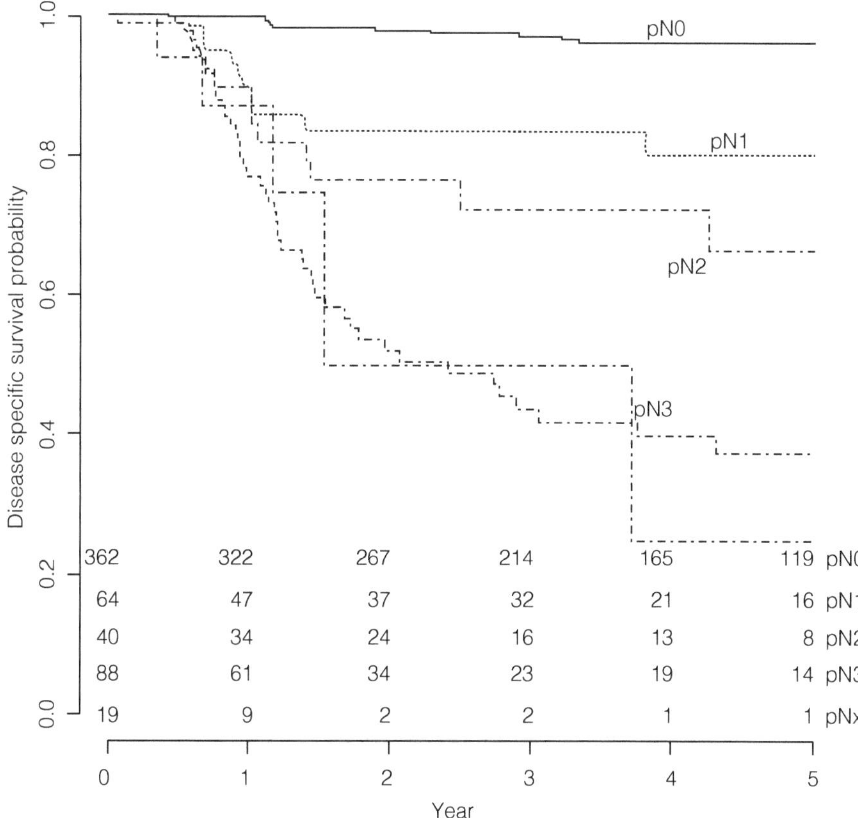

Fig. 9.4 Contemporary pN category CSS curves (Log rank $p<0.0001$). pN0: 96 % (95 %-CI 94–98); pN1: 80 % (95 %-CI 69–93); pN2: 66 % (95 %-CI 51–87); pN3: 37 % (95 %-CI 27–52)

Early detection and treatment of nodal metastases are essential, since the presence and extent of lymph node metastases are the most important prognostic factor in SCCp [16, 18]. This is exemplified by Ornellas et al. [21]. They have reviewed their long-term experience of patients with SCCp who have been treated surgically during a 46-year period. A total of 140 patients were staged pN0 and showed a 10-year CSS of 96 %. On the other hand, 111 patients were staged pN+ and had a survival of 35 % ($p<0.001$), regardless of pT category. The lack of discriminating value of pT category in this series also supports the safety of penile-preserving therapies.

Another explanation for the lack of discriminating value may be the definition of the T2 category. In the current TNM, no difference is made between extension into corpus spongiosum and corpus cavernosum, while several papers have shown that corpus cavernosum invasion has poorer prognostic outcome than corpus spongiosum involvement only [36, 37]. It was also shown that growth into the urethra, the criterion for T3/pT3 [36], had no discriminating value, compared to T2/pT2 tumors.

Our data also underscore the importance of the presence and extent of nodal involvement with survival [2, 4–6, 19, 20, 25], since the patients with extranodal extension have way worse survival when comparing them with node-positive patients without extranodal extension (HR 3.05, 95 % CI: 2.01–4.65).

Conclusion

Improvement of survival has been observed in cN0 patients with SCCp when adjusting for pathological T stage and grade; the most probable reason being the introduction of DSNB with early treatment of microscopic disease. In addition, an increase in penile-preserving therapies has not led to a decreased survival. Furthermore, ENE is highly associated with worse CSS in pN+ patients. In this group, other treatment strategies are needed, as no improvement was seen.

Acknowledgement This paper is based on two accepted papers: (1) Contemporary management of regional nodes in penile cancer: changes in survival? Rosa S. Djajadiningrat, Niels M. Graafland, Erik van Werkhoven, Wim Meinhardt, Axel Bex, Henk G. van der Poel, Hester H. van Boven, Renato A. Valdés Olmos, and Simon Horenblas, J Urol. 2014 Jan;191(1):68–73; and (2) Penile cancer: Penile sparing surgery does not affect survival? Rosa S. Djajadiningrat, Erik van Werkhoven, Wim Meinhardt, Axel Bex, Henk van der Poel, Bas van Rhijn, and Simon Horenblas, J Urol. 2013 Dec 24. pii: S0022-5347(13)06140–5. doi: 10.1016/j.juro.2013.12.038 [Epub ahead of print].

References

1. Lont AP, Gallee MPW, Meinhardt W, van Tinteren H, Horenblas S. Penis conserving treatment for T1 and T2 penile carcinoma: clinical implications of a local recurrence. J Urol. 2006;176(2):575–80; discussion 580.
2. Davis J, Schellhammer P, Schlossberg SM. Conservative surgical therapy for penile and urethral carcinoma. Urology. 1999;53(203):386–92.
3. Deem S, Keane T, Bhavsar R, El-Zawahary A, Savage S. Contemporary diagnosis and management of squamous cell carcinoma (SCC) of the penis. BJU Int. 2011;108(9):1378–92.
4. Pizzocaro G, Algaba F, Horenblas S, Solsona E, Van der Poel H, Watkin N. EAU penile cancer guidelines 2009. Eur Urol. 2010;57(6):1002–12.
5. Leijte JAP, Kroon BK, Valdés Olmos RA, Nieweg OE, Horenblas S. Reliability and safety of current dynamic sentinel node biopsy for penile carcinoma. Eur Urol. 2007;52(1):170–7.
6. Tanis PJ, Lont AP, Meinhardt W, Olmos RA, Nieweg OE, Horenblas S. Dynamic sentinel node biopsy for penile cancer: reliability of a staging technique. J Urol. 2002;168(1):76–80.
7. Lont AP, Horenblas S, Tanis PJ, Gallee MP, van Tinteren H, Nieweg OE. Management of clinically node negative penile carcinoma: improved survival after the introduction of dynamic sentinel node biopsy. J Urol. 2003;170(3):783–6.
8. Pizzocaro G, Nicolai N, Milani A. Taxanes in combination with cisplatin and fluorouracil for advanced penile cancer: preliminary results. Eur Urol. 2009;55:546–51.
9. Veeratterapillay R, Sahadevan K, Aluru P, Asterling S, Rao GS, Greene D. Organ-preserving surgery for penile cancer: description of techniques and surgical outcomes. BJU Int. 2012;2:1–4.

10. Berveiller P, Mir O, Veyrie N, Barranger E. The sentinel-node concept: a dramatic improvement in breast-cancer surgery. Lancet Oncol. 2010;11(9):906. Elsevier Ltd.
11. Morton DL, Bostick PJ. Will the true sentinel node please stand? Ann Surg Oncol. 1999;6(1):12–4.
12. Horenblas S. Lymphadenectomy in penile cancer. Urol Clin North Am. 2011;38(4):459–69, vi–vii. Elsevier Inc.
13. Srinivas V, Morse MJ, Herr HW, Sogani PC, Whitmore WF. Penile cancer: relation of extent of nodal metastasis to survival. J Urol. 1987;137(5):880–2.
14. Horenblas S, Van Tinteren H, Delemarre JF, Moonen LM, Lustig V, van Waardenburg EW. Squamous cell carcinoma of the penis. III. Treatment of regional lymph nodes. J Urol. 1993;149(3):492–7.
15. Leijte JAP, Kerst JM, Bais E, Antonini N, Horenblas S. Neoadjuvant chemotherapy in advanced penile carcinoma. Eur Urol. 2007;52(2):488–94.
16. Lont AP, Kroon BK, Gallee MPW, van Tinteren H, Moonen LMF, Horenblas S. Pelvic lymph node dissection for penile carcinoma: extent of inguinal lymph node involvement as an indicator for pelvic lymph node involvement and survival. J Urol. 2007;177(3):947–52; discussion 952.
17. Zhu Y, Zhang S-L, Ye D-W, Yao X-D, Dai B, Zhang H-L, et al. Prospectively packaged ilioinguinal lymphadenectomy for penile cancer: the disseminative pattern of lymph node metastasis. J Urol. 2009;181(5):2103–8. American Urological Association.
18. Ravi R. Correlation between the extent of nodal involvement and survival following groin dissection for carcinoma of the penis. Br J Urol. 1993;72(5 Pt 2):817–9.
19. Sánchez-Ortiz RF, Pettaway CA. The role of lymphadenectomy in penile cancer. Urol Oncol. 2004;22(3):236–44; discussion 244–5.
20. Pandey D, Mahajan V, Kannan RR. Prognostic factors in node-positive carcinoma of the penis. J Surg Oncol. 2006;93(2):133–8.
21. Ornellas AA, Kinchin EW, Nóbrega BLB, Wisnescky A, Koifman N, Quirino R. Surgical treatment of invasive squamous cell carcinoma of the penis: Brazilian National Cancer Institute long-term experience. J Surg Oncol. 2008;97(6):487–95.
22. Horenblas S, Van Tinteren H. Squamous cell carcinoma of the penis. IV. Prognostic factors of survival: analysis of tumor, nodes and metastasis classification system. J Urol. 1994; 151:1239–43.
23. Broders A. Squamous cell-epithelioma of the skin. Ann Surg. 1921;43(2):141–59.
24. Leijte JAP, Kirrander P, Antonini N, Windahl T, Horenblas S. Recurrence patterns of squamous cell carcinoma of the penis: recommendations for follow-up based on a two-centre analysis of 700 patients. Eur Urol. 2008;54(1):161–8.
25. Horenblas S, van Tinteren H, Delemarre JF, Boon TA, Moonen LM, Lustig V. Squamous cell carcinoma of the penis. II. Treatment of the primary tumor. J Urol. 1992;147(6):1533–8.
26. Horenblas S, Van Tinteren H, Delemarre JF, Moonen LM, Lustig V, Kröger R. Squamous cell carcinoma of the penis: accuracy of tumor, nodes and metastasis classification system, and role of lymphangiography, computerized tomography scan and fine needle aspiration cytology. J Urol. 1991;146(5):1279–83.
27. Kroon BK, Horenblas S, Estourgie SH, Lont AP, Valdés Olmos RA, Nieweg OE. How to avoid false-negative dynamic sentinel node procedures in penile carcinoma. J Urol. 2004;171(6):2191–4.
28. Pietrzak P, Corbishley C, Watkin N. Organ-sparing surgery for invasive penile cancer: early follow-up data. BJU Int. 2004;94(9):1253–7.
29. Sarin R, Norman A, Steel G, Horwich A. Treatment results and prognostic factors in 101 men treated for squamous carcinoma of the penis. Int J Radiat Oncol. 1997;38(4):713–22.
30. McDougal WS. Preemptive lymphadenectomy markedly improves survival in patients with cancer of the penis who harbor occult metastases. J Urol. 2005;173(3):681.
31. Zhu Y, Zhang SL, Ye DW, Yao XD, Jiang ZX, Zhou XY. Predicting pelvic lymph node metastases in penile cancer patients: a comparison of computed tomography, Cloquet's node, and disease burden of inguinal lymph nodes. Onkologie. 2008;31(1–2):37–41.

32. Graafland NM, Leijte JA, Valdés Olmos RA, Hoefnagel CA, Teertstra HJ, Horenblas S. Scanning with 18F-FDG-PET/CT for detection of pelvic nodal involvement in inguinal node-positive penile carcinoma. Eur Urol. 2009;56(2):339–45.
33. Sadeghi R, Gholami H, Zakavi SR, Kakhki VRD, Horenblas S. Accuracy of 18F-FDG PET / CT for diagnosing inguinal lymph node involvement in penile squamous cell carcinoma. Clin Nucl Med. 2012;37:436–41.
34. Al-Najar A, Alkatout I, Al-Sanabani S, Korda JB, Hegele A, Bolenz C, et al. External validation of the proposed T and N categories of squamous cell carcinoma of the penis. Int J Urol. 2011;11:312–6.
35. Zhu Y, Ye D-W, Yao X-D, Zhang S-L, Dai B, Zhang H-L. New N staging system of penile cancer provides a better reflection of prognosis. J Urol. 2011;186(2):518–23. American Urological Association Education and Research, Inc.
36. Leijte JA, Gallee M, Antonini N, Horenblas S. Evaluation of current TNM classification of penile carcinoma. J Urol. 2008;180(3):933–8; discussion 938.
37. Rees R, Freeman A, Borley N. PT2 penile squamous cell carcinomas: cavernosus vs. spongiosus invasion. Eur Urol Suppl. 2008;7(3):111 (abstract #63).
38. Sobin LH, Gospodarowicz MK, Wittekind C, editors, International Union Against Cancer (UICC). TNM classification of malignant tumors. 7th ed. Oxford: Wiley-Blackwell; 2009.

Chapter 10
Surgical Management of the Clinically Negative and Locally Advanced Inguinal Region in Patients with Squamous Penile Cancer

Curtis Pettaway and Lance Pagliaro

The presence and extent of metastasis to the inguinal region are the most important prognostic factors for survival among patients with squamous penile cancer. These findings affect the prognosis of the disease more than tumor grade, gross appearance, and morphologic or microscopic patterns of the primary tumor. Unlike many other genitourinary tumors, which mandate systemic therapeutic strategies once metastasis has occurred, lymphadenectomy alone can be curative and should be performed. The biology of squamous penile cancer is such that it exhibits a prolonged locoregional phase before distant dissemination, providing a rationale for the therapeutic value of lymphadenectomy. However, owing to the morbidity of traditional lymphadenectomy, especially among those patients with a clinically negative groin, contemporary controversial issues include (1) the selection of patients for lymphadenectomy vs. careful observation, (2) the types of procedures to correctly stage the inguinal region with low morbidity, and (3) multimodal strategies to improve survival among patients with bulky inguinal metastases. In this chapter, we will focus on the surgical evaluation and management of the inguinal region among penile cancer patients with either no palpable adenopathy or those with suspected or proven advanced regional metastases.

C. Pettaway, MD (✉)
Urology, Surgery Division, The University of Texas MD Anderson Cancer Center, 1515 Holcombe Blvd., Unit 1373, Houston, TX 77030, USA
e-mail: cpettawa@mdanderson.org

L. Pagliaro, MD
Department of Genitourinary Medical Oncology, The University of Texas MD Anderson Cancer Center, Houston, TX, USA

D.J. Culkin (ed.), *Management of Penile Cancer*,
DOI 10.1007/978-1-4939-0461-7_10, © Springer Science+Business Media New York 2014

Surgical Management of the Clinically Negative Inguinal Region

The reluctance to advocate automatic ilioinguinal lymphadenectomy in all patients with penile cancer stems from the substantial morbidity of the procedure. Early complications of phlebitis, pulmonary embolism, wound infection, flap necrosis, and permanent and disabling lymphedema of the scrotum and lower limbs were historically frequent after inguinal and ilioinguinal node Dissections [1, 2]. Postoperative complications have been reduced by improved preoperative and postoperative care; advances in surgical technique; plastic surgical consultation for myocutaneous flap coverage; and preservation of the dermis, Scarpa's fascia, and saphenous vein, as well as modification of the extent of the Dissection [3]. The relevant question then becomes, can a delayed therapeutic dissection effectively salvage cases of inguinal recurrence? If true, this would then only expose those patients with proven inguinal metastases to the morbidity of inguinal node dissection. However, Kroon et al. compared survival of 20 patients found to have positive lymph nodes subsequent to prophylactic dynamic sentinel node biopsy with that of 20 patients who underwent delayed inguinal dissection after proven nodal metastasis [4]. The 3-year survival for those patients whose positive nodes were detected during close surveillance was only 35 % vs 84 % for those undergoing early dissection ($p=0.0017$). Pathological evaluation of involved lymph nodes revealed extra nodal extension of cancer in 19 of 20 patients in the delayed group vs only 4 of 20 in the early group ($p=0.001$) [4]. Thus, despite careful follow-up, survival was adversely affected by the extent of cancer in the involved lymph nodes. Six series in the literature indicated improvement in survival for patients undergoing early vs delayed therapeutic Dissection [1, 4–8]. Furthermore, 5 of the 6 series showed that delayed therapeutic dissection can rarely salvage cases of recurrence. Taken together, these data suggest that a policy of early surgical inguinal staging gives greater assurance that surgery will be performed when the volume of metastasis is small (if present) and still highly curable.

Imaging Strategies in the Selection of Clinically Node-Negative (cN0) Penile Cancer Patients with Microscopic Metastases

Horenblas and associates compared the ability of physical examination, CT scan, and lymphangiography to assess the inguinal region in patients who were surgically staged or had prolonged follow-up [9].. In 102 patients with a 39 % prevalence of positive nodes, the sensitivity and specificity of physical examination were 82 and 79 %, respectively. Of note, both CT and lymphangiography were performed in patients who were thought to have metastases. The sensitivity of lymphangiography was only 31 %, but there were no false positives. Similarly, the sensitivity and specificity of CT scanning were 36 and 100 %, respectively. The combination of CT and lymphangiography performed simultaneously demonstrated equally poor sensitivity. Only one fifth of patients had positive nodes detected with either test. *Thus, CT scans are not recommended for staging the inguinal region among men with no palpable adenopathy*. However, they may be of use among the obese patients or those that have undergone a prior inguinal procedure where palpation may be less reliable.

Both ultrasound and PET/CT have been evaluated in small series of penile cancer patients that were cN0 and subsequently had an inguinal staging procedure to determine pathological nodal status [10, 11]. Kroon et al. evaluated inguinal ultrasound and selective fine needle aspiration among a cohort of penile cancer patients who subsequently underwent dynamic sentinel node biopsy [10]. Preoperative ultrasound detected only 9/23(39 %) proven groins with metastases. Ultrasound missed tumor deposits that were ≤2 mm in size. In another study from this group, 24 patients underwent PET/CT scans prior to DSNB [11]. Five were proven to have inguinal node metastases, but PET/CT only noted one of the 5 (20 %) to be positive. All false-negative tumor deposits were <10 mm [11]. Thus, current imaging techniques do not reliably allow the accurate detection of microscopic inguinal metastases from penile cancer.

Impact of Primary Tumor Histological Features on Predicting Occult Nodal Metastasis

Primary tumor pathological stage, grade, and the presence/absence of lymphovascular invasion are currently the most important factors that drive the decision to recommend an inguinal staging procedure for patients with penile cancer [12–15] and no palpable inguinal adenopathy. Figure 10.1 provides contemporary risk criteria for inguinal metastases and groupings based on pathological stage, grade, and the presence/absence of LVI. Patients with primary tumors exhibiting carcinoma in situ or verrucous carcinoma have little or no risk of metastasis. Only 2 cases of metastasis in association with carcinoma in situ have been reported, and none of 47 cases of penile verrucous carcinoma has been shown to metastasize [16–18]. Thus, patients with Tis and Ta penile cancer are included in the low-risk group for inguinal metastases [12]. In contrast, patients with corporeal invasion (stage pT2) in the penile tumor exhibit a high risk of metastasis. The average risk for inguinal metastasis among 225 patients in 7 different series was 59 % [19]. The risk for metastasis among patients exhibiting corporeal invasion was similar irrespective of whether palpable adenopathy was present. Stage T1 penile cancer exhibits involvement of the subepithelial connective tissue only and lacks involvement of the corpus spongiosum, corpora cavernosa, or urethra [12]. Similarly, staged tumors historically have been associated with a 4–14 % incidence of nodal metastasis [20, 21]. However, this finding is not universal as others have noted higher rates of metastases among patients presenting with pT1 primary tumors and initially negative nodes on clinical

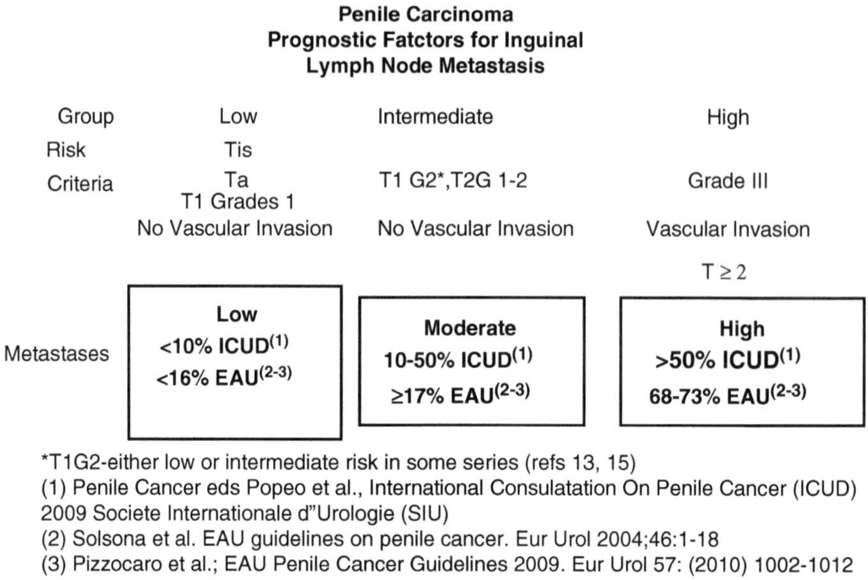

Penile Carcinoma
Prognostic Fatctors for Inguinal
Lymph Node Metastasis

Group	Low	Intermediate	High
Risk	Tis		
Criteria	Ta T1 Grades 1 No Vascular Invasion	T1 G2*,T2G 1-2 No Vascular Invasion	Grade III Vascular Invasion T ≥ 2
Metastases	**Low** **<10% ICUD(1)** **<16% EAU(2-3)**	**Moderate** **10-50% ICUD(1)** **≥17% EAU(2-3)**	**High** **>50% ICUD(1)** **68-73% EAU(2-3)**

*T1G2-either low or intermediate risk in some series (refs 13, 15)
(1) Penile Cancer eds Popeo et al., International Consulatation On Penile Cancer (ICUD) 2009 Societe Internationale d"Urologie (SIU)
(2) Solsona et al. EAU guidelines on penile cancer. Eur Urol 2004;46:1-18
(3) Pizzocaro et al.; EAU Penile Cancer Guidelines 2009. Eur Urol 57: (2010) 1002-1012

Fig. 10.1 Risk-adapted strategies to manage the inguinal region among patients with penile cancer and no palpable inguinal adenopathy. For reliable patients in the low-risk group, careful observation is recommended. Among patients in the intermediate- to high-risk group, an inguinal staging procedure is often recommended such as dynamic sentinel node biopsy or superficial inguinal dissection

assessment [22]. These data suggest that other variables within the penile cancer of the cohort of patients studied (i.e., tumor grade and presence of vascular invasion) may have modified the effect of tumor stage on metastasis [23]. Thus, there is consensus that patients exhibiting stage Ta, Tis, and T1 grade 1 tumors comprise a group at low risk for metastasis (i.e., 0–16 %). This finding is reflected in the EAU and Société Internationale d'Urologie/International Consultation on Urological Diseases guidelines as well as the 7th edition of the AJCC staging system [12, 13, 24, 25]. However, there is also consensus that patients who exhibit a high rate of microscopic metastasis should undergo an inguinal staging procedure. These patients have stage ≥ T2 primary tumor, T any stage tumors with poorly differentiated cancers or the presence of LVI. Metastases have been associated with these tumors in more than 50 % of cases [12, 13, 25]. Intermediate between these groups are tumors that do not fit into either category. For example, reported rates of metastasis vary from 9 to 44 % for T1 grade 2 tumors. Ficarra et al. developed the first penile cancer nomogram using data from 175 patients [15]. Based on tumor thickness and growth pattern, patients with T1 grade 2 tumors exhibited metastatic rates between 5 and 20 %. Thus, grade 2 tumors represent a heterogeneous group in which the histological criteria used to describe grade 2, and the presence or absence of other poor prognostic features ultimately determines metastatic risk [26]. Current risk groupings remain imprecise but do provide a ballpark estimate of metastatic risk among patients with invasive primary tumors and no palpable adenopathy. This estimate may be further refined as novel molecular markers are tested and incorporated into nomograms that are validated.

Expectant Management of the Inguinal Region

Compliant patients with primary tumors exhibiting carcinoma in situ (Tis), verrucous carcinoma (Ta), and stage T1 grade 1 tumors exhibit less than a 10 % incidence of positive lymph nodes overall and are optimal candidates for watchful waiting strategies [13, 25]. Recommendations for the management of T1 grade 2 tumors vary based on quoted rates of subsequent metastases. The former EAU guideline, while classifying such cases in the intermediate-risk group, recommended observation for T1 grade 2 tumors that lacked vascular invasion and exhibited a superficial growth pattern (i.e., absence of any other adverse features) [12]. This guideline was recently modified to recommend an inguinal staging procedure for this group of patients [13]. Given the low rate of metastases overall in a recent study of 9 % [27], we agree with the Société Internationale d'Urologie/International Consultation on Urological Diseases recommendation that these patients may also be considered for observation. All other cases should be considered for surgical staging. It is imperative for the patient and the physician to adhere to such follow-up agreements and be willing to intervene immediately if initial inguinal parameters change. Leijte et al. documented that only a third of patients with initially negative nodes but subsequently had an inguinal recurrence survived 5 years [28]. Modified inguinal procedures offer less invasive alternatives to traditional lymphadenectomy for patients with no palpable inguinal adenopathy but who are at significant risk for inguinal microscopic metastases.

Surgical Inguinal Staging Procedures for the Clinically Negative (cN0) Inguinal Field

Dynamic Sentinel Node Biopsy

DSNB offers the potential for precise localization of the sentinel node with the lowest morbidity of any surgical staging technique to our knowledge [28]. The goal of DSNB is to define where in the inguinal lymph node field the sentinel lymph node resides using a combination of visual (vital blue dyes) or gamma emission (handheld gamma probe) techniques at the time of surgery. Several studies evaluating the results of DSNB as a staging tool in penile cancer are now available. Kroon et al. described the use of a combination of preoperative lymphoscintigraphy and intraoperative intradermally injected blue dye in 123 patients with penile cancer [29] (Fig. 10.2). They identified a sentinel node in 98 % of patients, for a sensitivity rate of 82 % and a false-negative rate of 18 % (6 patients). Four of the 6 patients

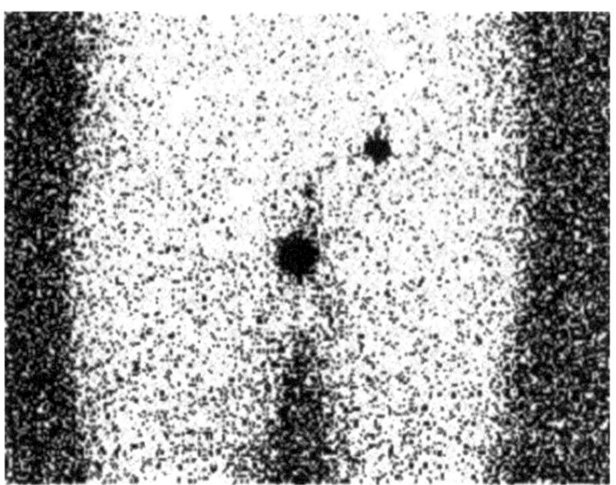

Fig. 10.2 A 67-year-old patient with stage T2N0M0 squamous carcinoma of the penis who previously underwent a partial penectomy and had a unilateral positive preoperative lymphoscintigraphy on the left side shown in anterior-posterior view

subsequently died of disease progression. Spiess et al. also reported a false-negative rate of 25 % among 31 patients undergoing DSNB [30]. In that study the sentinel node was found in the expected superomedial quadrant in 85 % of cases. However, it was detected in a more lateral location in 9 % of cases and in both locations in 6 % of cases. Kroon et al. subsequently instituted several changes, including (1) routine serial sectioning of the involved lymph nodes along with cytokeratin immunohistochemistry, (2) routine exploration of groins with low or no signal subsequent to preoperative or intraoperative studies, and (3) inguinal ultrasonography with FNA to detect subtle architectural changes (nonpalpable) in positive lymph nodes that could result in the redistribution of lymphatic flow [31].

In a multicenter update that included patients assessed with the modified DSNB protocol from 2 high-volume centers, Netherlands Cancer Institute and St. George's Hospital in London, the false-negative rate was 7 % (6 of 323 patients) [32]. Three of the 6 patients with recurrence (50 %) either died or had distant metastases. Thus, DSNB, when performed at high-volume centers using a standardized protocol, has an acceptable sensitivity, but deaths from penile cancer of patients with initial negative nodes still occurred [32]. This result limits the applicability of this strategy to larger centers with experienced surgeons and nuclear medicine specialists. Figure 10.3a demonstrates injection of isosulfan blue dye intradermally with blue dye noted in the penile shaft lymphatics. Subsequent to percutaneous identification of radioactivity over the specific inguinal area, an inguinal incision is created and the involved node(s) determined by either radioactive counts or blue staining are removed (Fig. 10.3b).

Superficial Complete Inguinal Dissection

A superficial inguinal complete dissection has been proposed as a staging tool for the patient without palpable inguinal lymphadenopathy. Superficial node dissection involves removal of those nodes superficial to the fascia lata. Subsequent to DSNB and superficial dissection, Spiess et al. showed lymphatic drainage in upper lymph node

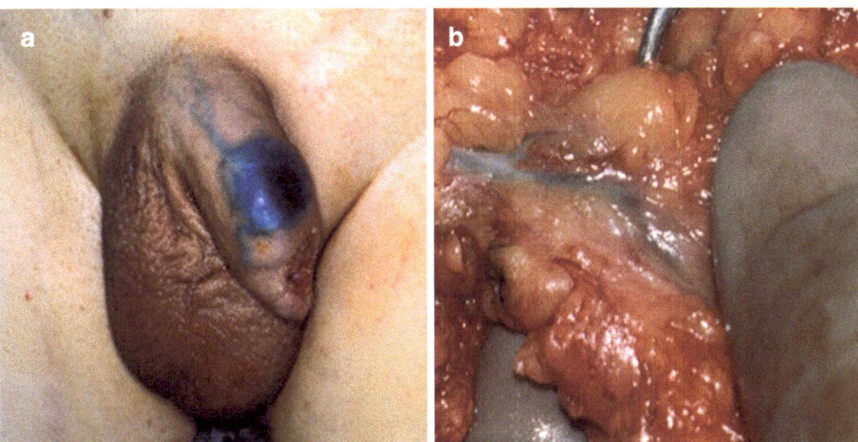

Fig. 10.3 Dynamic sentinel node biopsy (DSNB) for penile cancer. (**a**) Demonstration of the injection of isosulfan blue dye during DSNB at the site of the surgical scar from a previous partial penectomy and (**b**) subsequent demonstration of staining of lymphatic channels and sentinel node with DSNB

quadrants lateral and medial to the femoral vessels (see Fig. 10.1) [30]. Thus, a medial quadrant dissection or biopsy could produce false-negative findings. Leijte et al. reported similar findings when performing single-photon emission CT before DSNB [23]. A complete ilioinguinal lymphadenectomy (removal of those nodes deep to the fascia lata contained within the femoral triangle as well as the pelvic nodes) is then performed if the superficial nodes are positive at surgery on frozen section analysis.

The rationale for superficial dissection is that two series have shown no positive nodes deep to the fascia lata unless superficial nodes were also positive [33, 34]. Furthermore, Spiess et al. reported that of those patients with negative lymph nodes undergoing DSNB with completion of superficial dissection, none with a negative superficial dissection had recurrence at more than 3-year follow-up [30]. Thus, a superficial inguinal dissection should adequately identify microscopic metastases in patients with clinically normal inguinal examination findings without the need for a pelvic dissection if the inguinal nodes are negative. The disadvantage is the higher overall complication rate (12–35 %) compared to that of DSNB (5–7 %) [3, 29]. A superficial dissection provides more information than biopsy of a single node or group of nodes, and the possibility of not identifying the sentinel node is limited by removal of all potential first echelon nodes. The dissection is readily performed by any surgeon experienced in inguinal surgery without the need for specialized equipment. Figure 10.4 demonstrates some of the steps involved in performing a superficial inguinal dissection.

Laparoscopic/Robotic Inguinal Lymphadenectomy

Both the laparoscopic and robotic approaches to the inguinal region offer the potential of removing all of the inguinal lymph nodes at risk for disease while minimizing complications. The technical details of the contemporary procedure and early results have been described (see Fig. 10.5) [35–37]. To date the results of laparoscopic and robotic inguinal lymphadenectomy have been comparable to those of open inguinal lymph dissection with comparable node counts achieved in both. A single case of inguinal recurrence reported at 12- to 33-month follow-up, and minor complications in about 20 % of patients have been reported [3, 38]. However,

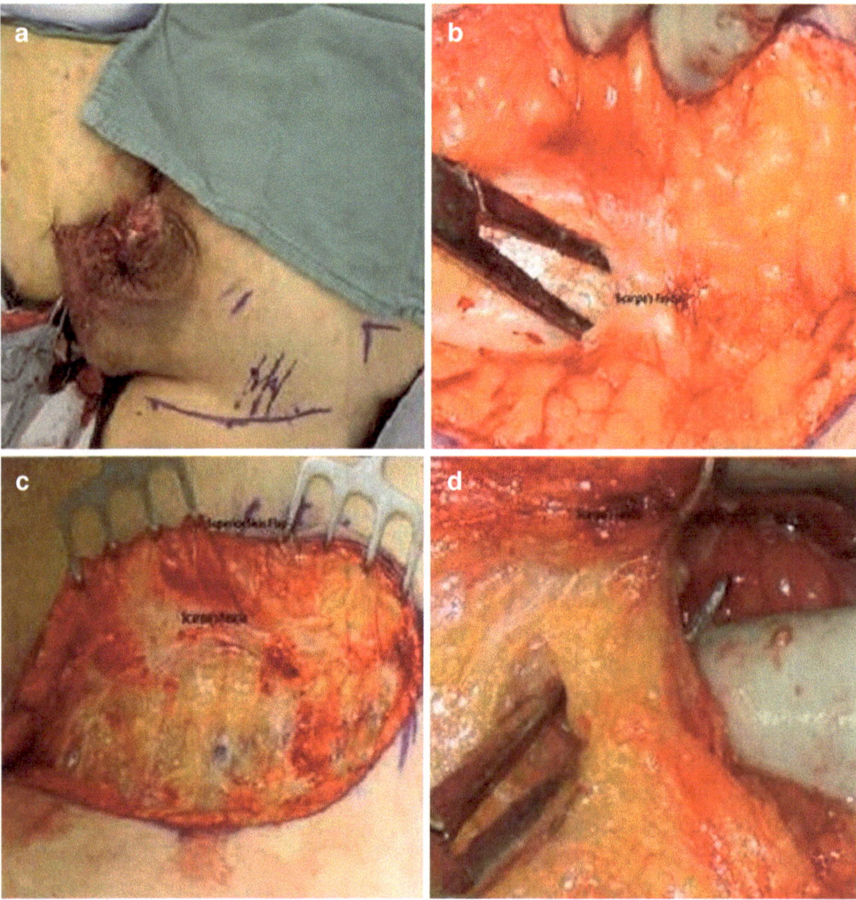

Fig. 10.4 Superficial inguinal lymph node dissection. (**a**) Left inguinal incision two fingerbreadths lateral to and inferior to pubic tubercle. Midpoint located over the femoral vessels. (**b, c**) Incision carried down to Scarpa's fascia and skin flaps raised just below the fascia. (**d**) With flap elevated nodes dissected from beneath the fascia to free the superior skin flap. (**e**) Left superomedial border of dissection identified by spermatic cord. (**f**) Inferior skin flap raised by dissecting Scarpa's fascia away from underlying nodes. (**g**) Self-retaining retractor placed and nodal tissue divided over the saphenous (SV) and femoral veins (FV) dividing specimens into medial and lateral packets. (**h**) Medial packet mobilized off the adductor longus (AL) fascia and the medial surface of saphenous and femoral veins. (**i**) Lateral packet nodes mobilized off the sartorius muscle fascia(s). (**j**) Completed superficial dissection. Sartorius (*right*) and adductor longus muscular fascia (*left*) are visualized as well as the femoral canal (FC) medial to the femoral vein (FV). Note that the femoral artery (FA) is not skeletonized by removing superficial nodes

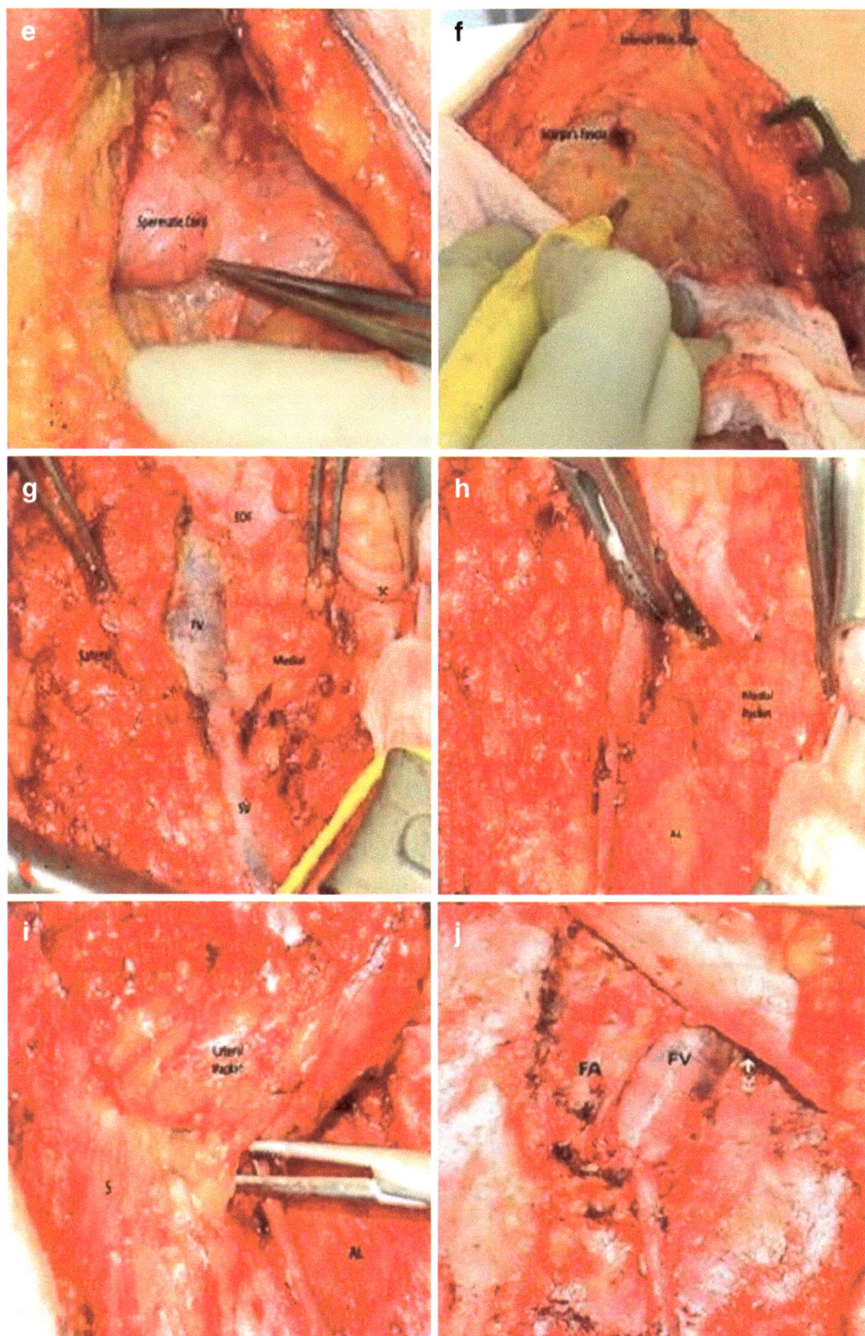

Fig. 10.4 (continued)

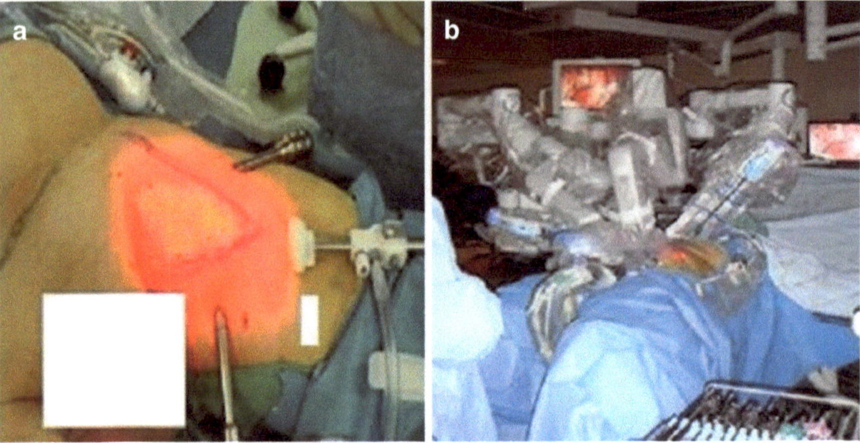

Fig. 10.5 Robotic-assisted inguinal lymphadenectomy (RAIL) for penile cancer. (**a**) Boundaries of the femoral triangle are marked based upon cutaneous landmarks. Camera port (c) located 3 cm below the apex of femoral with robotic ports (R) placed one handsbreadth diagonally proximal to the camera port. A 12-mm assistant port (not shown) is placed between the cameral port and one of the robotic ports. (**b**) Docking alignment for the RAIL procedure. The robotic surgical cart is docked on the opposite side of the table directly in line with the inguinal field to be explored

in one study using a laparoscopic approach with over 600 days of follow-up, Master et al. noted minor complications in 27 % of patients with major complications noted in 14.6 % [39]. These were mainly infectious in nature and were managed with intravenous antibiotics or incision and drainage. Of note among 41 dissections, there was only a single case of skin edge necrosis. Matin et al. using a robotic-assisted approach noted in a phase one pilot study that dissection was equivalent to an open approach in 18/19 (94.7 %) cases when verified by a second surgeon using an open incision to inspect the same groin [37]. Thus, these minimally invasive approaches, although promising, will require further validation with larger patient numbers and longer follow-up to better determine efficacy and complication rates.

Surgical Management of Advanced Regional Metastasis from Penile Cancer

Mobile Unilateral or Bilateral Inguinal Adenopathy

Penile cancer patients exhibiting inguinal metastases that are highly curable with surgery alone include those with one to two unilateral inguinal metastases with no evidence of extranodal extension (ENE) into the perinodal adipose tissue. In a recent series reported by Graafland et al., the 5-year cancer-specific survival among patients with three or more positive inguinal nodes, ENE, bilateral positive inguinal nodes, or proven pelvic metastases were 33, 42, 51, and 22 %, respectively, whereas those with two or less involved inguinal nodes, no ENE, unilateral metastases, and no pelvic metastases exhibited 74, 68, 80, and 72 %, respectively, 5-year cancer-specific survival [40]. Of note in their series, adjuvant radiation therapy was often used among patients with two or more positive inguinal nodes and ENE [40].

Given the adverse outcomes associated with poor-risk pathological findings, post inguinal lymphadenectomy predicting those patients destined to have such findings based upon preoperative clinical staging could be beneficial given the potential benefits of utilizing neoadjuvant chemotherapy to reduce the metastatic load prior to surgery [41, 42].Recently Graafland et al. described computerized tomography (CT) scan findings that were highly correlated with adverse pathological findings at surgery [43]. Among 30 patients with palpable adenopathy, CT scans were evaluated independently by two radiologists who were blinded to subsequent surgical pathology findings. CT parameters evaluated related to lymph node findings included short-axis diameter, central necrosis, indistinct margins, irregular nodal border, and infiltration of adjacent soft tissue. The investigators reported that among this cohort the CT scan findings of central necrosis or an irregular nodal border exhibited a sensitivity and specificity of 95 and 82 %, respectively, for predicting the presence of three or more positive inguinal nodes, ENE, or positive pelvic nodes. The latter is especially relevant as CT itself using size criteria alone for pelvic metastasis identified only 2 of 10 positive pelvic fields [43].

Preoperative fine needle aspiration (FNA) can also be utilized among patients with palpable inguinal adenopathy to define the presence of bilateral metastases. In addition among patients with abnormal pelvic CT scans, pelvic metastases can be confirmed by CT-directed biopsy. Saisorn et al. reported a 93 % sensitivity and 91 % specificity in 16 patients with palpable adenopathy (mean size 1.47 cm) undergoing FNA before lymphadenectomy [44]. Thus, among patients suspected to harbor potentially incurable inguinal metastases with surgery alone, preoperative imaging along with needle biopsy may assist in the selection of patients for neoadjuvant chemotherapy.

Bulky Adenopathy, Fixed Nodes, and Inguinal Tumor Recurrence

Treatment options for the patient with an unresectable groin mass consist of palliative surgery alone, up-front combination chemotherapy with surgical consolidation, radiotherapy, or chemoradiotherapy [45]. Ornellas et al. treated 39 patients with advanced penile cancer with palliative lymphadenectomy with reconstructive techniques to close soft tissues defects [46]. They reported that the procedures were associated with little morbidity or mortality and that there were improvements in short-term quality of life. However, it was noteworthy that only 4 of 39 patients (10 %) survived 12 months. One patient did survive, however, for 5 years [46].

Modern chemotherapy regimens have shown an overall response rate of 31–50 % [42, 47], with some responders showing a pathological complete response (i.e., no viable disease remaining at the time of surgical consolidation). To our knowledge there has only been one prospective neoadjuvant chemotherapy trial in penile cancer. The combination chemotherapy agents used were cisplatin, paclitaxel and ifosfamide. Of 30 patients with clinical N2-3 disease, 73 % underwent post-chemotherapy surgery, and 30 % were alive and free of recurrence at a median follow-up of 34 months. Two patients died of unrelated causes, such that the long-term progression-free survival rate approached 40 % [42]. Leijte et al. from Netherlands Cancer Institute have reviewed their experience with neoadjuvant chemotherapy in patients with initially "unresectable" penile cancer [41]. The series included 20 patients treated with five different regimens including (1) single-agent bleomycin; (2) bleomycin, vincristine, and methotrexate; (3) cisplatin and 5-fluorouracil; (4) bleomycin, cisplatin, and methotrexate; and (5) cisplatin and irinotecan. The objective responses were evaluable in 19 (one patient died due to bleomycin toxicity after 2 weeks) with 12 responses (63 %, 2 complete, 10 partial) [41]. Surgical procedures included treatment of the primary tumor as well as inguinal and pelvic dissections. Additional soft tissue resection including bone was sometimes required. Vascularized tissue flaps were used for inguinal reconstruction. Among 12 responders only 9 went to surgery, as two died of bleomycin-related complications while the third was deemed unfit for surgery [41]. Eight of nine responding patients taken to surgery (two were pT0) were free of disease with a median follow-up of 20.4 months. This is in contrast to three nonresponders who went to surgery for palliative intent. All three died within 4–8 months due to locoregional recurrence [41]. *The implications from the above studies suggest that response to chemotherapy together with an aggressive surgical procedure provides the optimal scenario for significant palliation or potentially cure.* Up-front surgical resection may provide palliation of pain or prevent erosion of tumor into the femoral vessels, but survival for more than a year is rare.

Technique for Post-Chemotherapy Ilioinguinal Lymphadenectomy

After completion of neoadjuvant chemotherapy and hematologic recovery, patients should be assessed for clinical evidence of response to chemotherapy based on clinical and radiologic parameters. Patients that are medically fit post-chemotherapy and have had an objective response to chemotherapy are optimal candidates for resection. We have previously described surgical techniques utilized in prior publications [3, 48, 49]. Of importance, surgical incisions were planned to allow for resection of grossly palpable or visible residual disease with negative surgical margins and to leave the normal surrounding tissue. Thus, a wide ellipse of normal skin was often included in the resected specimen (see Fig. 10.6a). The resected tissue also included the underlying lymph nodes between the lateral borders of the adductor longus and sartorius muscles, with complete removal of the muscular fascia, skeletonization of the femoral vessels, and en bloc resection of the saphenous vein (Fig. 10.6c–f). Ancillary procedures occasionally used to achieve negative margins, such as resection of the femoral vessels or abdominal wall, have previously been described [48, 49].

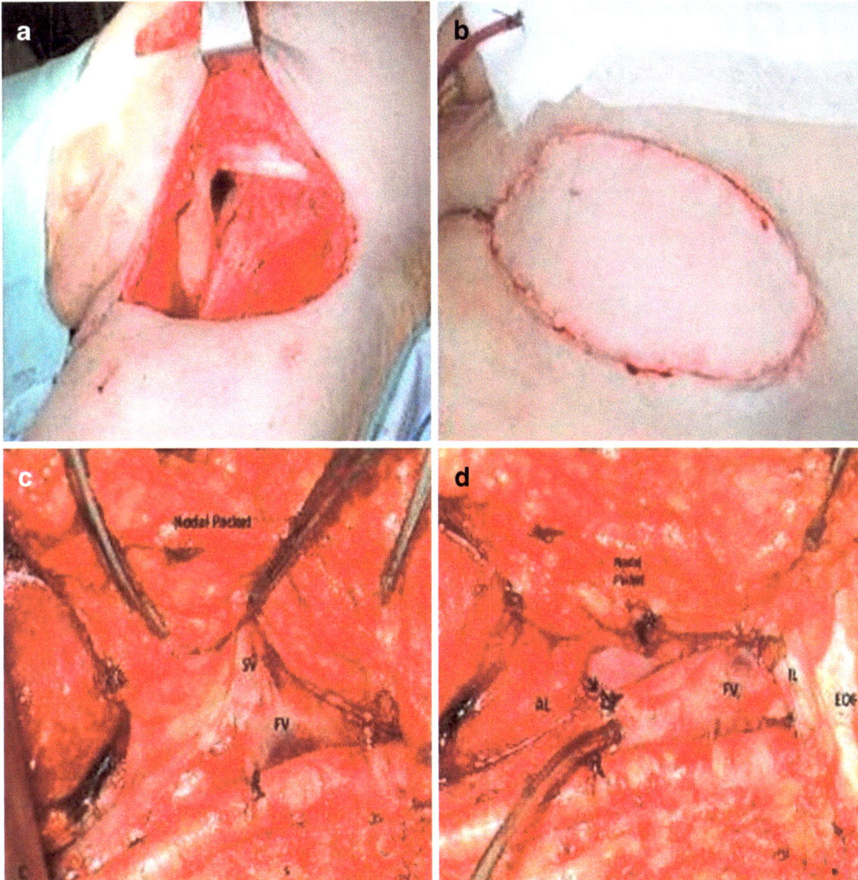

Fig. 10.6 Inguinal lymphadenectomy for regionally advanced penile cancer. (**a**) Wide skin ellipse of inguinal skin removed with en bloc superficial and deep inguinal Dissection. (**b**) Anterolateral thigh flap reconstruction of the skin defect. (**c**) Resection of superficial and deep inguinal nodes en bloc. Femoral sheath is excised, thus skeletonizing the femoral vessels. The saphenofemoral junction (SV, FV) is exposed to be ligated. (**d**) Saphenous vein ligated (*arrow*) and specimen mobilized towards inguinal ligament (IL). (**e**) Specimen divided at femoral canal between adductor longus muscle (AL) and the femoral vein (FV). (**f**) Completed superficial and deep dissection visualized landmarks which include the sartorius muscle(s), adductor longus muscle (AL), external oblique fascia (EOF), and spermatic cord (SC). (**g**) Sartorius muscle detached from its insertion to rotate over the femoral vessels to provide coverage

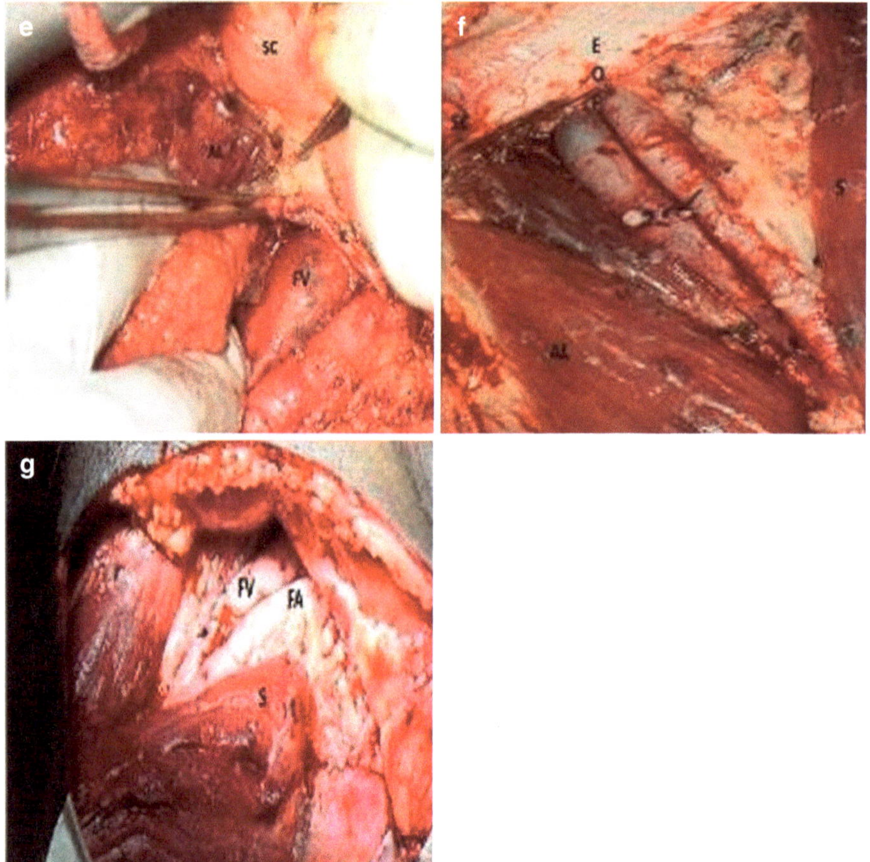

Fig.10.6 (continued)

Subsequently, an ipsilateral pelvic lymph node dissection was performed with the boundaries including the genitofemoral nerve laterally, the bladder medially, the ureters superiorly, and the Cloquet node within the femoral canal distally. Myocutaneous flap reconstruction by plastic surgeons was performed routinely to cover the exposed vasculature and to provide for rapid wound healing without tension. This may include transposition of the sartorius muscle, anterolateral thigh, or vertical rectus myocutaneous flap (Fig. 10.6b, g).

Perioperative care of such patients includes the use of prophylactic antibiotic therapy, deep venous thromboembolism prophylaxis (especially if immobilized due to myocutaneous flap reconstruction), and maintenance of closed suction drains until outputs are consistently less than 30 ml/day. The above procedures help in reducing the incidence of infection, venous thromboembolism, and seroma/abscess formation [3].

Data on surgical complications of post-chemotherapy surgery were reported with the results of the neoadjuvant clinical trial [42]. Adverse events were retrospectively scored, including hemorrhage, infection, edema (lower extremities, trunk, and genitalia), soft tissue necrosis, seroma, and/or abscess formation, and the need for secondary procedures to address adverse events. Acute and chronic complications were defined as those occurring within and after 30 days of the surgical resection, respectively, and are shown in Table 10.1. Overall the procedures were well tolerated among the cohort reported that underwent protocol-driven surgery. A single patient experienced a grade 4 episode of inguinal hemorrhage that was controlled with exploration. Other than this, the majority of episodes were related to infections requiring antibiotic therapy and mild to moderate scrotal and lower extremity edema and seroma formation [42].

While this chapter is focused on management of the inguinal region, we should briefly discuss the role of pelvic lymph node dissection and postoperative radiotherapy in the setting of advanced nodal disease. These topics are more fully discussed in other chapters. Patients in the prospective neoadjuvant clinical trial routinely underwent pelvic lymph node dissection on the involved side(s) [42]. It is unknown whether this contributed to observed progression-free survival or was of merely prognostic value by detecting residual disease. A randomized clinical trial would be informative on this question. Whether postoperative radiotherapy improves progression-free survival is also unproven. None of the patients in the prospective neoadjuvant study received adjuvant radiotherapy. With this strategy it is possible to use radiotherapy later in the event of recurrence for palliation. The potential benefit of adjuvant radiotherapy for patients at high risk of recurrence based on the extent of residual disease after neoadjuvant chemotherapy deserves further study.

Summary

Among patients with invasive penile cancer and no evidence of inguinal adenopathy, surgical decision making and procedures should focus on reliably detecting microscopic inguinal metastasis at the earliest possible timepoint among those patients that are truly node positive while minimizing complications among the truly node-negative cohort. DSNB is favorable in this regard but requires a dedicated team and specialized equipment and is best performed at specialized higher-volume centers. Superficial dissection with simultaneous frozen section analysis is an alternative strategy that is more readily accessible but has a higher complication rate than DSNB. In this regard laparoscopic/robotic techniques have been developed, but it remains to be determined whether they will be associated with a substantially lower complication rate when compared with superficial dissections. As the window for surgical cure of patients with inguinal metastases is relatively narrow, CT imaging and needle biopsy may allow us to detect those patients exhibiting palpable adenopathy who are at risk for failing surgical treatment alone. The feasibility and early efficacy of neoadjuvant chemotherapy suggests that such patients along with those exhibiting bulky inguinal metastases could benefit from this approach employed routinely. The relative benefits of this strategy as well as chemoradiation approaches in the definitive management of advanced penile cancer await further prospective clinical trials.

Table 10.1 Postsurgical complications among patients who completed four courses of neoadjuvant chemotherapy and then underwent lymphadenectomy ($N=22$)

Time of complication	Complication	Wound, noninfectious	Hemorrhage/bleeding, postoperative	Infection:skin	Edema: limb	Edema: trunk/ genital	Soft tissue necrosis	Seroma
Early (≤POD 30)	Grades 4–5	0 (0)	1 (4.5)[a]	0 (0)	0 (0)	0 (0)	0 (0)	0 (0)
	Grade 3	2 (9.1)	2 (9.1)	1 (4.5)	0 (0)	1 (4.5)	2 (9.1)	0 (0)
	Grades 1–2	3 (13.6)	0 (0)	0 (0)	6 (27.3)	2 (9.1)	2 (9.1)	1 (4.5)
Delayed (>POD 30)	Grades 4–5	0 (0)	0 (0)	0 (0)	0 (0)	0 (0)	0 (0)	0 (0)
	Grade 3	0 (0)	0 (0)	1 (4.5)	0 (0)	0 (0)	0 (0)	3 (13.6)
	Grade 1–2	0 (0)	0 (0)	2 (9.1)	5 (22.7)	2 (9.1)	0 (0)	0 (0)

Modified from Pagliaro et al. [42]

[a]One grade 4 hemorrhage was noted on postoperative day (POD) 2 and required operative intervention without further issue. All patients were assessed utilizing the Common Terminology Criteria version 3 Grade Assessment. Actual numbers followed by (%)

References

1. Johnson DE, Lo RK. Complications of groin dissection in penile cancer. Experience with 101 lymphadenectomies. Urology. 1984;24:312–4.
2. McDougal WS, Kirchner Jr FK, Edwards RH, et al. Treatment of carcinoma of the penis: the case for primary lymphadenectomy. J Urol. 1986;136:38–41.
3. Spiess PE, Hernandez MS, Pettaway CA. Contemporary inguinal node dissection: minimizing complications. World J Urol. 2009;27:205–12.
4. Kroon BK, Horenblas S, Lont AP, et al. Patients with penile carcinoma benefit from immediate resection of clinically occult lymph node metastases. J Urol. 2005;173:816–9.
5. Ravi R. Correlation between the extent of nodal involvement and survival following groin dissection for carcinoma of the penis. Br J Urol. 1993;72:817–9.
6. Srinivas V, Morse MJ, Herr HW, et al. Penile cancer: relation of extent of nodal metastasis to survival. J Urol. 1987;137:880–2.
7. Fosså SD, Hall KS, Johannessen MB, et al. Cancer of the penis. Experience at the Norwegian Radium Hospital 1974–1985. Eur Urol. 1987;13:372–7.
8. Fraley EE, Zhang G, Manivel C, et al. The role of ilioinguinal lymphadenectomy and significance of histological differentiation in treatment of carcinoma of the penis. J Urol. 1989;142:1478–82.
9. Horenblas S, van Tinteren H, Delemarre JF, et al. Squamous cell carcinoma of the penis: accuracy of tumor, nodes and metastases classification system and role of lymphangiography, computerized tomography scan, and fine needle aspiration cytology. J Urol. 1991; 146:1279–83.
10. Kroon BK, Horenblas S, Deurloo EE, et al. Ultrasonography-guided fine-needle aspiration cytology before sentinel node biopsy in patients with penile carcinoma. BJU Int. 2005;95:517–21.
11. Leijte JAP, Graafland NM, ZValdes Olmos RA, van Boven HH, Hoefnagel CA, Horenblas S. Prospective evaluation of hybrid 18 F-fluorodeoxyglucose positron emission tomography/ computed tomography in staging clinically node-negative patients with penile carcinoma. BJU Int. 2009;104(5):640–4.
12. Solsona E, Algaba F, Horenblas S, et al. EAU guidelines on penile cancer. Eur Urol. 2004;46:1–8.
13. Pizzocaro G, Algaba F, Horenblas S, et al. EAU penile cancer guidelines 2009. Eur Urol. 2010;57:1002.
14. Ficarra V, Zattoni F, Cunico SC, et al. Lymphatic and vascular embolizations are independent predictive variables of inguinal lymph node involvement in patients with squamous cell carcinoma of the penis: Gruppo Uro-Oncologico del Nord Est (Northeast Uro-Oncological Group) Penile Cancer data base data. Cancer. 2005;103:2507–16.
15. Ficarra V, Zattoni F, Artibani W, et al. Nomogram predictive of pathological inguinal lymph node involvement in patients with squamous cell carcinoma of the penis. J Urol. 2006;175:1700–4.
16. Johnson DE, Lo RK, Srigley J, et al. Verrucous carcinoma of the penis. J Urol. 1985;133:216–8.
17. Seixas ALC, Ornellas AA, Marota A, et al. Verrucous carcinoma of the penis: retrospective analysis of 32 cases. J Urol. 1994;152:1476–8.
18. Eng TY, Petersen JP, Stack RS, et al. Lymph node metastasis from carcinoma in situ of the penis: a case report. J Urol. 1995;153:432–4.
19. Pettaway CA, Lynch D, Davis J. Tumors of the penis. In: Wein AJ, Kavoussi LR, Novick AC, et al., editors. Campbell-Walsh urology. 9th ed. Philadelphia: WB Saunders; 2007. p. 959–92.
20. Solsona E, Iborra I, Ricós JV, et al. Corpus cavernosum invasion and tumor grade in the prediction of lymph node condition in penile carcinoma. Eur Urol. 1992;22:115–8.

21. Hall MC, Sanders JS, Vuitch F, et al. Deoxyribonucleic acid flow cytometry and traditional pathologic variables in invasive penile carcinoma: assessment of prognostic significance. Urology. 1998;52:111–6.
22. Theodorescu D, Russo P, Zhang ZF, et al. Outcomes of initial surveillance of invasive squamous cell carcinoma of the penis and negative nodes. J Urol. 1996;155:1626–31.
23. Leijte JA, Valdés Olmos RA, Nieweg OE, et al. Anatomical mapping of lymphatic drainage in penile carcinoma with SPECT-CT: implications for the extent of inguinal lymph node dissection. Eur Urol. 2008;54:885–90.
24. Edge SB, Byrd DR, Compton CC, et al. AJCC cancer staging manual. 7th ed. New York: Springer; 2010.
25. Pompeo ACL, Heyns CF, Abrams P. Penile cancer: International Consultation on Penile Cancer, Santiago, Chile. Montreal: Société Internationale d'Urologie (SIU); 2009.
26. Cubilla AL. The role of pathologic prognostic factors in squamous cell carcinoma of the penis. World J Urol. 2009;27:169–77.
27. Hughes BE, Leijte JAP, Kroon BK, et al. Lymph node metastasis in intermediate-risk penile squamous cell cancer: a two-centre experience. Eur Urol. 2010;57:688–92.
28. Leijte JAP, Kirrander P, Antonini N, et al. Recurrence patterns of squamous cell carcinoma of the penis: recommendations for follow-up based on a two-centre analysis of 700 patients. Eur Urol. 2008;54:161–8.
29. Kroon BK, Lont AP, Valdés Olmos RA, et al. Morbidity of dynamic sentinel node biopsy in penile carcinoma. J Urol. 2005;173:813–5.
30. Spiess PE, Izawa JI, Bassett R, et al. Preoperative lymphoscintigraphy and dynamic sentinel node biopsy for staging penile cancer: results with pathological correlation. J Urol. 2007;177:2157–61.
31. Kroon BK, Horenblas S, Estourgie SH, et al. How to avoid false-negative dynamic sentinel node procedures in penile carcinoma. J Urol. 2004;171:2191–4.
32. Leijte JAP, Hughes B, Graafland NM, et al. Two-center evaluation of dynamic sentinel node biopsy for squamous cell carcinoma of the penis. J Clin Oncol. 2009;27:3325–9.
33. Pompeo AC, Mesquita JL, Junior WA, et al. Staged inguinal lymphadenectomy (SIL) for carcinoma of the penis (CP). A 13 years prospective study of 50 patients. J Urol. 1995;153(suppl):246A, abstract 72.
34. Puras-Baez A, Rivera-Herrera J, Miranda G, et al. Role of superficial inguinal lymphadenectomy in carcinoma of the penis. J Urol. 1995;153(suppl):246A, abstract 71.
35. Sotelo R, Sánchez-Salas R, Carmona O, et al. Endoscopic lymphadenectomy for penile carcinoma. J Endourol. 2007;21:364–7.
36. Tobias-Machado M, Tavares A, Ornellas AA, et al. Video endoscopic inguinal lymphadenectomy: a new minimally invasive procedure for radical management of inguinal nodes in patients with penile squamous cell carcinoma. J Urol. 2007;177:953–7.
37. Matin SF, Cormier JN, Ward JF, Pisters LL, Wood CG, Dinney CP, Royal RE, Huang X, Pettaway CA. Phase 1 prospective evaluation of the oncological adequacy of robotic assisted video-endoscopic inguinal lymphadenectomy in patients with penile carcinoma. BJU Int. 2013;111(7):1068–74.
38. Sotelo R, Sanchez-Salas R, Clavijo R. Endoscopic inguinal lymph node dissection for penile carcinoma: the developing of a novel technique. World J Urol. 2009;27:213–9.
39. Master VA, Mohammad S, Jafri A, Moses K, Ogan K, Kooby D, Delman KA. Minimally invasive inguinal lymphadenectomy via endoscopic groin dissection: comprehensive assessment of immediate and long-term complications. J Urol. 2012;188:1176–80.
40. Graafland NM, van Boven HH, van Werkhoven E, Moonen LMF, Horenblas S. Prognostic significance of extranodal extension in patients with pathological node positive penile carcinoma. J Urol. 2011;184(4):1347–53.
41. Leijte JAP, Kerst JM, Bais E, Antonini N, Horenblas S. Neoadjuvant chemotherapy in advanced penile carcinoma. Eur Urol. 2007;52:488–94.
42. Pagliaro LC, Williams DL, Daliani D, Williams MB, Osai W, Kincaid M, Wen S, Thall P, Pettaway CA. Neoadjuvant paclitaxel, ifosfamide, and cisplatin chemotherapy for metastatic penile cancer: a phase II study. J Clin Oncol. 2010;28:3851–7.

43. Graafland NM, Teertstra HJ, Besnard PE, van Boven HH, Horenblas S. Identification of high risk pathological node positive penile carcinoma: value of preoperative computerized tomography imaging. J Urol. 2011;185:881–7.
44. Saisorn I, Lawrentschuk N, Leewansangtong S, Bolton D. Fine-needle aspiration cytology predicts inguinal lymph node metastasis without antibiotic pretreatment in penile carcinoma. BJU Int. 2006;97:1225–8.
45. Pettaway CA, Pagliaro L, Theodore C, Haas G. Treatment of visceral, unresectable, or bulky/unresectable regional metastases of penile cancer. Urology. 2010;76:S58–65.
46. Ornellas AA, et al. Surgical treatment of invasive squamous cell carcinoma of the penis: Brazilian National Cancer Institute long-term experience. J Surg Oncol. 2008;97(6):487–95.
47. Theodore C, Skoneczna I, Bodrogi I, Leahy M, Kerst JM, Collette L, Ven K, Marreaud S, Oliver RDT. A phase II multicentre study of irinotecan (CPT 11) in combination with cisplatin (CDDP) in metastatic or locally advanced penile carcinoma (EORTC PROTOCOL 30992). Ann Oncol. 2008;19:1304–7.
48. Bermejo C, Busby JE, Spiess PE, Heller L, Pagliaro LC, Pettaway CA. Neoadjuvant chemotherapy followed by aggressive surgical consolidation for metastatic penile squamous cell carcinoma. J Urol. 2007;177(4):1335–8.
49. Bevan-Thomas R, Slaton JW, Pettaway CA. Contemporary morbidity from lymphadenectomy for penile squamous cell carcinoma: The M. D. Anderson Cancer Center experience. J Urol. 2002;167:1638–42.

Chapter 11
Primary and Adjuvant Radiation Therapy in the Management of Penile Cancer

Özer Algan and Juanita Crook

Abbreviations

BT	Brachytherapy
CSS	Cause-specific survival/cancer-specific survival
DFS	Disease-free survival
EBRT	External beam radiation therapy
HDR	High dose rate
IMRT	Intensity-modulated radiation therapy
LC	Local control
LDR	Low dose rate
LN	Lymph node
OS	Overall survival
PDR	Pulsed dose rate
SCC	Squamous cell carcinoma

Introduction

Carcinoma of the penis is an uncommon tumor that is almost exclusively limited to uncircumcised men. In the United States, the incidence of penile cancer is low with an estimated 1,570 new cases and 310 deaths occurring from penile and other rare

Ö. Algan, MD (✉)
Department of Radiation Oncology, Stephenson Cancer Center,
University of Oklahoma Health Sciences Center,
800 NE 10th St., OKCC L100, Oklahoma City, OK 73104, USA
e-mail: oalgan@ouhsc.edu

J. Crook, MD, FRCPC
Department of Radiation Oncology, Cancer Center for the Southern Interior,
British Columbia Cancer Agency, University of British Columbia,
399 Royal Avenue, Kelowna, BC, Canada

D.J. Culkin (ed.), *Management of Penile Cancer*,
DOI 10.1007/978-1-4939-0461-7_11,

genital cancers in 2013 [2]. Compared to Western countries, the incidence of penile cancer is higher in other regions of the world such as India, China, Brazil, and Uganda [64, 65].

Over 95 % of penile cancers are squamous cell carcinomas (SCC), but other types include basal cell carcinoma, melanoma, sarcoma, and lymphoma. Subtypes of squamous cell carcinoma include classic, basaloid, verrucous, sarcomatoid, and adenosquamous carcinomas. Of these subtypes, verrucous tumors tend to have the best prognosis with the lowest risk of spread or local recurrence. Metastases to the penis from prostate cancer or lymphoma have been reported in the literature, although it is a rare occurrence [8, 29, 54]. The majority of tumors involving the penis are primary penile cancers with SCC histology.

At the time of presentation, up to 50 % of patients have inguinal lymph node involvement [7, 59, 63]. Because of the rich lymphatics and the central location of the penis, involvement is often bilateral. Traditionally, for early stage penile cancer, the gold standard has been surgical resection. Depending on the stage of the tumor, surgery provides local control rates in the range of 80–90 % [33, 49]. Local control decreases with increasing tumor size. The strongest prognostic factor for survival is nodal stage, but patients with low inguinal tumor burden (0–1 positive nodes, no extracapsular extension) still have a favorable outcome in 80 % of cases [27, 28, 35, 51, 72]. Despite these favorable outcomes, surgical intervention, and in particular penectomy, can have significant psychosocial impact on patients to the extent that suicides have been reported after penectomy [77]. Because of the quality of life and psychosocial impact of penectomy, various organ-preserving treatment options have been developed. These include glans-sparing surgery, laser therapy, brachytherapy, or external beam radiation therapy, among others. In this chapter, the role of radiation therapy in the management of patients with penile cancer will be reviewed.

Workup/Staging

Workup

Initial assessment involves a detailed physical examination. The location, appearance (exophytic vs. ulcerative), size, and depth of invasion for the lesion need to be carefully evaluated and documented. Examination of the inguinal region is required, as the presence of inguinal lymphadenopathy has a significant impact on prognosis, choice of treatment modality, and outcome. A biopsy is required to confirm the diagnosis of cancer as well as to assess the depth of invasion. Biopsy will also provide information about the grade of the tumor, as well as the presence or absence of lymphovascular invasion.

Various imaging studies including US, CT scan, PET/CT, and MRI scans have been used to evaluate the extent of disease (Fig. 11.1). Ultrasound can be used to

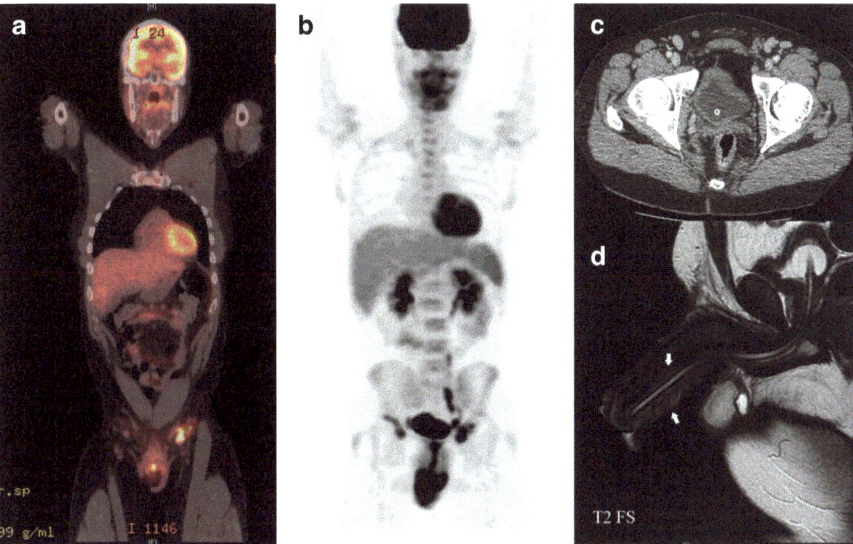

Fig. 11.1 Imaging studies including (**a**, **b**) PET/CT scan, (**c**) diagnostic CT scan, and (**d**) sagittal MRI scan of a patient with a suspected T3N3M0 penile cancer extending into the urethra and suspicious inguinal and iliac lymph nodes. PET/CT imaging (**a**, **b**) demonstrates increased FDG update in the region of the penis, as well as the bilateral inguinal and the left iliac region. Diagnostic CT scan (**c**) demonstrates inguinal lymphadenopathy. (**d**) MRI of the penis demonstrates a large mass extending into the urethra (*arrows*)

assess the depth of invasion of the primary tumor, but its role in evaluation of the inguinal regions, especially for clinically negative lymph nodes, is limited. CT scans have a limited role in evaluating the primary tumor and depth of invasion, but are often used to evaluate inguinal and pelvic lymph nodes, despite a high false-negative rate due to the inability to detect micrometastases in normal-sized nodes [34]. There is limited information in the use of PET/CT in penile cancer [36, 75, 78, 82], but a meta-analysis from 2012 suggested a pooled sensitivity and specificity of 81 and 92 %, respectively. The sensitivity was considerably better in clinically node-positive patients than in clinically node negative [75]. MRI may be best suited for evaluating the primary for depth of invasion as well as for the presence of multifocality [42]. MRI has similar spatial resolution as CT for imaging of clinically negative lymph nodes. The use of lymphotropic nanoparticle as a part of the MRI study may help overcome some of these limitations [84].

Staging

The two most common staging systems for penile cancer include the Jackson staging system [40] and the AJCC/UICC TNM staging system [20]. Both are shown in Table 11.1.

Table 11.1 Summary of the Jackson and the AJCC/UICC staging systems for penile cancer

Jackson staging system [40]			
Stage I	Cancer confined to glans or prepuce		
Stage II	Cancer invades into shaft or corpora		
Stage III	Operable inguinal lymph node metastasis		
Stage IV	Tumor invades adjacent structures or there are inoperable inguinal lymph nodes		
AJCC/UICC staging system, 7th edition [20]			
T0	No evidence of primary tumor		
Tis	Carcinoma in situ		
Ta	Noninvasive verrucous carcinoma		
T1a	Tumor invades subepithelial connective tissue without lymphovascular invasion and is not poorly differentiated		
T1b	Tumor invades subepithelial connective tissue with lymphovascular invasion or is poorly differentiated		
T2	Tumor invades corpus spongiosum or cavernosum		
T3	Tumor invades urethra		
T4	Tumor invades other adjacent structures		
N0	No palpable or visible enlarged inguinal lymph nodes		
N1	Palpable, mobile, single unilateral inguinal lymph nodes		
N2	Palpable, mobile, multiple or bilateral inguinal lymph nodes		
N3	Palpable, fixed, inguinal nodal mass or pelvic lymphadenopathy (unilateral or bilateral)		
M0	No distant metastases		
M1	Distant metastases		
Stage groupings			
Stage 0	Tis, Ta	N0	M0
Stage I	T1a	N0	M0
Stage II	T1b-T3	N0	M0
Stage IIIA	T1-3	N1	M0
Stage IIIB	T1-3	N2	M0
Stage IV	T4	Any N	M0
	Any T	N3	M0
	Any T	Any N	M1

Used with the permission of the American Joint Committee on Cancer (AJCC), Chicago, Illinois. The original source for this material is the AJCC Cancer Staging Manual, Seventh Edition (2010) published by Springer Science and Business Media LLC, www.springer.com

Since much of the literature for radiation therapy spans several decades, it is important to be aware of the differences in the older staging systems. The UICC TNM 3rd edition was published in 1978 and used tumor size and, to a lesser degree, depth of invasion as the main determinants of T-stage (T1, ≤2 cm and superficial; T2, >2 cm and ≤5 cm; T3, >5 cm or with deep invasion including urethra; and T4, invasion of adjacent structures) [39]. The main difference between the 3rd and 4th editions has been the change from size-based tumor staging to one based on the depth of invasion [30]. Since the 4th edition, there have not been any significant changes in the staging for penile cancer in the AJCC/UICC staging systems.

Prognostic Factors

The most important prognostic factors include the size and extent of the primary lesion, tumor grade, and the presence of inguinal and pelvic lymphadenopathy. The risk of nodal involvement increases with tumor size and depth of invasion [59]. Several studies have also demonstrated that tumor grade impacts the risk of local relapse and lymph node metastases as well as survival [11, 15, 61, 69, 77]. The most important factor predicting survival is the presence and extent of lymph node metastases. Because lymph node metastases tend to occur in a stepwise fashion, and skip metastases to the pelvis are uncommon, patients with early superficial inguinal metastases may not have significantly diminished outcome. However, as the inguinal lymphatic tumor burden increases or with the presence of pelvic node metastases, outcomes worsen significantly [45, 47, 48, 61, 70, 81, 86]. Other risk factors include the presence of vascular invasion and histologic subtype [22, 79].

Based on these risk factors, patients can be classified into risk groups. Various classification systems have been developed [10, 37, 38, 55, 70]. From a treatment outcome perspective, low risk would include patients with T1 tumors, low-grade histology, and negative inguinal lymph nodes. Locally advanced disease would include T3–T4 tumors; multiple, large, or matted inguinal lymph nodes; extracapsular extension; or extension to pelvic LNs. Various risk stratification systems have been developed to estimate the risk of pathologic inguinal node involvement in the setting of clinically negative nodes [38, 55, 70]. In general, patients with Tis, Ta, or T1G1 tumors are considered low risk and surveillance is recommended. Patients with T1G2 tumors are considered intermediate risk, and evaluation of additional risk factors such as the presence of perineural and lymphovascular invasion, tumor size, and depth of invasion is recommended to better estimate the risk of inguinal lymph node involvement. Any tumor greater than T1 or grade 2 is considered high risk and lymph node evaluation with either dynamic sentinel node biopsy or lymphadenectomy is recommended.

Treatment of Penile Cancer with Radiation Therapy

Radiotherapy allows the potential for organ-sparing in the management of early stage and locally advanced penile cancer. Although penectomy, either partial or complete, provides excellent local control, it is associated with considerable psychological and sexual morbidity [57, 60]. Because of this, there is a growing trend towards organ-sparing treatment as reflected in the updated European Association of Urology guidelines [80]. The purpose of using radiation therapy for organ sparing is to achieve similar treatment outcomes to penectomy while maintaining organ function and reducing morbidity [58].

For most early stage penile cancers, radiation treatment is performed with either brachytherapy or megavoltage treatment machines. The only exception to this may be a small superficial noninvasive tumor, which could potentially be treated with more superficial radiation therapy utilizing a hypofractionated regimen [12, 53]. This type of treatment should be reserved for carefully selected patients with early stage tumors, the majority of whom can be treated with organ-sparing surgical techniques or laser therapy. The choice between external beam radiation and brachytherapy depends on the location and size of the tumor as well as availability of equipment and expertise [12]. External beam radiation has the advantage of being more readily available and producing a more homogenous dose distribution with a larger margin around the tumor. Brachytherapy has the advantage of greater conformality and a shorter treatment time. Most of the published reports on brachytherapy have used either low dose rate (LDR) or pulsed dose rate (PDR) brachytherapy. PDR requires an automated afterloading system to deliver hourly pulses of radiation similar to what is delivered in 1 h of continuous LDR and as such is considered radiobiologically equivalent.

In more advanced penile cancers, a combined modality approach is recommended. The management of the primary tumor depends on size and location. For smaller, distal primary tumors, organ-preserving treatment may still be an option. For larger tumors, surgery is recommended. Partial penectomy may be possible for more distal lesions, especially if sufficient penile length can be spared to allow direction of the urinary stream. For more proximal tumors extending into the membranous urethra, or large tumors where complete resection is not possible, a combined modality approach is recommended. Neoadjuvant therapy may reduce the tumor burden sufficiently to make surgery feasible. If surgery is not an option, then treatment can be completed with radiation therapy alone or combined with chemotherapy. The data for chemoradiation therapy in the setting of advanced penile cancer is limited [4], but an international cooperative trial is being developed through the International Rare Cancers Initiative. Chemoradiation has been used in other lower pelvic tumors including vulvar cancer and anal cancer as well as other nonpelvic sites such as head and neck, lung, and gastrointestinal malignancies. Likewise, the role of adjuvant radiation therapy is unclear, but a number of studies have utilized adjuvant RT in the setting of positive margins or positive lymph nodes, especially if multiple lymph nodes or lymph nodes with extracapsular extension are present [11, 45].

Prior to any penile irradiation, with either external beam or brachytherapy, circumcision should be performed to expose the lesion to allow full evaluation and also to prevent treatment side effects [4, 12, 52]. The irradiated foreskin is prone to fibrosis, contracture, and subsequent phimosis.

Management of the Primary with Radiation Therapy

There are no randomized studies comparing outcomes between various treatment modalities. Most reports are single institution series with a limited number of patients.

Brachytherapy

The data for brachytherapy comes from various institutions across the world including Canada, France, India, and Brazil and includes treatments using low dose rate iridium (Ir-192) wires or strands, pulsed dose rate automated afterloading, or fractionated high dose rate treatments. Table 11.2 summarizes the literature evaluating the use of brachytherapy. For patients undergoing low dose rate brachytherapy, the 5-year local control rates range from 73 to 86 % [9, 15, 17–19, 43, 52, 74, 81, 83]. Both the prescribed total dose and the hourly dose rate vary from study to study, with the most common prescription dose being 60 Gy delivered at 0.40–0.60 Gy per hour. Factors affecting local control include tumor stage, grade, depth of invasion, and needle spacing [15, 19, 43, 69, 74]. Local control decreases with increasing stage, increasing grade, and increasing depth of invasion. Local control is improved with wider needle spacing secondary to the resulting larger margin and greater depth of treatment in accordance with the Paris system.

The penile preservation rate for patients undergoing LDR brachytherapy ranges from 68 to 88 % at 5 years. The most commonly reported side effects from brachytherapy include soft tissue ulceration and meatal stenosis. As shown in Table 11.2, the risk of nonhealing ulceration varies from 3 to 26 % and the risk of stenosis varies from 7 to 47 %. Factors associated with worsening toxicity include higher brachytherapy dose rate, larger tumor size/volume of implant, and higher total treatment dose [18, 23, 52, 83].

The 5-year overall survival (OS), cause-specific survival (CSS), and disease-free survival (DFS) range from 50 to 90 %, 84 to 92 % (5–10 years), and 43 to 63 %, respectively, depending on the tumor stage and risk group (Table 11.2). Despite the lower disease-free survival rates, there is no significant impact on cancer-specific survival because of the high rates of successful surgical salvage for tumor recurrence. Factors affecting survival include tumor extension into the corpus callosum, nodal stage, Jackson stage, and histologic subtype [81].

Several authors have published results of LDR brachytherapy. Crook et al. reported on 67 patients with squamous cell carcinoma of the penis, including tumor size up to 5 cm. Thirty-five percent of the patients had well-differentiated tumors, 43 % were moderately differentiated, and the rest were poorly differentiated. All were initially clinically node negative. Treatment consisted of 2- or 3-plane implant using predrilled Lucite templates. The radiation was delivered using either LDR iridium 192 wire or an automated afterloading unit administering hourly pulses of 0.50–0.65 Gy (PDR), for a total dose of 60 Gy over 4–5 days. The PDR regimen delivered the same hourly dose as classic LDR brachytherapy and several studies have suggested equivalence in terms of the delivered biological effective dose [3, 24]. The 5- and 10-year freedoms from local failure rates were 87.3 and 72.3 %. At a median follow-up of 48 months, 8 patients had local failures, all of whom underwent salvage surgery. The 5- and 10-year penile preservation rates were 87 and 67.3 %, respectively. In patients who required surgical salvage, the prior course of brachytherapy did not impair healing. On univariate analysis, needle spacing was

Table 11.2 Treatment results with brachytherapy

Author	*N*	FU (months)	Patient population	Treatment	Dose (Gy)	CSS (5 years)	DFS (5 years)	Reg failure	Local control	Penile preservation rate	Complications
Chaudhery et al. [9]	23	24 (4–117)	7 T1 7 T2 9 recurrent	LDR BT Int	50 (40–60)	–	–	–	70 % (8 years)	70 % (8 years)	No necrosis 2/23 stenosis
Crook et al. [15]	67	48 (4–194)	52 % T1	LDR BT Int	60	83.6 %	71 % 5 years	11 regional or DM	87.3 % (5 years)	88 (5 years)	12 % necrosis
			33 % T2 Select T3				59 % 10 years (RFS)		72.3 % (10 years)	67 % (10 years)	9 % stenosis
Daly et al. [17]	22	–	6 T1 14 T2 2 T3	LDR BT Int	–	3/22 DOD	–	–	1 local failure	19/22	2 necrosis 47 % stenosis
Delannes et al. [19]	51	65 (12–144)	17 T1 28 T2 6 T3, 8 LN+	LDR BT Int	50–65	85 %		12 %	86 % (crude)	75 %	23 % necrosis 45 % stenosis
DeCrevoisier et al. [18]	144	68 (6–348)	N0 or Nx	LDR BT Int	65	92 % (10 years)	78.5 % (10 years)	11 % 10 years, 6 % DM	80 % (10 years)	72 % (10 years)	26 % necrosis 29 % stenosis
Kiltie et al. [43]	31	61.5	27 stage I, 4 stage II	LDR BT Int	63.5	85.4 %	85.4 %	7/31 pt	81 %	75 %	8 % necrosis 44 % stenosis
Mazeron et al. [52]	50	(36–96)	9 T1, 27 T2, 14 T3; 5 LN+	LDR BT Int	60–70	79 %	63 %	–	78 % crude	74 %	3 % necrosis, 16 % stenosis
Rozan et al. [74]	184	139	–	LDR BT Int	59 (mean)	88 % (5 years) 88 % (10 years)	78 % 5 years 67 % 10 years	–	85 %	76 %	21 % necrosis 45 % stenosis

Soria et al. [81]	102	111	69 stage I, 17 stage II, 15 stage III	35 BT 35 LE+BT, 32 others	61–70	72 % (5 years) 66 % (10 years)	56 % 5 years 42 % 10 years	–	89 % CR 4.1 % PR 4 % others	68 % (brachy grp)	1 necrosis 1 stenosis
Suchaud et al. [83]	53	> 10 years	7 T1 32 T2 15 T3 16 LN+	LDR BT Int	–	–	–	–	11 penile recur	31/53 pt	15 severe complication (necrosis or stenosis)
Akimoto et al. [1]	15	84	8 T1 5 T2 2 T3	HDR BT mold	32–74	1 pt DOD	–	–	80 %	73 %	–
Neave et al. [56]	44	–	–	24 mold BT 20 EBRT	–	–	–	–	–	Similar	13 % stenosis (BT) 10 % stenosis (EBRT)
Petera et al. [66]	10	20	Early penile cancer	HDR BT	BID 3Gy × 18	–	100 %	–	100 %	100 %	No necrosis No stenosis

All results are at 5 years unless otherwise noted

FU is median follow-up time. *LE* local excision, *BT* brachytherapy, *OS* overall survival, *CSS* cause-specific survival, *DFS* disease-free survival, *DM* distant metastases, *DOD* dead of disease the only significant factor affecting local control. For every unit increase in needle spacing, there was a 52 % reduction in local recurrence. A total of 11 patients developed regional or distant metastases. All patients with regional recurrence underwent lymph node dissection and two patients also received radiotherapy for multiple positive nodes or extracapsular disease. The 5- and 10-year relapse-free survival rates were 71 and 59 %, respectively. Approximately one-third of recurrences occurred after 5 years. Tumor grade was the only factor significant for RFS on univariate analysis. The 5- and 10-year CSS in this series were both 84 % [15].

DeCrevoisler et al. reported on 144 patients clinically N0 or Nx treated with brachytherapy alone. Brachytherapy consisted of an LDR "hypodermic needle technique" using iridium wires. The median prescribed dose was 65 Gy delivered at a dose rate of 0.4 Gy/h. The median implant volume was 22 cc. The 10-year local recurrence rate was 20 %. Late recurrences, occurring after 8 years, were noted in 20 % of patients. When taking salvage into account, the 10-year local control rate was 86 % and the 10-year penile preservation rate was 72 %. The treatment volume greater than 22 cc (relative risk 1.02, p value 0.005) and reference isodose rate greater than 0.6 Gy/h (relative risk 9.17, p value 0.008) were associated with increased risk of toxicity on multivariate analysis. They recommended using a needle spacing of 15 mm. A total of seven patients required surgery for necrosis. The 10-year overall and cause-specific survival rates were 65 and 92 %, respectively [18].

Mazeron et al. reported on 50 patients treated with LDR brachytherapy using Ir-192 wires with a prescribed dose of 60–70 Gy. Local control was achieved in 39 of 50 patients. Two of eleven recurrences occurred after 5 years. In the 11 patients that developed a local recurrence, 10 underwent salvage surgery, and 7 were salvaged successfully for an overall local control rate of 46 of 50. At the time of last follow-up, 74 % of the patients were disease-free with penile preservation. In their series, three patients developed necrosis, two of whom required partial amputation, and eight patients developed meatal stenosis, three of whom required surgery. They noted increased risk of stenosis in patients with local control when they were treated to doses greater than 63 Gy (41.7 % vs. 53.8 %, p value not significant). At last follow-up, 74 % were free of disease with conservation of penile morphology and function. Twenty-one percent of patients died of their disease for a 5-year CSS of 79 %. They recommended brachytherapy for patients with noninvasive or moderately invasive SCC of the penis 4 cm or less in size. Preimplant circumcision was recommended to reduce the risk of treatment-related side effects [52].

One of the largest series in the literature was the cooperative report by Rozan et al. in 1995, with a total of 259 patients, 184 of whom were treated with brachytherapy alone. The mean brachytherapy dose for this group of patients was 63 Gy. The 5-year local control and penile preservation rates were 85 and 76 %, respectively. Increasing size and depth of invasion significantly reduced local control. The addition of surgery or external beam RT did not improve local control when compared to brachytherapy alone. There was a 53 % late complication rate for the entire patient population, some of whom also received surgery (56 patients) or external beam radiation therapy (26 patients) as a part of their definitive treatment. Overall,

65 patients developed necrosis and 79 patients developed stenosis. The 10-year overall survival rate and cause-specific survival rates were 52 and 88 %, respectively. The nodal status impacted CSS [74].

There are few studies evaluating the use of non-LDR equivalent treatments such as fractionated medium dose rate (MDR) or high dose rate (HDR) brachytherapy treatments [1, 56, 66]. Akimoto et al. [1] reported on 15 patients treated with an HDR mold technique to a dose of 32–74 Gy given at an average dose rate of 2.00 Gy/h. At a median follow-up of 7 years, they reported an 80 % local control rate and a 73 % penile preservation rate. Overall, 1 of 15 patients died from their disease. Petera et al. [66] reported on 10 patients with early penile cancer treated with HDR brachytherapy using a breast interstitial template. The prescribed dose was 54 Gy given in 18 fractions using twice-a-day treatment regimen. At a median FU of 20 months, they reported a 100 % local control rate and a 100 % penile preservation rate with no incidence of necrosis or severe stenosis. All implants were single plane and these results may not be transferrable to multiplane larger volume implants.

Various conclusions can be drawn from these studies. Brachytherapy provides excellent local control, in the range of 80 %, with an associated high organ preservation rate of 65–80 %. For those patients that develop a local recurrence, surgical salvage is often successful, resulting in ultimate local control and cause-specific survival rates that are comparable to primary surgery. Although the presence of high-grade tumor can impact prognosis and increase the risk of inguinal metastases, it is not a contraindication for brachytherapy when appropriate treatment to the inguinal region is also delivered. Even though the majority of recurrences are early, in approximately 20–30 % of patients, recurrences will occur after 5 years [15, 18, 52]. This emphasizes the importance of continued long-term follow-up.

IMRT/EBRT

The results of external beam radiation in the management of primary penile cancer are shown in Table 11.3. The local control rates range from 50 to 70 % and penile preservation varies from 55 to 66 % for invasive cancers. Factors predicting worse local control include a total dose less than 60 Gy, daily fraction size less than 2 Gy, and an overall treatment time greater than 45 days [77, 86]. The assessment of regional control is more difficult, since some of the studies included patients with positive inguinal lymph nodes. This issue will be discussed in more detail in the next section.

The survival results for patients treated with external beam radiation therapy are shown in Table 11.3. For invasive cancers, the 5-year OS rates range from 57 to 88 %. In subset analysis, the overall survival rates for T1 N0 or T2 N0 disease are as high as 90–100 %. For invasive cancer, the cause-specific rate varies from 66 to 96 %. The necrosis and stenosis rates reported with external beam radiation therapy are in the range of 1–12 % for necrosis and 6–29 % for stenosis.

Table 11.3 Treatment outcomes with external beam radiation therapy

Author	*N*	FU (months)	Patient population	Rx	RT dose	CSS (5 years)	DFS (5 years)	Regional control (5 years)	Local control (5 years)	Penile preservation rate (5 years)	Complications
Azrif et al. [5]	41	54	37 T1 4 T2 1 LN+	EBRT	50–52.5Gy in 16 fx	96	51 % (RFS)	88 %	62 %	62 %	8 % necrosis 29 % stenosis
Gotsadze et al. [26]	155	78 (3–168)	51 T1 N0 73 T2 N0 10 T3 N1 2 T2 N1 10 T2 N2 1 T2 N3, and 2 T3 N2	EBRT	40–60Gy to primary 30–50Gy to groins	88 %	–	–	65 %	65 %	1 % necrosis 7 % stenosis
McLean et al. [53]	26	116 (84–168)	19 T1 4 T2 2 T3 1 T4 7 LN pos	EBRT	25/10–60/25	69 %	15/26	–	61.5 %	66 %	27 % unspecified
McLean et al. [53]	11	116	In situ SCC	EBRT	25/10–60/25	100 %	100 %	–	100 %	100 %	–
Mistry et al. [54]	18[a]/65	62	13 T1 3 T2 1 T3	EBRT	50/20–55/16	85 %[b]	63 % (RFS)	–	63 %	66 % crude	2 pt necrosis 1 pt stenosis
Neave et al. [56]	20	36 min	–	EBRT	50–55Gy in 20–22 fx	58 %	–	–	69.7 %	–	10 % stenosis
Ozsahin et al. [61]	33[a]/60	62 (6–450)	–	EBRT	52	53 % 10 years	–	36 % (LRC)	44 %	52 %	10 % stenosis

Ravi et al. [73]	128[a]/285	83	65 T1 50 T2 39 T3	EBRT	50–60	–	84 % (for entire grp)	–	65 % RT alone (additional 33 % salvage)	–	6 % necrosis 24 % strictures
Sarin et al. [77]	59[a]/101	62 (2–264)	79 T1 19 LN+ 2 DM	EBRT	60/30 (40–78.4)	66 % 5 years, 57 % 10 years	–	35/59	60 % 5 years 55 % 10 years	55 % (10 years)	3 % necrosis 14 % stenosis
Zouhair et al. [86]	23[a]/41	70	12 T1 24 T2 4 T3 1Tx 12 LN+	EBRT	60/30 (45–74)	–	63 % relapsed	48 % 5 years 33 % 10 years (LRC)	57 % 5 years 39 % 10 years	36 % entire grp 18 % RT grp	10 % stenosis

All results are at 5 years unless otherwise noted

FU is median follow-up time. *EBRT* external beam radiation therapy, *CSS* cause-specific survival, *DFS* disease-free survival

[a]Subset of patients from the entire study population treated with external beam RT

[b]Number read from graph

Ravi et al. reported on 285 patients between 1959 and 1988, 120 of whom had positive inguinal lymph nodes. A subset of 128 of these patients were treated with external beam radiation, including deep x-rays in 28, cesium 137 in 61, and cobalt 60 x-ray unit in 45 patients. A wooden jig was used for positioning of all patients, and either a single AP field or opposed fields were used. The treatment dose was 50–60 Gy to the primary. For patients with large pelvic lymph nodes (>4 cm), 40 Gy in 4 weeks was given preoperatively, followed by lymphadenectomy. The inguinal region was, otherwise, managed with primary lymphadenectomy. With a median follow-up of 83 months, the 5-year local control rate with RT alone was 65 %. An additional 33 % of patients were salvaged with either total or partial penectomy. The local recurrence rate for T1 tumors was 12 %, for T2 was 25 %, for T3 was 50–55 %, and for T4, local failure occurred in 2 of 2 patients. The significant complication rate included 6 % necrosis and 24 % urethral strictures. The overall survival in this group of patients was over 90 % for T1 and T2 tumors and 50–60 % for T3 and T4 tumors. The authors recommended RT alone for T1 and T2 tumors and surgical treatment with or without adjuvant radiation therapy for T3/T4 tumors [73].

Gotsadze et al. reported on 155 patients treated with external beam radiation therapy over four decades. Fifty-one patients had T1 N0 disease, and 73 had T2N0 disease. The remainder had positive lymph nodes. All patients were treated to the primary and the inguinal lymph nodes on a cobalt 60 treatment unit. Radiation dose was 50–60 Gy in 2 Gy fractions to the primary and 30–50 Gy to the bilateral inguinal LNs using a single AP field. Overall, 63 % achieved a complete response. Efficacy of radiation therapy was associated with tumor stage, with CR in 89.4 % of T1 disease compared to 53.5 % for T2 and 8.3 % for T3 ($p<0.05$). Local recurrence occurred in 15 patients. Nine of 10 local recurrences were salvaged with surgical resection and 2 of 5 patients with both local and inguinal recurrences were salvaged with surgery. The overall penile preservation rate was 64.5 %. The 5- and 10-year cause-specific survival rates were 85 and 82 %, respectively [26].

Ozsahin reported on a series of 60 patients, 29 of whom received definitive radiation therapy. Treatment consisted of external beam alone in 21 patients, external beam with a brachytherapy boost in 7 patients, and brachytherapy alone in 1 patient. The treatment volume included the regional nodes in 19 patients. The median dose to the penis was 52 Gy (range 26–74.5 Gy) given in 1.8–2.0 Gy fractions. The brachytherapy boost consisted of 15–25 Gy using LDR brachytherapy with Ir-192 wire at a dose rate of 0.50–1.00 Gy/h. In their analysis, 4 patients that refused postoperative RT were included in the radiation group. Local failure was noted in 19 of the 33 patients, at a median of 14 months. The higher recurrence rate was related to the low prescribed dose for the primary tumor. Regardless, 73 % of patients who developed local recurrence were successfully salvaged with surgery. Local control with penile preservation was 39 %, but the overall penile preservation rate was 52 % when organ-sparing salvage surgery was taken into account. Ten percent developed severe urethral stenosis. The treatment modality (surgery vs. EBRT) appeared to impact local control but not cause-specific survival. The 10-year CSS for patients treated with definitive RT with salvage surgery for local recurrence and primary surgery with or without adjuvant postoperative RT was 56 and 53 %, respectively ($p=0.16$) [61].

Azrif et al. reported on 41 patients treated with a hypofractionated radiation therapy regimen. Thirty-seven patients had T1 tumors, and 4 had T2. One patient had positive lymph nodes. Treatment consisted of external beam radiation to a dose of 50–52 Gy in 16 fractions over 22 days using a 4 MV linear accelerator. The local control rate and penile preservation rates were both 62 %. All patients developing a local recurrence were salvaged with surgery. They noted an 8 % penile ulceration rate and a 29 % urethral stenosis rate. No patient required a penectomy for necrosis. The 5-year overall survival rate was 88 % and CSS was 96 %.

There are very limited reports evaluating the use of adjuvant therapy to the primary after surgical resection. The most common indications for postoperative radiation therapy to the penis include close or positive margins or deep invasion. However, in the setting of limited data, treatment recommendations need to be individualized.

It is difficult to summarize the results for external beam radiation therapy in the treatment of penile cancer. In general, patients selected for external beam radiation therapy tend to have either more advanced disease or poorer health and are therefore not surgical candidates. The external beam radiation literature contains more heterogeneous patient populations and treatment techniques, especially since the series span several decades over which time there have been vast technological improvements in radiation therapy. Techniques have progressed from using kV and cobalt units to high-energy linear accelerators with CT-based treatment planning. This permits planning and delivery of radiation in a more conformal 3-dimensional fashion, especially with the use of techniques such as intensity-modulated radiation therapy. Similarly, the ability to verify patient setup has improved with the use of on-board imagers and cone beam CT scans. These advances are likely to be associated with improved treatment outcomes and reduced side effects from external beam radiation therapy.

Management of Inguinal and Pelvic LNs

Treatment of the regional lymph nodes remains controversial. The pattern of lymphatic spread goes from the superficial inguinals to the deep inguinals to the pelvic lymph nodes, with skip metastases being uncommon. The risk of LN involvement is dependent on the tumor size, grade, depth of invasion, and the presence of perineural or lymphovascular invasion [21, 35, 71, 79]. Because of the midline location, lymphatic spread can occur to either side of the inguinal region. For clinically negative inguinal lymph nodes, the risk of micrometastases can be as much as 40 % [32], depending on tumor size, grade, and associated prognostic factors. If left untreated, these lymph nodes will significantly affect treatment outcome [44]. In patients with palpable LNs, approximately 50 % will be metastatic and 50 % reactive [62].

Nodal evaluation techniques include radiographic imaging, fine needle aspiration, dynamic sentinel node biopsy (DSNB), and formal inguinal dissection. For clinically node-negative patients, risk stratification is recommended. DSNB may be an option although proper technique is imperative. Initial reports suggested a false-negative rate up to 40 % [67]. However, the use of newer techniques and the addition of scintigraphy with sulfur-labeled colloid in more recent reports suggest a reduction of the false-negative rate to 0–20 % [36, 85].

Because lymphatic spread occurs in a stepwise fashion, for low-risk early stage penile cancer with clinically negative inguinal lymph nodes, observation of the groins is recommended. For moderately or poorly differentiated tumors, or more advanced T-stages, pathologic staging of the lymph nodes with either dynamic sentinel lymph node biopsy or modified inguinal lymph node dissection (ILD) is recommended [71]. Lymph node dissection is also recommended for patients with clinically positive lymph nodes [6] [55].

Pathologically negative nodes do not require additional prophylactic treatment of the inguinal regions [9, 52, 55, 70, 74]. For patients with early pathologic N1 disease, there is some data to suggest that for a small single positive inguinal lymph node with no extracapsular extension, the risk of regional recurrence after lymph node dissection is small, and no further therapy is indicated. This would be similar to the finding for SCC in certain gynecologic cancers such as vulvar cancer [31]. However, when the inguinal tumor burden is greater, adjuvant radiation therapy is recommended. Similarly, adjuvant radiation therapy would be recommended for N2/N3 disease or extracapsular extension, where the risk of regional recurrence exceeds 30 % [25, 50].

There is no need to treat the pelvis if the inguinal lymph nodes are negative since skip metastases are uncommon. In the presence of two or more inguinal lymph nodes, the risk of pelvic lymph node involvement can be as high as 56 % [80], and thus, the pelvis should be included in the regional treatment fields unless there has been a negative pelvic lymph node dissection.

For unresectable nodal disease, neoadjuvant therapy is recommended. This can be in the form of chemotherapy [71], radiotherapy [73], or concurrent chemoradiotherapy. The study by Ravi et al. included 38 patients that received preoperative radiation for lymph nodes greater than 4 cm. At the time of surgery, only three patients demonstrated perinodal infiltration and only one patient (3 %) developed an inguinal recurrence [73]. The study by Ozsahin et al. [61] included 18 patients with clinically positive inguinal lymph nodes. Eleven patients were treated with surgery plus radiation therapy and 7 patients received radiation alone. Two patients developed regional recurrence in each group, for a crude regional recurrence rate of 18 % vs. 29 % favoring lymph node dissection followed by adjuvant radiation.

For patients with low nodal tumor burden involving only the superficial inguinal lymph nodes, the 5-year OS can be as high as 80 % [25], but this decreases to 10–20 % for bilateral or pelvic LN involvement and 10 % in the presence of extracapsular extension [62]. These results underline the need for aggressive nodal treatment. When treating the regional lymph nodes, a dose of 45–50 Gy in 5 weeks with a boost to known areas of gross disease or extracapsular extension is recommended.

The surgical salvage rate for regional recurrence is lower, but salvage is still possible with aggressive therapy. Aggressive treatment of regional recurrence is warranted since uncontrolled regional disease can have a significant impact on quality of life because of lymphedema, pain, and decreased range of motion [27].

Radiation Treatment Technique

Brachytherapy

The goal of brachytherapy in treating the primary cancer is to deliver a high dose to a limited volume so as to maintain a high likelihood of cure with an acceptable risk for side effects. Generally, brachytherapy is recommended for tumors less than 4 cm. Various different techniques and doses have been described in the literature. Also in 2013, the American Brachytherapy Society–Groupe Europeen de Curietherapie–European Society of Therapeutic Radiation Oncology (ABS-GEC-ESTRO) published their consensus statement on the use of brachytherapy for penile cancer [16]. The majority of studies used afterloading catheters placed in accordance with the Paris system of dosimetry [68]. Prior to needle/catheter placement, a Foley catheter is inserted to localize the urethra and decrease the potential for a brachytherapy catheter transecting the urethra. Although single-plane implants may be used for small superficial lesions, this is generally discouraged. For the majority of the penile cancers, a 2- or 3-plane implant is appropriate (Fig. 11.2). The recommended spacing between the needles is 12–18 mm and depends on the volume of the implant [16]. The use of a pair of templates ensures uniform needle spacing and parallelism as the dose can change rapidly with a 1–2 mm variation in spacing. The needles should be placed in a fashion to allow for a 1 cm margin around the tumor, and an exterior set of needles, outside of the penis, can be used to ensure adequate coverage of the tumor surface.

A Styrofoam collar can be placed at the base of the penis to distance the implanted sources from the surrounding normal tissue (Fig. 11.3). A thin layer of lead can be placed underneath the collar to further shield the surrounding normal tissues. For low dose rate brachytherapy, the prescription dose is 60 Gy given at a continuous dose rate of 0.40–0.60 Gy/h. When pulsed dose rate brachytherapy is used, then hourly pulses of radiation, equivalent to the hourly dose rate of an LDR implant, are delivered [3, 16, 24].

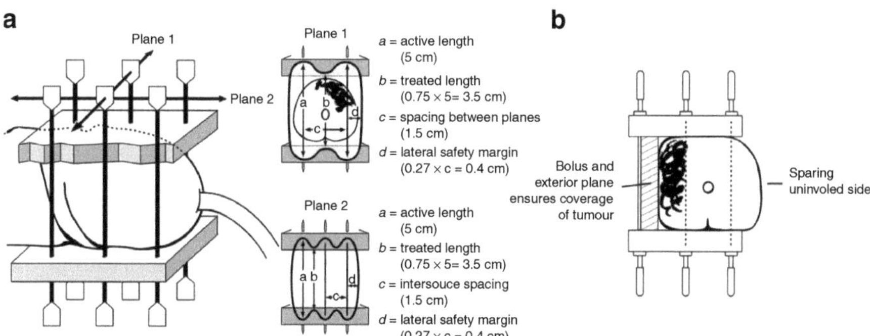

Fig. 11.2 Schematic for prostate brachytherapy. (**a**) A two-plane six-needle implant showing the isodose coverage according to the Paris system. (**b**) An implant demonstrating the use of bolus to fill the gap between an exterior plane of needles and the penile surface (Reprinted from Crook et al. [16]. Copyright 2013, with permission from Elsevier)

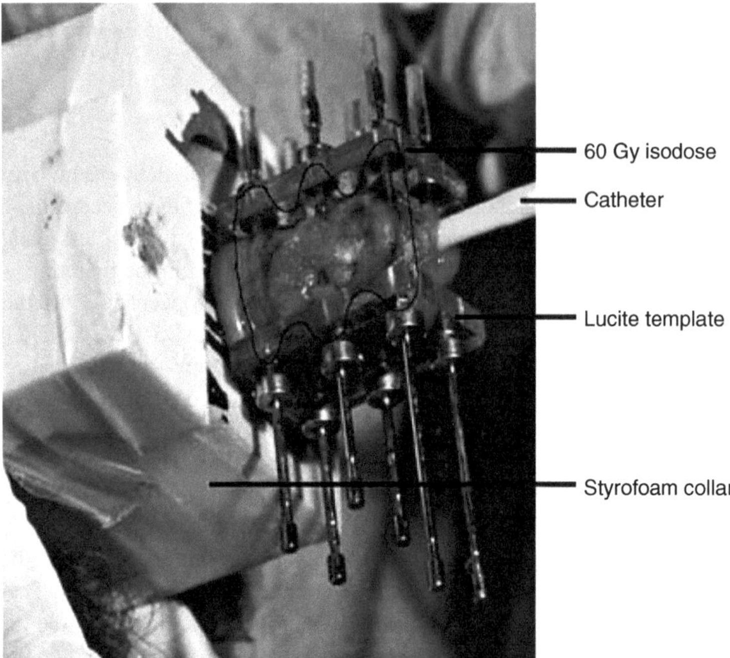

Fig. 11.3 Interstitial brachytherapy using a 2-plane, 6-needle implant in accordance with the Paris system. A Styrofoam collar provides distance from the implant to limit the dose to surrounding normal tissues. The addition of a lead plate behind the Styrofoam collar will provide additional shielding (From Crook et al. [15], with kind permission from Springer Science and Business Media)

From a technical perspective, HDR brachytherapy is similar to LDR brachytherapy. The recommended needle spacing for HDR is 10–12 mm [16]. Because of HDR treatments' ability to vary the dose at different dwell positions along each catheter, the exact spacing of needles is less crucial. CT-based planning with 3-dimensional reconstruction of the individual catheters, target volume, and surrounding normal tissues, including urethra and skin, is mandatory. Similar to LDR brachytherapy, a Foley catheter is used to identify the urethra for dose restriction. Generally, treatments are delivered twice daily, with at least 6 h between treatments. There are no clearly established dose regimens for HDR brachytherapy. Petera et al. prescribed a dose of 54 Gy, given in 3 Gy fractions, twice daily. At a median follow-up time of 20 months, they reported 100 % penile preservation with no cases of necrosis or severe stenosis, but all implants were single plane and the same excellent results may not be seen with larger volume or multiplane implants [66]. The ABS-GEC-ESTRO report also presented unpublished dose regimens including 38.4 Gy total dose given in 3.2 Gy fraction size over 6 days using a BID regimen with no necrosis seen. The authors noted that necrosis was a complication after doses of 42–45 Gy given in 12 fractions over 6 days, but that these doses may be tolerable if close attention is paid to dose homogeneity and the volume receiving 125 % (V_{125}) of the prescribed dose. They recommended keeping the V_{125} under 40 % and the V_{150} (volume receiving 150 % of the prescribed dose) to 20 %. To decrease the risk of urethral strictures, they recommended limiting the urethral V_{115} to less than10 % and the urethral V_{90} to less than 95 % of the urethral volume [16]. Caution is advised with the use of HDR for penile cancer as published clinical data is lacking.

IMRT/EBRT

External beam radiation therapy requires a setup that allows treatment of the full thickness of the penis while preventing incidental irradiation of surrounding normal tissues. Various techniques including the use of a Perspex block, wax mold, or water baths have been developed to achieve this goal.

The tissue block system uses a 10×10–15×15cm wax or Perspex block [53, 77, 86] constructed in two halves with a central cutout in order to encompass the penis. The patient is placed supine on the treatment table. The two halves are placed around the penis, and the penis is supported in the vertical position within the central cutout. The entire length of the penis is treated. The material used to create the block acts as bolus to ensure adequate dosage of the skin surface. As the treatments progress, edema may necessitate modification to the chamber. If a wax chamber is used, then this will require construction of a new block. Another disadvantage of wax is that the penis is not visible through the block, and the block must be snug enough to ensure that the penis does not retract. Perspex blocks [77] are constructed in a similar fashion but can be pre-made with various different central cutout sizes. This will allow the changing of blocks if significant swelling develops. Also, the transparent block allows for verification of penile position

Systems utilizing the water bath technique [76] require treatment of patients in the prone position. Patients are lying either on Styrofoam slabs with a cutout in the region of the pelvis or on a special plate with a central cutout that is attached to the patient couch top. Using this system, Perspex blocks with central openings of various sizes can be attached to the tabletop plate. This cylinder can be filled with lukewarm water to act as bolus (Fig. 11.4) [46].

Generally, two opposed fields are used with various dose fractionation regimens ranging from 35 Gy in 10 fractions to 60 Gy in 25 fractions to 74 Gy in 37 fractions. The most commonly used doses are in the range of 60–66 using standard fractionation size of 2 Gy. Because penile cancer originates on the skin, the skin surface must receive the full dose. Due to the rarity of penile cancer, and the lack of large trials, treatment needs to be individualized.

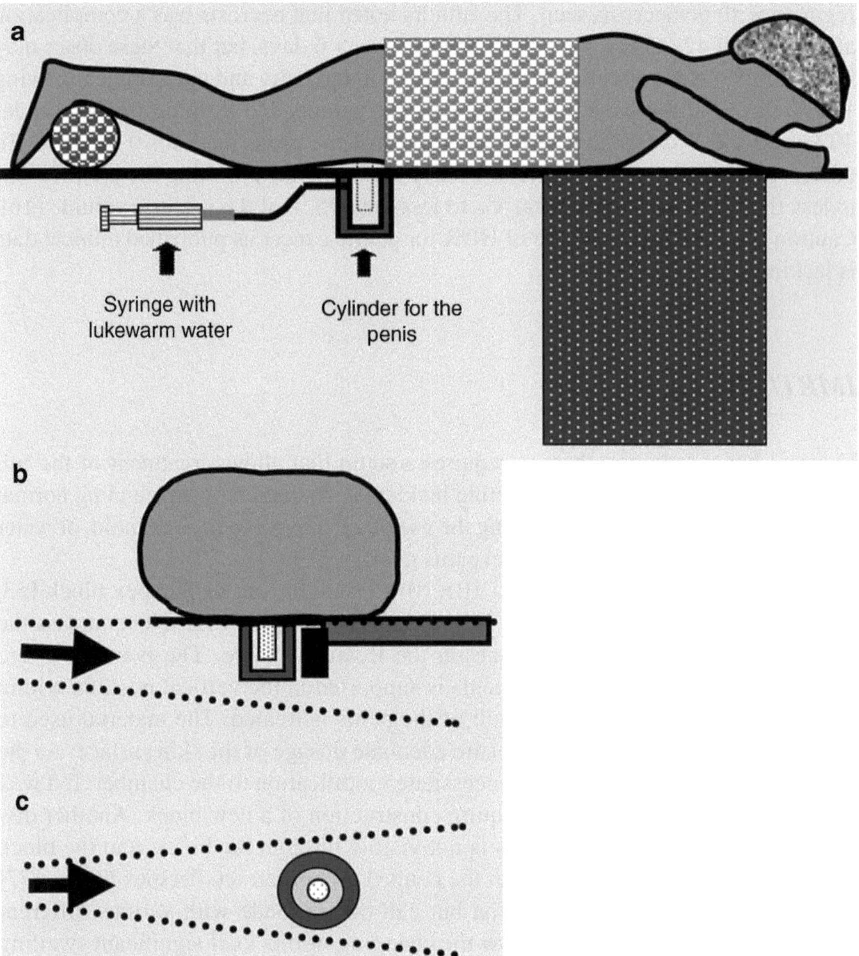

Fig. 11.4 Patient setup for external beam radiation therapy using the water bath system. Patient lying in the prone treatment position. (**a**) Side view, (**b**) axial view, (**c**) coronal view. Note the nondivergent field edge along to base of the penis (**b**), to reduce the radiation dose to surrounding normal tissue (Reprinted from Lofroth et al. [46], Copyright 2004 with permission from Elsevier)

Treatment Technique for the Inguinal and Pelvic LNs

There is no standard approach for treatment of the regional lymphatics. The technique will depend on the clinical and dosimetric expertise and the treatment modalities available. In the reported studies for treatment of inguinal nodes, the most common techniques are AP fields alone or AP:PA fields. However, many of these reports involved treatment prior to the advent of CT simulation and 3D treatment planning. Prescribing to a set depth, such as 3 cm, can result in underdosing secondary to variation in the depth of the nodes due to body habitus [41]. Other techniques for treating the inguinal region include the use of electron fields or AP:PA fields. Margins need to be individualized but volumes should encompass both the superficial and the deep inguinal nodes. When the pelvic lymph nodes are included in the target volume, an IMRT treatment technique can cover the inguinal and pelvic lymph nodes while limiting the dose to the surrounding normal tissues. Doses in the range of 45–50.4 Gy are used for treatment of areas with suspected microscopic disease. A further boost to a total dose in the range of 60–70 Gy, depending on the extent of disease, is recommended for areas with gross residual tumor.

Normal Tissue Effects

Treatment-related side effects depend on the region treated and the regimen used. For treatment of the primary, severe skin reaction is the most common acute side effect. With brachytherapy, the skin reaction generally peaks 2–3 weeks after treatment. With external beam radiation therapy, the skin reaction generally starts 2–3 weeks into treatment and progressively worsens as the treatment continues. A proactive approach to skin care is essential. This includes good hygiene in the treated region, warm baths, and ointments, including those containing antibiotics and/or vit. E, as indicated [14]. In addition, a loose Telfa or other nonstick dressing can provide a protective layer around the inflamed skin. Other acute side effects include irritative urinary symptoms secondary to urethritis.

The most commonly reported late effects are soft tissue necrosis and meatal stenosis. For brachytherapy, ulceration occurs 6–18 months after treatment but can occur later [19]. The risk of necrosis increases with doses over 60 Gy [74]. Causative factors can include trauma or cold exposure [14, 15]. Initial conservative management is recommended, including the use of creams containing antibiotic, steroids, and/or vit. E. In severe cases or when healing is prolonged, hyperbaric oxygen can be very beneficial. Whenever feasible, hyperbaric oxygen should be tried prior to amputation. The risk of necrosis is lower with external beam radiation therapy when compared to brachytherapy (Tables 11.2 and 11.3).

Urethral/meatal stenosis tends to occur within the first couple of years after completion of therapy. For patients receiving brachytherapy, the proximity of the needles to the urethra is associated with an elevated risk of stenosis. This is more of an issue for LDR brachytherapy as opposed to PDR or HDR brachytherapy, where the individual dwell positions can be optimized to limit the radiation dose to the urethra. For external beam radiation therapy, the risk of urethral stenosis is associated with fraction size, with fraction sizes >2 Gy resulting in increased rates of urethral stenosis. Usually, urethral/meatal stenosis can be managed with repeat dilatations in the physician's office or with self-dilatation with a meatal dilator [14].

Maintenance of erectile function depends on the length of penile shaft irradiated. Sexual function appears to be preserved more frequently after brachytherapy than external radiotherapy because of the more limited treatment volume [13, 19, 52, 77]. Other less common late effects include balanitis (swelling of the foreskin or tip of the penis), penile pain, telangiectasia, or changes in pigmentation.

When radiation therapy includes the treatment of the inguinal and pelvic lymph nodes, then additional side effects can occur due to irradiation of the femoral head and hip joint, small bowel, and skin. Parts of the bladder and rectum may also be implicated. Acute side effects include skin reaction in the groin region, irritative bowel symptoms, and urinary symptoms. Potential long-term side effects include lymphedema in the lower extremities, arthritic changes in the hip joints, and small bowel obstruction. However, with the use of IMRT and with proper treatment planning, the likelihood of these late complications is low, especially when compared to older treatment techniques.

Summary

For patients with early stage (T1N0, T2N0) penile cancer, radiation therapy, either in the form of brachytherapy or external beam radiation therapy, offers an organ-preserving treatment option with high rates of local control and penile preservation. For patients that develop a local recurrence, surgical salvage rates are such that there is little impact on cause-specific survival. In the setting of more advanced disease, a combined modality approach is recommended. For patients with involved lymph nodes, especially multiple, or with extracapsular extension, adjuvant radiation to the regional lymph nodes is recommended. Secondary to the limited number of cases and absence of large clinical trials, treatment needs to be individualized.

References

1. Akimoto T, Mitsuhashi N, Takahashi I, Yonome I, Takahashi M, Hayakawa K, et al. Brachytherapy for penile cancer using silicon mold. Oncology. 1997;54(1):23–7.
2. American Cancer Society. Cancer facts and figures, 2013. http://www.cancer.org/research/cancerfactsfigures/cancerfactsfigures/cancer-facts-figures-2013; 2013.
3. Armour EP, White JR, Armin A, Corry PM, Coffey M, DeWitt C, et al. Pulsed low dose rate brachytherapy in a rat model: dependence of late rectal injury on radiation pulse size. Int J Radiat Oncol Biol Phys. 1997;38(4):825–34.
4. Auvert J, Roubach L. Cancer of the penis. 1989. Ann Urol (Paris). 1994;28(6–7):318–29.
5. Azrif M, Logue JP, Swindell R. External beam radiation therapy in T1-2 N0 penile carcinoma. Clin Oncol (R Coll Radiol). 2006;18:320–5.
6. Bouchot O, Rigaud J. Penis tumours: techniques and indications. Ann Urol (Paris). 2004;38(6):285–97.
7. Burgers JK, Badalament RA, Drago JR. Penile cancer. Clinical presentation, diagnosis and staging. Urol Clin North Am. 1992;19:247–56.
8. Celebi MM, Venable DD, Nopajaroonsri C, Eastham JA. Prostate cancer metastatic only to the penis. South Med J. 1997;90(9):959–61.
9. Chaudhary AJ, Ghosh S, Bhalavat RL, Kulkarni JN, Sequeira BV. Interstitial brachytherapy in carcinoma of the penis. Strahlenther Onkol. 1999;175(1):17–20.
10. Chaux A, Cubilla AL. Stratification systems as prognostic tools for defining risk of lymph node metastasis in penile squamous cell carcinomas. Semin Diagn Pathol. 2012;29(2):83–9.

11. Chen MF, Chen WC, Wu CT, Chuang CK, Ng KF, Chang JT. Contemporary management of penile cancer including surgery and adjuvant radiotherapy: an experience in Taiwan. World J Urol. 2004;22(1):60–6.
12. Crook J. Radiation therapy for cancer of the penis. Urol Clin North Am. 2010;37(3):435–43.
13. Crook J, Grimard L, Tsihlias J, Morash C, Panzarella T. Interstitial brachytherapy for penile cancer: an alternative to amputation. J Urol. 2002;167(2 Pt 1):506–11.
14. Crook J, Jezioranski J, Cygler JE. Penile brachytherapy: technical aspects and post implant issues. Brachytherapy. 2010;9(2):151–8.
15. Crook J, Ma C, Grimard L. Radiation therapy in the management of the primary penile tumor: an update. World J Urol. 2009;27(2):189–96.
16. Crook JM, Haie-Meder C, Demanes DJ, Mazeron JJ, Martinez AA, Rivard MJ. American Brachytherapy Society-Groupe Europeen de Curietherapie-European Society of Therapeutic Radiation Oncology (ABS-GEC-ESTRO) consensus statement for penile brachytherapy. Brachytherapy. 2013;12:191–8.
17. Daly NJ, Douchez J, Combes PF. Treatment of carcinoma of the penis by iridium 192 wire implant. Int J Radiat Oncol Biol Phys. 1982;8(7):1239–43.
18. de Crevoisier R, Slimane K, Sanfilippo N, Bossi A, Albano M, Dumas I, et al. Long-term results of brachytherapy for carcinoma of the penis confined to the glans (N- or NX). Int J Radiat Oncol Biol Phys. 2009;74(4):1150–6.
19. Delannes M, Malavaud B, Douchez J, Bonnet J, Daly NJ. Iridium-192 interstitial therapy for squamous cell carcinoma of the penis. Int J Radiat Oncol Biol Phys. 1992;24(3):479–83.
20. Edge SB, Byrd DR, Compton CC, editors. AJCC (American Joint Committee on Cancer) cancer staging manual. 7th ed. New York: Springer Science; 2010.
21. Ficarra V, Zattoni F, Artibani W, Fandella A, Martignoni G. Nomogram predictive of pathological inguinal lymph node involvement in patients with squamous cell carcinoma of the penis. J Urol. 2006;175:2103–8.
22. Ficarra V, Zattoni F, Cunico SC, Galetti TP, Luciani L, Fandella A, et al. Lymphatic and vascular embolizations are independent predictive variables of inguinal lymph node involvement in patients with squamous cell carcinoma of the penis: Gruppo Uro-Oncologico del Nord Est penile cancer database data. Cancer. 2005;103:2507–16.
23. Fortier P, Maylin C, Gerbaulet A, Zeller J, Touraine R. Iridium 192 interstitial radiotherapy of carcinoma of the penis. Carcinologic results, dermatologic evaluation. Ann Dermatol Venereol. 1979;106(5):465–8.
24. Fowler JF, Van Limbergen EF. Biological effect of pulsed dose rate brachytherapy with stepping sources if short half-times or repair are present in tissues. Int J Radiat Oncol Biol Phys. 1997;37:877–83.
25. Franks KN, Kancherla K, Sethugavalar B, Whelan P, Eardley I, Kiltie AE. Radiotherapy for node positive penile cancer: experience of the Leeds teaching hospitals. J Urol. 2011; 186(2):524–9.
26. Gotsadze D, Matveev BP, Zak B, Mamaladze VT. Is conservative organ-sparing treatment of penile carcinoma justified? Eur Urol. 2000;38(3):306–12.
27. Graafland NM, Moonen LM, van Boven HH, van Werkhoven E, Kerst JM, Horenblas S. Inguinal recurrence following therapeutic lymphadenectomy for node positive penile carcinoma: outcome and implications for management. J Urol. 2011;185(3):888–93.
28. Graafland NM, van Boven HH, van Werkhoven E, Moonen LM, Horenblas S. Prognostic significance of extranodal extension in patients with pathological node positive penile carcinoma. J Urol. 2010;184(4):1347–53.
29. Griffin JH, Wheeler Jr JS, Olson M, Melian E. Prostate carcinoma metastatic to the penis: magnetic resonance imaging and brachytherapy. J Urol. 1996;155(5):1701–2.
30. Hermanek P, Sobin L. Penis. In: Hermanek P, editor. TNM classification of malignant tumours. 4th ed. Berlin: Springer; 1987. p. 130–132.
31. Homesley HD, Bundy B, Sedlis A, Adcock L. Radiation therapy versus pelvic node resection for carcinoma of the vulva with positive groin nodes. Obstet Gynecol. 1986;68:733–40.

32. Horenblas S. Lymphadenectomy for squamous cell carcinoma of the penis. Part 1: diagnosis of lymph node metastasis. Br J Urol Int. 2001;88:467–72.
33. Horenblas S, van Tinteren H, Delemarre JF, Boon TA, Moonen LM, Lustig V. Squamous cell carcinoma of the penis. II. Treatment of the primary tumor. J Urol. 1992;147(6):1533–8.
34. Horenblas S, van Tinteren H, Delemarre JF, Moonen LM, Lustig V, Kroger R. Squamous cell carcinoma of the penis: accuracy of tumor, nodes and metastasis classification system, and role of lymphangiography, computerized tomography scan and fine needle aspiration cytology. J Urol. 1991;146(5):1279–83.
35. Horenblas S, van Tinteren H, Delemarre JF, Moonen LM, Lustig V, van Waardenburg EW. Squamous cell carcinoma of the penis. III. Treatment of regional lymph nodes. J Urol. 1993;149(3):492–7.
36. Hughes B, Leijte J, Shabbir M, Watkin NA, Horenblas S. Non-invasive and minimally invasive staging of regional lymph nodes in penile cancer. World J Urol. 2009;27(2):197–203.
37. Hughes BE, Leijte JAP, Kroon BK, Shabbir MA, Swallow TW, Heenan SD, et al. Lymph node metastasis in intermediate-risk penile squamous cell cancer: a two-centre experience. Eur Urol. 2010;57(4):688–92.
38. Hungerhuber E, Schlenker B, Karl A, Frimberger D, Rothenberger KH, Stief CG, et al. Risk stratification in penile carcinoma: 25-year experience with surgical inguinal lymph node staging. Urology. 2006;68(3):621–5.
39. International Union Against Cancer Committee on TNM Classification. Penis. In: Harmer E, editor. TNM classification of malignant tumours. 3rd ed. Geneva: The Union; 1978. p. 126–8.
40. Jackson SM. The treatment of carcinoma of the penis. Br J Surg. 1966;53:33–5.
41. Kalidas H. Influence of inguinal node anatomy on radiation therapy techniques. Med Dosim. 1995;20(4):295–300.
42. Keyes O, Minhas S, Allen C, Harc C, Freeman A, Ralph D. The role of magnetic resonance imaging in the local staging of penile cancer. Eur Urol. 2007;51:1313–9.
43. Kiltie AE, Elwell C, Close HJ, Ash DV. Iridium-192 implantation for node-negative carcinoma of the penis: the Cookridge Hospital experience. Clin Oncol (R Coll Radiol). 2000;12(1):25–31.
44. Kroon BK, Horenblas S, Lont AP. Patients with penile carcinoma benefit from immediate resection of clinically occult lymph node metastases. J Urol. 2005;173:816–9.
45. Langsenlehner T, Mayer R, Quehenberger F, Prettenhofer U, Langsenlehner U, Pummer K, et al. The role of radiation therapy after incomplete resection of penile cancer. Strahlenther Onkol. 2008;184(7):359–63.
46. Lofroth P-O, Bergstrom P, Forsmark C, Karlsson N-O, Franzen L. Penis holder for external radiation treatment. Radiother Oncol. 2004;71(1):115–6.
47. Lont AP, Kroon BK, Gallee MP, van Tinteren H, Moonen LM, Horenblas S. Pelvic lymph node dissection for penile carcinoma: extent of inguinal lymph node involvement as an indicator for pelvic lymph node involvement and survival. J Urol. 2007;177(3):947–52.
48. Lopes A, Hidalgo GS, Kowalski LP, Torloni H, Rossi BM, Fonseca FP. Prognostic factors in carcinoma of the penis: multivariate analysis of 145 patients treated with amputation and lymphadenectomy. J Urol. 1996;156(5):1637–42.
49. Loughlin KR. Surgical management of penile cancer: the primary lesion. Br J Urol Int. 2006;97:655–67.
50. Marconnet L, Rigaud J, Bouchot O. Long-term followup of penile carcinoma with high risk for lymph node invasion treated with inguinal lymphadenopathy. J Urol. 2010;186(6):2227–32.
51. Marconnet L, Rigaud J, Bouchot O. Long-term followup of penile carcinoma with high risk for lymph node invasion treated with inguinal lymphadenopathy. J Urol. 2010;183(6):2227–32.
52. Mazeron JJ, Langlois D, Lobo PA, Huart JA, Calitchi E, Lusinchi A, et al. Interstitial radiation therapy for carcinoma of the penis using iridium 192 wires: the Henri Mondor experience (1970–1979). Int J Radiat Oncol Biol Phys. 1984;10(10):1891–5.
53. McLean M, Akl AM, Warde P, Bissett R, Panzarella T, Gospodarowicz M. The results of primary radiation therapy in the management of squamous cell carcinoma of the penis. Int J Radiat Oncol Biol Phys. 1993;25(4):623–8.

54. Mistry T, Jones RW, Dannatt E, Prasad KK, Stockdale AD. A 10-year retrospective audit of penile cancer management in the UK. BJU Int. 2007;100(6):1277–81.
55. National Comprehensive Cancer Network. Penile cancer, version 1.2013 2013 [4 June 2013]. Available from: http://www.nccn.org/professionals/physician_gls/pdf/penile.pdf.
56. Neave F, Neal AJ, Hoskin PJ, Hope-Stone HF. Carcinoma of the penis: a retrospective review of treatment with iridium mould and external beam irradiation. Clin Oncol (R Coll Radiol). 1993;5(4):207–10.
57. Opjordsmoen S, Fossa SD. Quality of life in patients treated for penile cancer. A follow-up study. Br J Urol. 1994;74(5):652–7.
58. Opjordsmoen S, Waehre H, Aass N, Fossa SD. Sexuality in patients treated for penile cancer: patients' experience and doctors' judgement. Br J Urol. 1994;73(5):554–60.
59. Ornellas AA, Kinchin EW, Nobrega BL, Wisnescky A, Kolfman N, Quirino R. Surgical treatment of invasive squamous cell carcinoma of the penis: Brazilian National Cancer Institute long-term experience. J Surg Oncol. 2008;97:487–95.
60. Ornellas AA, Seixas AL, Marota A, Wisnescky A, Campos F, de Moraes JR. Surgical treatment of invasive squamous cell carcinoma of the penis: retrospective analysis of 350 cases. J Urol. 1994;151(5):1244–9.
61. Ozsahin M, Jichlinski P, Weber DC, Azria D, Zimmermann M, Guillou L, et al. Treatment of penile carcinoma: to cut or not to cut? Int J Radiat Oncol Biol Phys. 2006;66(3):674–9.
62. Pagliaro LC, Crook J. Multimodality therapy in penile cancer: when and which treatments? World J Urol. 2009;27(2):221–5.
63. Pandey D, Mahajan V, Kannan RR. Prognostic factors in node-positive carcinoma of the penis. J Surg Oncol. 2006;93:133–8.
64. Parkin DM, Muir CS. Cancer incidents in five continents. Comparability and quality of data. IARC Sci Publ. 1992;120:45–173.
65. Parkin DM, Whelan SL, Ferlay J, Teppo L, Thomas DB. Cancer incidence in five continents. Lyon: International Agency for Research on Cancer; 2002. Contract No.: 155.
66. Petera J, Sirak I, Kasaova L, Macingova Z, Paluska P, Zouhar M, et al. High-dose rate brachytherapy in the treatment of penile carcinoma–first experience. Brachytherapy. 2011;10(2):136–40.
67. Pettaway CA, Pisters LL, Dinney CP, Jularbal F, Swanson DA, von Eschenbach AC, et al. Sentinel lymph node dissection for penile carcinoma: the M. D. Anderson Cancer Center experience. J Urol. 1995;154(6):1999–2003.
68. Pierquin B, Dutrex A, Paine C. The Paris system in interstitial radiation therapy. Acta Radiol Oncol. 1978;17:33.
69. Piva L, Nicolai N, Di Palo A, Milani A, Merson M, Salvioni R, et al. Therapeutic alternatives in the treatment of class T1N0 squamous cell carcinoma of the penis: indications and limitations. Arch Ital Urol Androl. 1996;68(3):157–61.
70. Pizzocaro G, Algaba F, Horenblas S, Solsona E, Tana S, Van Der Poel H, et al. EAU penile cancer guidelines 2009. Eur Urol. 2010;57(6):1002–12.
71. Pizzocaro G, Piva L, Nicolai N. Treatment of lymphatic metastasis of squamous cell carcinoma of the penis: experience at the National Tumor Institute or Milan. Arch Ital Urol Androl. 1996;68(3):169–72.
72. Ravi R. Correlation between the extent of nodal involvement and survival following groin dissection for carcinoma of the penis. Br J Urol. 1993;75(5 Pt 2):817–9.
73. Ravi R, Chaturvedi HK, Sastry DV. Role of radiation therapy in the treatment of carcinoma of the penis. Br J Urol. 1994;74(5):646–51.
74. Rozan R, Albuisson E, Giraud B, Donnarieix D, Delannes M, Pigneux J, et al. Interstitial brachytherapy for penile carcinoma: a multicentric survey (259 patients). Radiother Oncol. 1995;36(2):83–93.
75. Sadeghi R, Gholami H, Zakavi SR, Kakhki VR, Horenblas S. Accuracy of 18F-FDG PET/CT for diagnosing inguinal lymph node involvement in penile squamous cell carcinoma: systemic review and meta-analysis of the literature. Clin Nucl Med. 2012;37(5):436–44.
76. Sagerman RH, Yu WS, Chung CT, Puranik A. External-beam irradiation of carcinoma of the penis. Radiology. 1984;152(1):183–5.

77. Sarin R, Norman AR, Steel GG, Horwich A. Treatment results and prognostic factors in 101 men treated for squamous carcinoma of the penis. Int J Radiat Oncol Biol Phys. 1997;38(4):713–22.
78. Schlenker B, Scher B, Tiling R, Siegert S, Hungerhuber E, Gratzke C, et al. Detection of inguinal lymph node involvement in penile squamous cell carcinoma by 18F-Flurodeoxyglucose PET/CT: a prospective single-center study. Urol Oncol. 2012;30(1):55–9.
79. Slaton JW, Morgenstern N, Levy DA, Santos MWJ, Tamboli P, Ro JY, et al. Tumor stage, vascular invasion and the percentage of poorly differentiated cancer: independent prognosticators for inguinal lymph node metastasis in penile squamous cell cancer. J Urol. 2001;165(4):1138–42.
80. Solsona E, Algaba F, Horenblas S, et al. EAU guidelines on penile cancer. Eur Urol. 2004;46:1–8.
81. Soria JC, Fizazi K, Piron D, Kramar A, Gerbaulet A, Haie-Meder C, et al. Squamous cell carcinoma of the penis: multivariate analysis of prognostic factors and natural history in monocentric study with a conservative policy. Ann Oncol. 1997;8(11):1089–98.
82. Souillac I, Rigaud J, Ansquer C, Marconnet L, Bouchot O. Prospective evaluation of 18F-Fluorodeoxyglucose positron emission tomography-computerized tomography to assess inguinal lymph node status in invasive squamous cell carcinoma of the penis. J Urol. 2012;187(2):493–7.
83. Suchaud JP, Kantor G, Richaud P, Mage P, Lamarche P, Dilhuydy JM, et al. Brachytherapy of cancer of the penis. Analysis of a series of 53 cases. J Urol (Paris). 1989;95(1):27–31.
84. Tabatabaei S, Harisinghani M, DMcDougal WS. Regional lymph node staging using lymphotropic nanoparticle enhanced magnetic resonance imaging with ferumox-tran-10 in patients with penile caner. J Urol. 2005;174(3):923–7.
85. Tanis PJ, Lont AP, Meinhardt W, Olmos RA, Nieweg OE, Horenblas S. Dynamic sentinel node biopsy for penile cancer: reliability of staging technique. J Urol. 2002;168(1):76–80.
86. Zouhair A, Coucke PA, Jeanneret W, Douglas P, Do HP, Jichlinski P, et al. Radiation therapy alone or combined surgery and radiation therapy in squamous-cell carcinoma of the penis? Eur J Cancer. 2001;37(2):198–203.

Chapter 12
Chemotherapy in Penile Cancer

Chris Protzel and Oliver W. Hakenberg

Advanced penile cancer is characterized by a very poor prognosis. Systemic spread in penile cancer is as yet not curable at all. Chemotherapy in different variations has shown limited response rates in advanced cancer, and its role is therefore palliative in systemically advanced disease, but it has a curative potential in a multimodal approach in limited disease [1]. Since squamous cell cancer is highly aggressive, all chemotherapy regimens for penile cancer have considerable toxicity and carry the risk of very relevant side effects. In addition, many patients with penile cancer are elderly which increases the risk of cardiac or pulmonary toxicity of chemotherapy. Thus, a relevant number of treatment-associated deaths have been reported in published penile cancer chemotherapy series [2, 3]. Finally, the incidence of penile cancer is low, and there is a limited number of reported penile cancer chemotherapy series in the literature and all of those report small patient numbers. As a consequence, there is a large number of different chemotherapy regimens which have been tried and are still being used which emphasizes the fact that there is yet no "best" chemotherapy for penile cancer and that most patients are not cured by it [4]. However, some advances have been made.

This chapter provides an overview of the principles of chemotherapy for penile cancer and the current options and limitations of therapeutic applications.

C. Protzel, MD (✉) • O.W. Hakenberg, MD, PhD
Department of Urology, University of Rostock,
E. Heydemann Str. 6, Rostock 18055, Germany
e-mail: chris.protzel@med.uni-rostock.de

D.J. Culkin (ed.), *Management of Penile Cancer*,
DOI 10.1007/978-1-4939-0461-7_12,

Principles of Chemotherapy in Penile Cancer

Targets and Effects of Antineoplastic Treatment

Today, there are two main mechanisms of action of pharmacological antineoplastic treatment. One is an unspecific action directed against proliferating cells – classical chemotherapy – and the second is the "targeted therapy." The latter uses the so-called smart drugs which can specifically target receptors or pathways which are activated in neoplastic cells.

Classical chemotherapy drugs used in penile cancer all interfere with DNA or RNA during the transition of the cell cycle and cell division and eventually induces apoptosis of the neoplastic cells. Alkylating agents (cisplatin/carboplatin, ifosfamide) induce cross-linking and damage of DNA strands; they do not depend on the cells being in a specific phase of the cell cycle for their mechanism of action. Topoisomerase inhibitors (irinotecan, topotecan, etoposide) interfere with the DNA replication (phase G2 of the cell cycle). Antimetabolites (5-fluorouracil, gemcitabine) interfere with DNA and RNA synthesis (in the S phase of the cell cycle). Antibiotic chemotherapeutics (bleomycin, mitomycin) induce DNA/RNA cross-linking and thereby apoptosis (phases G1, G2, M of the cell cycle). Finally, the vinca alkaloids and taxanes (vinblastine, paclitaxel/docetaxel) inhibit the mitosis by disturbing microtubule formation (M phase of the cell cycle).

Some targeted therapeutics which have been used in penile cancer are monoclonal antibodies directed against growth receptors such as EGFR (panitumumab) or Her (dacomitinib) or tyrosine kinase inhibitors such as sunitinib.

Side Effects

All drugs used for antineoplastic treatment induce toxicity and result in unspecific side effects which are common and some specific side effects which are less common but often more harmful. Chemotherapeutic drugs inhibit cell proliferation in all replicating organ systems, and therefore, nonspecific and common side effects occur in the bone marrow, the gastrointestinal tract, and the skin. Effects on the hematopoietic system result in neutropenia which may be severe and lead to neutropenic fever or septicemia, thrombopenia which may result in occult or overt bleeding associated with minor trauma, and long-lasting anemia which commonly leads to treatment-associated fatigue. Gastrointestinal side effects due to loss of mucosal regeneration can become manifest as stomatitis, dysphagia, diarrhea, and gastrointestinal bleeding episodes. Effects on the skin are manifest as alopecia and perioral stomatitis. These common side effects occur usually in all patients to some degree, but individual tolerance and resilience are highly variable. Specific prophylactic and therapeutic measures are available to treat these toxicities which otherwise can be life-threatening in some cases.

The specific toxicities associated with the different chemotherapeutic drugs used for penile cancer such as nephrotoxicity or pulmonary toxicity are discussed below with the different treatment regimens which may be used.

Targeted drugs are known for allergic reactions, diarrhea, and skin toxicity (e.g., hand-foot syndrome with tyrosine kinase inhibitors).

Counteracting Treatment Resistance

Neoplastic tissue may be or become resistant to some or many antineoplastic drugs. Resistance may be inherent (primary) or it may develop (secondary/acquired). Mechanisms of resistance relate to the specifics of drug metabolism (uptake, efflux, detoxification) as the drugs must be incorporated into the cells for their effect to occur. Other mechanism of resistance may be enhanced DNA repair in the neoplastic tissue, deregulation of apoptotic pathways, and modification or mutations of drug targets.

Recently, the potential importance of primary resistance against chemotherapy and radiation by some tumor stem cells has been shown. The tumor microenvironment will also have an influence; some neoplastic cells may survive in special "niches" as minimal residual disease (MRD) which later on will proliferate with some degree of resistance against the previously effective chemotherapy.

Treatment strategies are directed at counteracting the development of chemotherapy resistance. The classical approach is to use combination chemotherapy in combinations of several drugs with different mechanisms of action. More recent approaches include the integration of smart drugs (such as the anti-integrin alpha-4 antibody natalizumab, the restoration of p53, the inhibition of cell cycle checkpoints, or the targeted inhibition of DNA repair).

Clinical Situations for the Application of Chemotherapy in Penile Cancer

Several approaches for chemotherapy in penile cancer have been examined in clinical trials [1]. The *neoadjuvant* approach refers to its use in clinically lymph node-positive disease after sufficient local treatment of the primary tumor. The neoadjuvant chemotherapy is intended to reduce or eliminate neoplastic lymph node disease and must be followed by a radical salvage lymph node dissection of the groins and/or the pelvic regional nodes. This approach holds some promise and can lead to curative results in patients in whom disease is actually limited to regional lymphatic spread.

Adjuvant chemotherapy refers to the clinical situation where treatment is given after complete surgical treatment either in locally advanced, clinically node-negative patients or after inguinal lymphadenectomy with histologically positive nodes. Such adjuvant treatment should also be considered following neoadjuvant treatment for node-positive patients in whom salvage lymphadenectomy has shown viable residual metastatic disease.

Palliative treatment of penile cancer in patients with overt systemic metastatic disease aims at slowing down disease progression [1, 3]. The results of palliative chemotherapy in penile cancer are extremely poor, and it should always be critically assessed whether best supportive care is not the better option for a given patient.

The available data for chemotherapy in penile cancer is very limited and usually only applies to first-line chemotherapy; there are virtually no data for effective second-line chemotherapy (see below) which again emphasizes the fact that chemotherapy has very limited efficacy in progressive penile cancer.

Chemotherapy Regimens with Proven Efficacy in Penile Cancer

Monotherapy

The activity of several chemotherapy agents used as monotherapy in penile cancer was initially reported in case reports and small patient series, with very moderate response rates. These reports concerned cisplatin, bleomycin, and methotrexate which have all since become classical components of combination chemotherapy regimens used for penile cancer. With monotherapy, the reported response rates were 15–27 % for cisplatin, 20–21 % for bleomycin, and 0–62 % for methotrexate [5–9]. For methotrexate monotherapy, one case of a complete remission has been reported for high-dose treatment [10]. The relevant and often limiting specific toxicities were pulmonary fibrosis with bleomycin (one treatment-related death reported) and severe hematological toxicity with the use of cisplatin.

Monotherapy is no longer an option for first-line chemotherapy in penile cancer as combination treatment is much more effective.

Dual-Drug Regimens

The frequently used combination of cisplatin and 5-fluorouracil (5-FU) was initially described by Hussein et al. and Shammas et al. in the early 1990s [11, 12]. 960–1,000 mg/m^2 5-FU was given on days 1–5 and 100 mg/m^2 cisplatin on day 1 in a typical 3-week schedule. Partial responses were reported for two of eight patients. The authors reported septicemia in two patients and an increase in serum creatinine in three patients, while nausea and vomiting were frequently seen, i.e., in all patients [12].

Cisplatin/methotrexate chemotherapy has been reported in case reports only. One penile cancer patient has been reported with a long-term survival of 84 months after receiving 100 mg/m^2 cisplatin plus 200 mg/m^2 methotrexate for inguinal node and bone metastases [13].

More recently, the taxanes paclitaxel and carboplatin as well as irinotecan have been used for penile cancer. Paclitaxel/carboplatin (80–200 mg/m^2/AUC 6, respectively) in a neoadjuvant application resulted in one partial response and one stable disease [14]; in one case report a significant regression was seen after three paclitaxel/carboplatin cycles with a reduced dosage (75 mg/m^2/AUC3, respectively) [15]. The side effects of this dual combination treatment are usually relatively mild, and its advantage is that in contrast to cisplatin, this carboplatin-based regimen can be given to patients with impaired renal function [16].

The cisplatin/irinotecan combination (80 mg/m^2 on day 1/60 mg/m^2 on days 1, 8, 15, respectively) was examined in an EORTC protocol. Two patients achieved a complete remission with a calculated overall response rate of 30.8 %. The reported side effects were mild with grade 3 diarrhea in three cases and grade 4 neutropenia with fever in two cases.

Triple-Drug Regimens

The first triple-agent regimen series was reported by Dexeus et al. in 1991 [17]. 14 patients were treated with cisplatin (20 mg/m^2 on days 2–6), methotrexate (200 mg/m^2 on days 1, 15), and bleomycin (10 mg/m^2 on days 2–6) in a 3-week schedule. Dexeus et al. reported favorable response rates for 10/14 patients including two complete remissions. Based on this small series, the so-called Dexeus regimen with cisplatin, bleomycin, and methotrexate became the standard chemotherapy protocol for penile cancer for many years. However, later evaluations of this regimen have not been able to confirm the high response rate originally reported by Dexeus et al.; furthermore, treatment-related toxicity of this regimen is high. Thus, Haas et al. in a series of 40 patients thus treated reported five complete and eight partial responses in 40 patients in a dose-modified regimen (cisplatin 75 mg/m^2 on day 1; methotrexate 25 mg/m^2 on days 1 and 8; and bleomycin 10 mg/m^2 on days 1 and 8) with considerably more toxicity and a treatment-related mortality rate of 12.5 % [2]. Similarly, severe toxicity and treatment-related deaths were reported for this regimen by other series as well [3, 18, 19]. Deaths due to toxicity were all associated with bleomycin-induced interstitial pneumonitis. Other side effects reported were deep venous thrombosis, pulmonary embolism, and neutropenia-associated infections with grade 4 hematological toxicity reported in 24/45 treatment in five cycles [3]. Another frequently seen side effect of cisplatin was an increase in serum creatinine reported in 15–33 % of patients.

A different approach to the penile cancer combination chemotherapy treatment was reported by Pizzocaro and Piva in 1988 with vincristine (1 mg/m^2 day 1), bleomycin (15 mg/m^2 days 1, 2), and methotrexate (30–50 mg/m^2 day 3) in a 1-week schedule in a very small series [20]. Response was seen in three of the five patients but with severe toxicity as well with one treatment-associated death due to bleomycin pneumonitis with fatal pulmonary embolus.

A new approach became available with the advent of the taxanes which had been successfully used in patients with squamous cell carcinoma of the head and neck. Pizzocaro et al. described the first series of cisplatin/5-FU plus a taxane in 2008 [21]. The regimen with paclitaxel 120 mg/m^2 on day 2, cisplatin 50 mg/m^2 on days 1 and 2, and 5-FU 1,000 mg/m^2 on days 2–5 showed a high activity in patients with advanced or recurrent penile cancer with a clinical response reported for five of the six patients and rather mild toxicity (at most grade 2 hematotoxicity). This so-called Pizzocaro regimen has since been widely used.

Bermejo et al. reported the results of a triple regimen with ifosfamide instead of 5-FU. The combination of paclitaxel 175 mg/m^2 on days 1–5 and 20 mg/m^2 cisplatin and ifosfamide 1,200 mg/m^2 on days 1–3 resulted in a clinical response in 4 of the 5 patients treated [14]. The same regimen was used by Pagliaro et al. who have published the largest neoadjuvant chemotherapy study in penile cancer so far [22]. The same regimen with the same dosage was used in 30 patients with bulky inguinal nodal disease and resulted in partial responses in 15/30 patients and three patients with histologically confirmed complete remission. Following salvage inguinal lymphadenectomy, 9/30 patients in this series achieved long-term survival.

Other Agents

Interferon was used for penile cancer in a neoadjuvant trial as well as in advanced cases in combination with cisplatin (cisplatin 20 mg/m^2 (days 1–5) plus 5×10^6 IU interferon alpha-2b (days 1–5) and on 3 days in weeks 2–4) in a 4-week schedule. The reported toxicity was relatively mild (anemia in five and renal impairment in three patients). The clinical response was poor without long-term efficacy [23].

Target drugs have also been used in a few cases so far. Zhu et al. reported one partial response and four patients with stable disease under either sunitinib or sorafenib monotherapy [24]. Necchi et al. have reported one case of successful panitumumab treatment in a patient with multilocular cutaneous metastases from penile cancer who achieved a substantial partial remission [25]. The same group of authors have recently completed a series of ten patients with panitumumab monotherapy whereby three patients are reported to have achieved a complete remission (personal communication).

Current Standards for Penile Cancer Chemotherapy

Standards in penile cancer chemotherapy are somewhat difficult to define since the data available are very limited. However, the efficacy of several drugs has been clearly established and the treatment in a triple-drug regimen seems to be the most effective in first-line application.

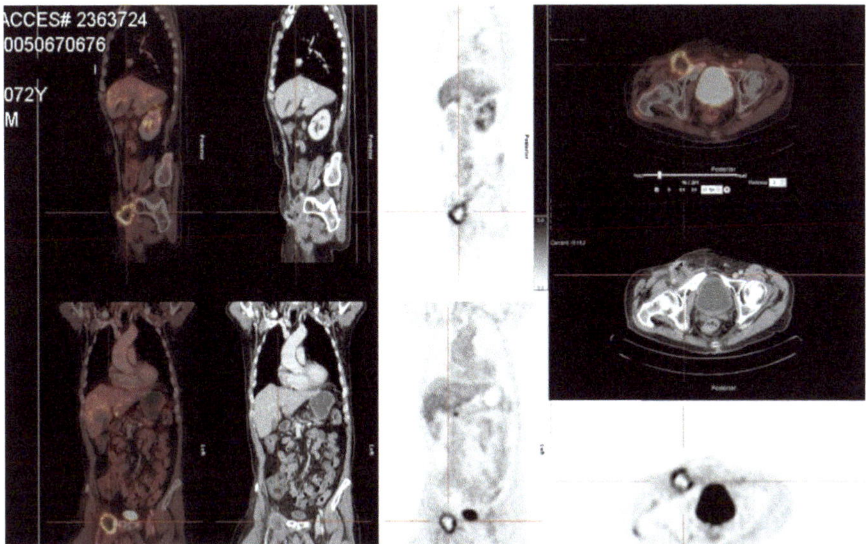

Fig. 12.1 Response of neoadjuvant chemotherapy for fixed inguinal lymph nodes in the right groin showing central necrosis

The clinical situation with potentially the most benefit for the patient to be gained is currently the neoadjuvant treatment of clinically node-positive patients after sufficient local treatment of the primary tumor followed by salvage lymphadenectomy. An example is shown in Fig. 12.1.

Neoadjuvant Treatment

Leijte et al., in a retrospective case series, reported a clinical response in 12 out of 19 patients after neoadjuvant chemotherapy with different dual- or triple-drug regimens (vincristine/bleomycin/methotrexate, cisplatin/bleomycin/methotrexate, cisplatin/5-FU or cisplatin/irinotecan) [19]. Following salvage lymphadenectomy eight patients achieved long-term survival. Pagliaro et al. used neoadjuvant paclitaxel/cisplatin/ifosfamide chemotherapy in 30 patients and reported a clinical response in 15 with histologically confirmed complete remissions in three cases and long-term survival in nine [22]. Pizzocaro et al. reported neoadjuvant paclitaxel/cisplatin/5-FU chemotherapy for three patients with a clinical response in all three cases [21]. Relevant studies for neoadjuvant chemotherapy are summarized in Table 12.1.

Thus, the recent studies published on neoadjuvant chemotherapy all report a favorable response to this multimodal treatment in advanced penile cancer with overt regional lymph node metastasis (mostly bulky or fixed inguinal lymph nodes). This concept is also supported by the favorable reports of neoadjuvant

Table 12.1 Neoadjuvant chemotherapy

Drug	Regimen	No. of cycles	No. of patients	Response	Complete response	Treatment-related death	Median survival (months)	Reference
Cisplatin Methotrexate Bleomycin	20–30 mg/m², days 2–5 200 mg/m², day 1 15 mg/m², days 2–5; 3 week	4	10	6		2	n.d.	Leijte et al. [19]
Vinblastine Methotrexate Bleomycin	1 mg/m², day 1 30–50 mg/m², day 3 15 mg/m², days 1, 2; 2 week	12	5	3		1	n.d.	Leijte et al. [19]
Paclitaxel Cisplatin Ifosfamide	175 mg/m², days 1 20 mg/m², days 1–3 1,2 g/m², days 1–3; 3 week	4	30	15	3	0	30	Pagliaro et al. [22]
Paclitaxel Cisplatin 5-FU	120 mg/m², day 1 50 mg/m², days 1, 2 1,000 mg/m², days 2–5; 3 week	2	3	3	2	0	11	Pizzocaro et al. [21]
Cisplatin Irinotecan	80 mg/m² day 1 60 mg/m² days 1, 8, 15; 4 week	4	7	2 4 stable	1	0	n.d.	Theodore et al. [26]

Abbreviations: *n.d.* no data, *n.r.* not reached

chemotherapy in lymph node-positive disease in head and neck cancers as well as in bladder and testicular cancer. There are so far no reports on neoadjuvant chemotherapy for large and advanced primary penile cancer tumors.

Regimens for Neoadjuvant Chemotherapy

Efficacy has been reported for the triple combinations of paclitaxel/cisplatin/ifosfamide [22] as well as paclitaxel/cisplatin/5-FU [21]. Whether one is better than the other cannot be decided. In order to reduce the toxicity of cisplatin, we use a modified "Pizzocaro regimen" whereby the cisplatin dose is delivered in aliquots over 5 days.

For neoadjuvant treatment, three cycles should be given, and the clinical response assessed either clinically (regional lymph nodes) or by imaging studies. If the disease is unresponsive, the treatment should be discontinued or changed after two cycles.

Side Effects

Toxicity will be common and is relevant. *Cisplatin* induces neutropenia and thrombopenia and is nephro- and neurotoxic (inner ear); it also has some cardiotoxicity and can lead to symptomatic coronary artery spasms as well as ischemic heart manifestations. *Paclitaxel* is known for allergic reactions, neurotoxicity, and often considerable alopecia. The most pronounced and often clinically impressive toxicity of *ifosfamide* is neurotoxicity with an encephalopathy; it is also nephrotoxic and can induce a hemorrhagic cystitis and diarrhea. *5-Fluorouracil* carries some cardiotoxicity and often induces diarrhea.

Adjuvant Treatment

The rationale for adjuvant chemotherapy treatment is that lymph node-positive patients are at risk of harboring micrometastatic disease elsewhere so that radical surgical treatment of the regional lymph nodes alone will not be curative.

Pizzocaro et al. used adjuvant chemotherapy in patients with lymph node-positive disease after radical inguinal lymphadenectomy and retrospectively compared that cohort with a historical series without adjuvant chemotherapy. The 5-year survival rate in the adjuvant chemotherapy group was 82 % and had been only 37 % in the historical control group [27]. In that series with adjuvant chemotherapy, none of the pN1 patients later developed metastatic disease. In contrast to this, Franks et al. reported a recurrence rate of 17 % for pN1 patients after adjuvant radiotherapy [28].

Pizzocaro et al. also published a series of 12 patients with adjuvant vincristine/bleomycin/methotrexate treatment [20] and reported one disease recurrence.

Hakenberg et al. reported adjuvant chemotherapy treatment with cisplatin/bleomycin/methotrexate in eight patients with four long-term disease-free survivals but one treatment-associated death due to bleomycin toxicity [3]. Noronha et al. reported a larger series of 19 patients with adjuvant cisplatin/paclitaxel or carboplatin/paclitaxel chemotherapy with six locoregional recurrences [29]. Studies for adjuvant chemotherapy are shown in Table 12.2.

Thus, based on the favorable results of the retrospective analysis of Pizzocaro et al, adjuvant chemotherapy is advisable after radical inguinal lymphadenectomy in lymph node-positive patients as it has the potential to be curative and improve long-term survival rates. The current penile cancer guidelines of the European Association of Urology therefore recommend adjuvant chemotherapy for all patients with more than one lymph node metastasis (>pN1) [27]. However, in our opinion, adjuvant chemotherapy should be considered for all patients with lymph node-positive disease and should be a definite must in patients who underwent lymphadenectomy for locoregional recurrence after surveillance management.

Regimens for Adjuvant Chemotherapy

Pizzocaro et al. used vincristine/bleomycin/methotrexate or cisplatin/5-FU in the adjuvant setting [27], Noronha et al. used cisplatin/paclitaxel or carboplatin/paclitaxel [29]. The adjuvant use of the Dexeus regimen described by Hakenberg et al. is too toxic and should no longer be used. Since the combination of cisplatin/paclitaxel/ifosfamide has been reported with remarkable response rates combined with relatively mild toxicity, this regimen is an alternative in the adjuvant setting.

Side Effects

Again, toxicity will occur. For *vincristine*, neurotoxicity (optical nerve), constipation, and polyuria may be expected. *Bleomycin* is known to cause considerable pulmonary toxicity which can sometimes be fatal with the induction of a fibrous pneumonitis as well as vasculitis (Raynaud's syndrome) and dermatitis. Bleomycin should not be given to patients with preexisting pulmonary disease. *Methotrexate* can also induce a fibrotic pneumonitis, but to a much lesser extent than bleomycin, it carries some nephro- and hepatotoxicity and can induce toxic cutaneous reactions (exanthema, pruritus, stomatitis) as well as diarrhea.

Palliative Treatment

The prognosis of penile cancer patients with advanced metastatic disease is extremely poor and no cure is possible.

Table 12.2 Adjuvant chemotherapy

Drug	Regimen	No. of cycles	No. of patients	Progression	Treatment-related death	Mean remission time (months)	Reference
Vinblastine	1 mg/m^2, day 1	12	12	1	0	42	Pizzocaro et al.[20]
Methotrexate	30–50 mg/m^2, day 3						
Bleomycin	15 mg/m^2, days 1, 2; 1 week						
Cisplatin	20 mg/m^2, days 2–6	6	8	4	1	26	Hakenberg et al. [3]
Methotrexate	200 mg/m^2, days 1, 15, 22						
Bleomycin	10 mg/m^2, days 2–6; 4 week						
Cisplatin/Carboplatin	75 mg/m^2, day 1	4	19	6	1	16.2 (median)	Noronha et al. [29]
Paclitaxel	175 mg/m^2, days 1; 3 week						

Complete remissions of distant metastases have only been described in singular case reports [25]. In the largest penile cancer chemotherapy series of Haas et al. with 40 patients, complete responses were achieved in 5/40 and partial responses in eight with the Dexeus regimen (cisplatin/bleomycin/methotrexate) in a phase II multi-institutional study [2]. However, no patient with distant organ metastases achieved a complete response, while two patients with pulmonary metastases showed a partial response. One patient with a retroperitoneal lymph node metastasis showed complete response. The median duration of the response in that study was 16 weeks with an estimated median progression-free survival of 14 weeks. Of the 40 patients treated in that study, 36 died during follow-up with 31 deaths due to disease and 5 due to treatment toxicity. Corral et al. reported 21 patients in a phase II trial with complete response seen in 4/21 patients (one patient with distant metastases) and partial responses in eight patients [18]. The median duration of the complete responses was 20.9 months, for the partial responses 3.8 months only. In that series, all patients died of the disease with a median survival after a complete response of 32.7 months and after a partial response of 15.8 months. Nonresponders had a median survival of 6.7 months. In the study of Hakenberg et al, all five patients with M1 disease showed stable disease under the Dexeus regimen (cisplatin/bleomycin/methotrexate) [3]. However, after chemotherapy all patients showed immediate disease progression and died of the disease after a mean of 5 months. Hussein et al. reported partial responses in five patients with advanced penile carcinomas under cisplatin/5-FU dual drug chemotherapy, but all five patients died of disease after a median of 13.4 months [11]. The combination cisplatin/irinotecan was used in 19 patients with advanced disease in a recent EORTC trail with a reported response rate of 32 % (one complete remission and five partial responses) [26]. Data for palliative chemotherapy is summarized in Table 12.3.

Thus, there are neither good results nor clear indications for palliative chemotherapy in advanced and systemically metastatic penile cancer. The indication should be carefully considered depending on the patient circumstances and wishes. A response should be evaluated early and treatment discontinued if there is no or only minor response. Treatment evaluation may incorporate PET-CT scanning which has been reported to be very useful in the staging of head and neck squamous cell carcinoma, but only limited data are available for its utility in penile cancer. If stable disease can be achieved by chemotherapy with acceptable toxicity, treatment continuation should be considered discussing the aims and potential benefits with the patient. The alternative in view of the prognosis is best supportive care with quickly progressive disease.

Regimens for Palliative Chemotherapy

The combinations of cisplatin/paclitaxel/ifosfamide or cisplatin/paclitaxel/5-FU can be considered for patients with a performance score suggesting that toxicity will be tolerable. Carboplatin/paclitaxel carries less toxicity and is an alternative in

Table 12.3 Advanced disease

Drug	Regimen	No. of cycles	No. of patients	Response	Complete response	Treatment-related death	Median survival (months)	Reference
Cisplatin	20 mg/m^2, days 2–6		14	10	2	0	n.d.	Dexeus et al. [17]
Methotrexate	200 mg/m^2, days 1, 15, 22							
Bleomycin	10 mg/m^2, days 2–6; 4 week							
Cisplatin	75 mg/m^2, day 1	6	40	13	5	5	28	Haas et al. [2]
Methotrexate	25 mg/m^2, days 1, 8							
Bleomycin	10 mg/m^2, days 1, 8; 3 week							
Cisplatin	20 mg/m^2, days 2–6	4	21	12	4	1	32.7 (CR)	Corral et al. [18]
Methotrexate	200 mg/m^2, days 1, 15, 22						15.8 (PR)	
Bleomycin	10 mg/m^2, days 2–6; 4 week							
Cisplatin	20 mg/m^2, days 2–6	6	5	5 stable	0	1	17.9	Hakenberg et al. [3]
Methotrexate	200 mg/m^2, days 1, 15, 22							
Bleomycin	10 mg/m^2, d 2–6; 4 week							
Cisplatin	100 mg/m^2, day 1	4	5	5	0	0	15	Hussein et al. [11]
5-FU	960 mg/m^2, days 2–5							
Cisplatin	50 mg/m^2, days 1, 2	5	3	2	1	0	n.r.	Pizzocaro et al. [21]
5-FU	1,000 mg/m^2, days 2–5							
Paclitaxel	120 mg/m^2, day 1							
Cisplatin	80 mg/m^2 day 1	4	21	6	1	0	n.d.	Theodore et al. [26]
Irinotecan	60 mg/m^2 days 1, 8, 15; 4 week			4 stable				

Abbreviations: *n.d.* no data, *n.r.* not reached

patients who are older and have already more comorbidity or impaired renal function. There are no data on potential efficacy of targeted therapies as a basis for their use as an effective palliative treatment.

Second-Line Chemotherapy

There are extremely few reports on second-line chemotherapy in penile cancer. Di Lorenzo et al. reported a phase II trial of paclitaxel monotherapy (175 mg/m^2) in progressive disease after a failed previous chemotherapy. A partial response was seen in 5 of 25 patients treated, and the median progression-free survival with second-line chemotherapy was 11 weeks, the median survival for responders 32 weeks [30].

Regarding the experimental use of targeted therapies as a second-line treatment, Zhu et al. reported six patients with either sunitinib or sorafenib treatment after progression under primary chemotherapy; one partial response and four patients with stable disease were reported [24]. There is one case report describing a complete response to panitumumab second-line treatment for cutaneous metastases [25] and unpublished results of the same group reporting two complete responses, one partial responses, and two stable diseases in 10 patients with panitumumab second- or third-line treatment (Necchi, personal communication).

Future Perspectives

The main role of chemotherapy in penile cancer at present lies in the neoadjuvant and adjuvant application in lymph node-positive patients in conjunction with surgery. In that situation chemotherapy as an element in the multimodal approach can be curative and is therefore of utmost value but is at present in that role underused. Previously used regimens have been rather toxic, and the recently developed alternatives are more favorable in that respect. The regimen, the dosage, and the timing of applications should be tailored to the patients health status and comorbidities.

For systemically metastatic patients, chemotherapy is at present palliative and can at best prolong life for several months. The potential reduction in quality of life due to toxicity must be weighed against that due to progressing disease and that is often not possible.

For the future we have to find more effective treatment regimens hopefully incorporating targeted therapies with proven efficacy in penile cancer. Perhaps, more research into the molecular mechanisms of penile cancer will generate potential targets and prognostic markers for chemoresistance that would then be useful for treatment decisions. For those aims to be achievable, we need better collaboration in large multicenter international trials in order to generate meaningful data for better treatment of penile cancer. For example, the multi-ERBB inhibitor dacomitinib is under examination in an ongoing clinical trial for advanced penile cancer. Trials in head and neck squamous cell cancer have shown promising results for radiochemotherapy with the use of radiosensitizers such as capecitabine; this might also be an option for clinical investigation.

However, until we are successful in performing very large multicenter international trials in penile cancer, progress in chemotherapy will be rather slow.

References

1. Protzel C, Hakenberg OW. Chemotherapy in patients with penile carcinoma. Urol Int. 2009;82(1):1–7.
2. Haas GP, Blumenstein BA, Gagliano RG, Russell CA, Rivkin SE, Culkin DJ, Wolf M, Crawford ED. Cisplatin, methotrexate and bleomycin for the treatment of carcinoma of the penis: a Southwest Oncology Group study. J Urol. 1999;161(6):1823–5.
3. Hakenberg OW, Nippgen JB, Froehner M, Zastrow S, Wirth MP. Cisplatin, methotrexate and bleomycin for treating advanced penile carcinoma. BJU Int. 2006;98(6):1225–7.
4. Protzel C, Ruppin S, Milerski S, Klebingat KJ, Hakenberg OW. The current state of the art of chemotherapy of penile cancer: results of a nationwide survey of german clinics. Urologe A. 2009;48:1495–8.
5. Ahmed T, Sklaroff R, Yagoda A. An appraisal of the efficacy of bleomycin in epidermoid carcinoma of the penis. Anticancer Res. 1984;4(4–5):289–92.
6. Ahmed T, Sklaroff R, Yagoda A. Sequential trials of methotrexate, cisplatin and bleomycin for penile cancer. J Urol. 1984;132(3):465–8.
7. Maiche AG. Adjuvant treatment using bleomycin in squamous cell carcinoma of penis: study of 19 cases. Br J Urol. 1983;55(5):542–4.
8. Sklaroff RB, Yagoda A. Methotrexate in the treatment of penile carcinoma. Cancer. 1980;45(2):214–6.
9. Sklaroff RB, Yagoda A. Cis-diamminedichloride platinum II (DDP) in the treatment of penile carcinoma. Cancer. 1979;44(5):1563–5.
10. Garnick MB, Skarin AT, Steele Jr GD. Metastatic carcinoma of the penis: complete remission after high dose methotrexate chemotherapy. J Urol. 1979;122(2):265–6.
11. Hussein AM, Benedetto P, Sridhar KS. Chemotherapy with cisplatin and 5-fluorouracil for penile and urethral squamous cell carcinomas. Cancer. 1990;65(3):433–8.
12. Shammas FV, Ous S, Fossa SD. Cisplatin and 5-fluorouracil in advanced cancer of the penis. J Urol. 1992;147(3):630–2.
13. Kattan J, Culine S, Droz JP, Fadel E, Court B, Perrin JL, Wibault P, Haie-Meder C. Penile cancer chemotherapy: twelve years' experience at Institut Gustave-Roussy. Urology. 1993;42(5):559–62.
14. Bermejo C, Busby JE, Spiess PE, Heller L, Pagliaro LC, Pettaway CA. Neoadjuvant chemotherapy followed by aggressive surgical consolidation for metastatic penile squamous cell carcinoma. J Urol. 2007;177(4):1335–8.
15. Joerger M, Warzinek T, Klaeser B, Kluckert JT, Schmid HP, Gillessen S. Major tumor regression after paclitaxel and carboplatin polychemotherapy in a patient with advanced penile cancer. Urology. 2004;63(4):778–80.
16. Protzel C, Klebingat HJ, Hakenberg OW. Treatment of advanced penile cancer. Do we need new methods for chemotherapy? Urologe A. 2008;47(9):1229–32.
17. Dexeus FH, Logothetis CJ, Sella A, Amato R, Kilbourn R, Fitz K, Striegel A. Combination chemotherapy with methotrexate, bleomycin and cisplatin for advanced squamous cell carcinoma of the male genital tract. J Urol. 1991;146(5):1284–7.

18. Corral DA, Sella A, Pettaway CA, Amato RJ, Jones DM, Ellerhorst J. Combination chemotherapy for metastatic or locally advanced genitourinary squamous cell carcinoma: a phase II study of methotrexate, cisplatin and bleomycin. J Urol. 1998;160(5):1770–4.
19. Leijte JA, Kerst JM, Bais E, Antonini N, Horenblas S. Neoadjuvant chemotherapy in advanced penile carcinoma. Eur Urol. 2007;52(2):488–94.
20. Pizzocaro G, Piva L. Adjuvant and neoadjuvant vincristine, bleomycin, and methotrexate for inguinal metastases from squamous cell carcinoma of the penis. Acta Oncol. 1988;27(6b):823–4.
21. Pizzocaro G, Nicolai N, Milani A. Taxanes in combination with cisplatin and fluorouracil for advanced penile cancer: preliminary results. Eur Urol. 2009;55:546–51.
22. Pagliaro LC, Williams DL, Daliani D, Williams MB, Osai W, Kincaid M, Wen S, Thall PF, Pettaway CA. Neoadjuvant paclitaxel, ifosfamide, and cisplatin chemotherapy for metastatic penile cancer: a phase II study. J Clin Oncol. 2010;28(24):3851–7.
23. Mitropoulos D, Dimopoulos MA, Kiroudi-Voulgari A, Zervas A, Dimopoulos C, Logothetis CJ. Neoadjuvant cisplatin and interferon-alpha 2B in the treatment and organ preservation of penile carcinoma. J Urol. 1994;152(4):1124–6.
24. Zhu Y, Li H, Yao XD, Zhang SL, Zhang HL, Shi GH, Yang LF, Yang ZY, Wang CF, Ye DW. Feasibility and activity of sorafenib and sunitinib in advanced penile cancer: a preliminary report. Urol Int. 2010;85(3):334–40.
25. Necchi A, Nicolai N, Colecchia M, Catanzaro M, Torelli T, Piva L, Salvioni R. Proof of activity of anti-epidermal growth factor receptor-targeted therapy for relapsed squamous cell carcinoma of the penis. J Clin Oncol. 2011;29(22):e650–2.
26. Theodore C, Skoneczna I, Bodrogi I, Leahy M, Kerst JM, Collette L, Ven K, Marreaud S, Oliver RD. A phase II multicentre study of irinotecan (CPT 11) in combination with cisplatin (CDDP) in metastatic or locally advanced penile carcinoma (EORTC PROTOCOL 30992). Ann Oncol. 2008;19:1304–7.
27. Pizzocaro G, Piva L, Bandieramonte G, Tana S. Up-to-date management of carcinoma of the penis. Eur Urol. 1997;32(1):5–15.
28. Franks KN, Kancherla K, Sethugavalar B, Whelan P, Eardley I, Kiltie AE. Radiotherapy for node positive penile cancer: experience of the Leeds teaching hospitals. J Urol. 2011;186(2):524–9.
29. Noronha V, Patil V, Prabhash K. Role of paclitaxel and platinum based adjuvant chemotherapy in high risk penile cancer. Urol Ann. 2012;4(3):150–3.
30. Di Lorenzo G, Federico P, Buonerba C, Longo N, Carteni G, Autorino R, Perdona S, Ferro M, Rescigno P, DAniello C. Paclitaxel in pretreated metastatic penile cancer: final results of a phase 2 study. Eur Urol. 2011;60(6):1280–4.

Index

D.J. Culkin (ed.), *Management of Penile Cancer*,
DOI 10.1007/978-1-4939-0461-7, © Springer Science+Business Media New York 2014

R

S

T

U

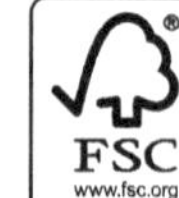

MIX
Papier aus verantwortungsvollen Quellen
Paper from responsible sources
FSC® C105338

If you have any concerns about our products,
you can contact us on
ProductSafety@springernature.com

In case Publisher is established outside the EU,
the EU authorized representative is:
Springer Nature Customer Service Center GmbH
Europaplatz 3, 69115 Heidelberg, Germany

Printed by Libri Plureos GmbH
in Hamburg, Germany